A Manual of Chinese Herbal Medicine

T0297027

A MANUAL OF
Chinese Herbal
Medicine

Principles and Practice
for Easy Reference

WARNER J-W. FAN, M.D.

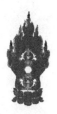

SHAMBHALA
Boston & London
1996

Shambhala Publications, Inc.
Horticultural Hall
300 Massachusetts Avenue
Boston, Massachusetts 02115

Printed in the United States of America
♾ This edition is printed on acid-free paper that meets the
American National Standards Institute Z39.48 Standard.
Distributed in the United States by Random House, Inc.,
and in Canada by Random House of Canada Ltd

Library of Congress Cataloging-in-Publication Data
Fan, Warner J-W., 1939–
    A manual of Chinese healing herbs: principles and practice for
  easy reference / by Warner J-W. Fan.
        p. cm.
    ISBN 1-57062-937-4
      1. Herbs—Therapeutic use.   2. Medicine, Chinese.   I. Title.
    RM666.H33F36   1996   95-39612
    615'.321'0951—dc20   CIP

BVG 01

For Fong-Bing, Maggie, and Ken

and

in memory of my parents

Contents

Preface

Traditional Chinese herbal medicine has been practiced for millennia. Through the years an enormous amount of data has been accumulated, and this has become a treasure trove of information about potentially very important drugs.

This book presents traditional Chinese herbal medicine with the aim of making its principles easily accessible to a general readership. The most important basic concepts, such as Yin, Yang, and Qi, cannot be translated, as no English terms come close to their meanings and connotations. For example, Qi (pronounced *chee*) has been translated by others as "air" or "breath." As shown in the text, this is clearly not adequate. What would "the breath (or air) of the ginseng root" mean? Also, a number of ordinary words that are used here in a very technical sense—for example, Heat, Wind, Wood, Metal—are capitalized. I have elected to retain the term *meridian* because it is widely recognized in connection with acupuncture. I have also resisted drawing close analogies to specific concepts and hypotheses of modern orthodox medicine, because such parallels can distort the Chinese concepts and impede understanding.

Various elements of Chinese medicine have become popular in many parts of the world, and some herbs have become very commonplace, to the point of being used much like a tonic. This casual use can be dangerous, and it was one of my motivations for writing this book.

The idea of this book was conceived while I was in medical school. Initially, it was to be a translation of *Introduction to Chinese Medicine* by Baiwei Qin, but over the years my interest became much broader, especially in comparing traditional Chinese medicine with contemporary pediatrics. In preparing this book I have drawn from many sources and have in my own way woven the information into a coherent whole. The Select Bibliography lists the main references used, except for Bensky and Barolet's *Formulas and Strategies* text, which became known to me only after my manuscript was completed. For the convenience of students, I have added Bensky and Barolet's translated formula names to my index, cross-referencing them to the formula names as I have translated them.

The text is organized into two parts and an appendix.

Part One contains a description of the basic concepts and principles of Chinese medicine. The fundamental concepts of Yin-Yang and the five elements are treated in detail, because proper understanding of these is essential for using the rest of the book. The bodily functions from the Chinese medical perspective are then elucidated and the causes of disease examined, followed by a general study of the methods and principles of diagnosis. Next follows a description of the principles of herbal pharmacology, the study of drugs. The part closes with a chapter on the approaches to treatment.

Part Two contains a number of compendia. The first two, chapters 7 and 8, list all the common diseases, one chapter by cause and the other by organ. Chapter 9 lists the common symptoms produced by these diseases. Chapter 10 covers therapeutics, the application of drugs. Finally, chapters 11 and 12 are compendia listing commonly used drugs in Chinese medicine and the formulas of the commonly used compound prescriptions. Unlike the chapters in Part One, these compendia are designed as reference material to be consulted as the need arises. The appendix contains case summaries derived from the Chinese medical literature that are intended as illustrations of the application of the principles of diagnosis and treatment.

Acknowledgments

Dr. Kou-Ping Yu originally intended to be co-translator, but his duties as oncologist at Kaiser-Permanente Hospitals prevented that; he gave me much encouragement and read my first draft. Mrs. John Young also gave me much encouragement and procured for me some rare, centuries-old Chinese medical books. My brother-in-law, Derek Ko, also procured for me a number of very useful references, including the *Encyclopedic Dictionary of Chinese Medicines* compiled by the Jiangsu New School of Medicine. James and Mary Louise O'Brien were like parents to me during my college and medical school years at Stanford University, and their broad cultural perspective inspired my interest in my own cultural heritage. Without Professor Howard Sachar of George Washington University and his wife, Eliana Sachar, this book would never have seen the light of day. The same is true of Shambhala Publications, especially Kendra Crossen. To all these people I owe more than gratitude. Any shortcomings, however, are entirely my responsibility.

A Manual of Chinese Herbal Medicine

Introduction

Chinese medicine developed as a mixture of fundamental concepts derived from philosophy and empirical observation and based on many centuries of trial and error. The *Book of Changes* (*Yijing* 易经) describes a cosmology based on the concept of Yin 阴 and Yang 阳. The concept of Yin-Yang pervades all Chinese intellectual thinking and is fundamental to the understanding of Chinese medicine. Yin and Yang are the two opposing forces of the "negative" and the "positive." All phenomena in the universe derive from the confrontation and interaction of these two forces. Thus, the heavens are Yang, the earth Yin; the sun is Yang, the moon Yin; daylight is Yang, night Yin; fire is Yang, water Yin; the exterior of the body is Yang, the interior Yin; and so forth. Just as night and day succeed and suppress each other, so do Yin and Yang—yet one cannot do without the other. Although in appearance and function Yin and Yang seem mutually opposing, yet they are mutually tolerant, even mutually stimulatory. Yin and Yang must therefore be properly balanced and harmonious.

Within this framework of Yin-Yang, Chinese medicine further uses the theory of the five elements (wuxing 五行) to describe the various processes in the body and its interactions with the environment. The five elements are Wood, Fire, Earth, Metal, and Water. Each element represents properties that have been found very useful in characterizing certain functions of nature and of the body. Thus:

> Wood (mu 木) is straight; it characterizes the liver, anger, acid taste, and windy weather.

Fire (huo 火) rises; it characterizes the heart, joy, bitter taste, and hot weather.

Earth (tu 土) is quiet and solid; it characterizes the spleen, melancholy, sweet taste, and damp weather.

Metal (jin 金) is luminous and firm; it characterizes the lung, grief, acrid taste, and dry weather.

Water (shui 水) is fluid and descendent; it characterizes the kidney, fear, salty taste, and cold weather.

As with Yin-Yang, these five elements are also interrelated in a stimulatory and an inhibitory manner. Wood stimulates Fire, Fire stimulates Earth, Earth stimulates Metal, Metal stimulates Water, Water stimulates Wood. Similarly, Wood inhibits Earth, Earth inhibits Water, Water inhibits Fire, Fire inhibits Metal, and Metal inhibits Wood. Each element both stimulates and is stimulated by another, and similarly each element both inhibits and is inhibited by another.

Health is maintained when Yin and Yang are in harmonious balance; similarly with the five elements. Disease results when either system becomes unbalanced. Many factors can cause disease, and they are broadly grouped into the external causes, the internal causes, and the unclassified causes (which are neither external nor internal). There are six external causes: Wind (feng 风), Heat (shu 暑), and Fire (huo 火) are Yang in nature, whereas Dampness (shi 湿), Cold (han 寒), and Dryness (gan 干) are Yin in nature. Invasion by Wind or Heat may damage Yin, whereas invasion by Dampness, Cold, or Dryness may damage Yang. Superficially similar conditions may result if some internal factor causes a deficiency of Yin or Yang. Thus, deficiency of Yin may produce symptoms of Heat; similarly, deficiency of Yang may produce symptoms of Cold. The important internal causes are the seven passions, Phlegm (dan 痰), food and drink, and the parasites. Excessive passion can damage an organ characterized by the same element as the passion. For example, excessive anger can damage the liver, excessive joy can damage the heart, excessive melancholy can damage the spleen, excessive grief can damage the lung, and excessive fear can damage the kidney.

Diseases produce symptoms, which manifest the dysfunction of the body. For example, when Heat injures the exterior body, the patient develops chills and fever, excessive perspiration, dryness of the lips and throat, and sometimes shortness of breath. If Heat specifically affects the urinary bladder, there will be bladder pain, frequent need to urinate but in only very small amounts, and pain while urinating. Most symptoms, however, can be produced by different diseases. Fever is one of the most common symptoms that prompt patients to visit their physicians, and fever may be a symptom of diseases due to Heat, diseases due to Cold, diseases due to Yin deficiency, diseases due to excess Yang, and other diseases. Since the presence of symptoms indicates the presence of an illness, by analyzing the symptoms presented by a patient, the physician is able to deduce the nature of the patient's illness. But most symptoms can result from a number of different diseases, and most diseases produce a variety of symptoms. Consequently, the analysis of all the patient's symptoms can become a very complicated endeavor.

Fortunately, the accumulated experience of many thousands of physicians through many centuries has produced a number of effective approaches to simplify this task. The most popular of these is the method called diagnosis by the eight fundamentals (bagang 八纲). The eight fundamentals are Yin-Yang, exterior-interior, Cold-Heat, and weakness-strength. Using this framework allows the physician to determine (1) whether the illness is due to a Yin or a Yang disease; (2) which part of the body is principally affected, the exterior or the interior; (3) whether the disease is of the nature of Cold or of Heat; and (4) whether it is due to strength of the cause or to weakness of the bodily functions. By following the principles of the eight fundamentals in observing the total person, one should arrive at a diagnosis without too much difficulty.

Having made the diagnosis, the physician must next treat the patient to eliminate the illness and its symptoms, and to restore the person's Yin-Yang to its balanced state. Chinese medicine uses principally herbal drugs. Chinese drugs exhibit properties called nature (Qi 气, pronounced *chee*) and taste (Wei 味). The nature of drugs falls into four categories: hot, warm, cool, and cold. The taste falls into five categories: acid, bitter, sweet, acrid, and salty. Drugs of hot or warm nature are Yang drugs, as are drugs of acrid or sweet taste. Drugs of cool or cold nature are Yin drugs, as are drugs of acid, bitter, or salty taste. Each drug has a nature and one or more tastes. The combination and interplay of the nature and the taste, as well as other properties, determine the efficacy of the drug. Because most illnesses are complex, it is usually necessary for the physician to select several herbs and blend them into a compound drug. Most Chinese prescriptions are of compound drugs, and the collective experience of the ages has produced a large number of such formulas that are very useful.

By its nature, Chinese medicine is holistic in its approach to the patient. Not only must the Yin-Yang of the body be restored to balance, but the body must also be in harmony with the outside environment. The wise physician therefore takes into account all aspects of the situation at hand—the season, the weather, and the habitat; the patient's mood, emotions, and personal habits; and the diseased organ or region. This approach is also important in the prevention of disease, because thorough understanding encourages harmonizing the body with the environment as well as maintaining harmony within the body, thereby minimizing the risk of illness.

PART ONE

Basic Principles

1

Fundamental Concepts

A. *Yin-Yang* (阴阳)

The theory of Yin-Yang derives from the ancients' observation of natural phenomena and is a metaphysical concept used to explain these phenomena. The ancients perceived that the myriad objects and images of the universe all manifest the opposing aspects of the negative and positive, thereby establishing the principle of Yin-Yang. Every object or process, however small or large, can be understood in terms of Yin-Yang.

Thus, the heavens are Yang, the earth Yin; the sun is Yang, the moon Yin; daylight is Yang, night Yin; fire is Yang, water Yin; and so forth. All changes in the universe are a reflection of the confrontation of these two forces and their synthesis. Yin and Yang are normally harmonious and balanced. To preserve bodily health, this unity is essential, not only within the body but also in the environment, so that the inside is in harmony with the outside. Furthermore, as one expands, the other decreases; as one shrinks, the other rises. Expansion and growth, contraction and recession—these processes indicate that Yin and Yang are mutually interdependent and at the same time mutually restrictive. Thus, in appearance and function, Yin and Yang are mutually opposing, yet mutually tolerant, even mutually stimulatory.

Within Yin-Yang there is Yin-Yang—that is, there is Yin within Yin and Yang within Yin, and there is Yang within Yang and Yin within Yang. To illustrate, day is Yang and night is Yin; but during the day, the forenoon is Yang within Yang, whereas the afternoon is Yin within Yang; and the evening before midnight is Yin within Yin, whereas the night after midnight is Yang within Yin. The visceral organs are Yin, but among them, the Fu (腑) organs are Yang, and the Zang (脏) organs are Yin. Among the Zang organs, however, the heart and lung are Yang, whereas the liver, spleen, and kidney are Yin. Furthermore, the heart is Yang within Yang, whereas the lung is Yin within Yang; the liver is Yang within Yin, the kidney is Yin within Yin, and the spleen is extreme Yin within Yin. (See diagram.)

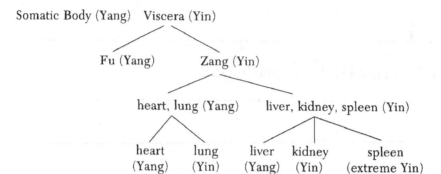

Similarly with drugs: nature is Yang, taste Yin; strong taste is Yin within Yin, delicate taste is Yang within Yin; strong nature is Yang within Yang, weak nature is Yin within Yang.

Chinese medicine applies this principle to the fundamental problems of medicine. It forms the backbone of Chinese medical understanding, linking together normal and abnormal processes, diagnosis, treatment, and the *materia medica*. The practice of Chinese medicine is impossible without a thorough understanding of Yin-Yang.

1. Normal Processes. Chinese medicine recognizes that the principle of Yin-Yang underlies the bodily functions. In general, Yang is active and aggressive, while Yin is quiescent and conservative. Yang protects the bodily strength, while Yin conserves the inner vitality. Yang represents the somatic structures: the skin, the skeleton, the muscles and sinews, and so on; Yin represents the viscera (internal organs). The Zang viscera serve to house the vital forces and are Yin; the Fu viscera govern digestion and transport and are Yang. The upper position is Yang while the lower position is Yin; the sides are Yang while the middle is Yin. Blood is Yin and Qi is Yang; substance is Yin and function is Yang.

Yin	Yang
substance	function
material	activity
conservative	aggressive
quiescent	active
viscera	somatic body
middle	sides
blood	Qi

2. *Abnormal Processes.* Regional and superficial afflictions are Yang, internal afflictions Yin. Heat-induced diseases are Yang; Cold-induced diseases are Yin. When function is weakened, as in shortness of breath, apathy, cold intolerance, fatigue, or lethargy, it is generally due to Yang insufficiency. When matter is deficient, such as blood deficiency, emaciation, or spontaneous seminal emission, it is generally due to Yin insufficiency. On such a basis, illnesses are separated into four categories: Yang deficiency, Yin deficiency, Yang excess, and Yin excess. To generalize, everything that advances or excites or tends toward Heat belongs to Yang; whereas everything that recedes or submerges or tends toward Cold belongs to Yin. In skin conditions, for example, Yang disorders are generally inflamed, whereas Yin disorders are generally pallid and cool.

	Yin	Yang
Deficiency	interior Heat	exterior Cold
	deficient matter	weakened function
Excess	interior Cold	exterior Heat
	interior illnesses	exterior illnesses

Since Yin and Yang are mutually opposing, when one weakens the other may become excessive. Thus, Chinese medicine has the following additional categories:

    a. Yin excess due to Yang deficiency,
    b. Yang excess due to Yin deficiency,
    c. Yang deficiency due to Yin excess, and
    d. Yin deficiency due to Yang excess.

The clinical application of Yin-Yang in Chinese medicine is rooted in practical observations, so that a thorough understanding requires considerable bedside experience. Thus, fever is Yang; but fever may be of the exterior or the interior, or due to deficiency or strength—hence, fever due to exposure to Wind is treated by inducing diaphoresis; fever due to pus-producing inflammation is treated by internal dissipation; fever due to Fire in the liver is treated by cooling and reduction; fever due to exhaustion is treated by restoration. In the case of perspiration caused by deficiency: daylight is a time of Yang, so that deficiency-perspiration in daytime is due to insufficiency of Yang and is treated with Yang drugs; night is a time of Yin, so that deficiency-perspiration at night is due to insufficiency of Yin and is treated with drugs that restore blood and Yin.

3. *Diagnosis.* In evaluating the pulse, three categorical pairs of opposites are recognized: (a) the rate may be slow or rapid, (b) the pulse may be felt at the superficial or the deep level, and (c) the pulse may

be smooth or impeded. Rapid, superficial, and smooth pulses are Yang; slow, deep, and impeded pulses are Yin. Alterations in the body of the tongue reflect alterations in the blood, so that a red tongue indicates Heat in the blood and belongs to Yang, whereas a pallid tongue indicates blood deficiency or Cold in the blood and belongs to Yin. Alterations in the tongue coating (shetai 舌苔) generally reflect stomach and intestinal processes; a dry, yellow coating is Yang, whereas a moist, white coating is Yin.

	Yin	Yang
Pulses	slow, deep, impeded	rapid, superficial, smooth
Tongue	pallid	red
Skin	pale, cool	inflamed

4. *Treatment.* The main concept of treatment is that when Yang goes to excess, Yin becomes insufficient; when Yin grows excessive, Yang becomes insufficient. Excess Yang produces Heat, excess Yin produces Cold; however, extreme Cold may show Heat symptoms and extreme Heat may show Cold symptoms. The physician therefore also treats Yin in Yang diseases, and Yang in Yin diseases; from Yin he draws out Yang, from Yang he draws out Yin.

In straightforward deficiency of Yin or Yang, treatment is relatively simple. In Yin or Yang deficiency resulting respectively from Yang or Yin excess, on the other hand, one must take into consideration not only the immediate symptoms but also the underlying process. For example, for accumulation of abdominal fluid, treatment consists of warming the circulation and gradual induction of diuresis—warming the circulation aids Yang, and diuresis dissipates the accumulated water resulting from Yang deficiency. Again, thirst is treated by cooling the stomach and generating fluids—cooling the stomach controls Heat while fluid generation restores fluid that has been depleted because of Yang excess.

5. *Therapeutics.* Chinese drugs are classified principally according to their nature and taste, nature being Yang and taste Yin. The four natures are further grouped into Yin (cold and cool) and Yang (warm and hot). Similarly, of the five tastes, acid, bitter, and salty are Yin, whereas acrid and sweet are Yang. Furthermore, drugs that are fragrant and can strengthen the stomach are also Yang drugs; those that can nourish and restore the liver and kidney are also Yin drugs.

B. *The Five Elements* (Wuxing 五行)

In addition to the theory of Yin-Yang, Chinese medicine also uses the theory of the five elements to explain the various processes in the body. The five elements are Wood, Fire, Earth, Metal, and Water. Like Yin-Yang, they are metaphysical concepts used to explain the qualities of the body parts. Thus:

Wood (mu 木). Its inherent efficacy is proper and straight; its disposition is gentle; its use is to straighten the crooked; its development is luxuriant.

Fire (huo 火). Its inherent efficacy is to ascend and bloom; its disposition is rapid and hurried; its use is to burn; its development is diverse and myriad.

Earth (tu 土). Its inherent efficacy is quiet and solid; its disposition is docile and peaceful; its use is to bring down the excessively high; its development is full and fulfilling.

Metal (jin 金). Its inherent efficacy is luminous and clear; its disposition is firm and strong; its use is to disperse; its development is unyielding and parsimonious.

Water (shui 水). Its inherent efficacy is inward and clear; its disposition is fluid and descendent; its use is free and over-flowing; its development is solid and congealed.

The application of the theory of the five elements in Chinese medicine is based on the characteristics of the elements, using them to classify the various activities of nature as well as the body. The major classification scheme is shown in the table.

	Wood	Fire	Earth	Metal	Water
Geographic location	east	south	center	west	north
Season	spring	summer	midsummer	fall	winter
Weather	windy	hot	wet, damp	dry	cold
Taste	acid	bitter	sweet	acrid	salty
Facial opening	eyes	tongue	mouth	nose	ears
Bodily parts	sinews	vessels	flesh	skin	bones
Zang organs	liver	heart	spleen	lung	kidney
Disease location	neck	chest	spine	shoulders	flank
Emotion	anger	joy	pensiveness	grief	fear

When applied to the disease processes of the various organs, the theory basically advocates that when Wood is pent up, relieve the obstruction; when Fire is pent up, dissipate it; when Earth is pent up, overpower it; when Metal is pent up, excrete it; when Water is pent up, reduce it. This is no more and no less than promoting the smooth functioning of each according to its properties in order to restore its inherent efficacy.

The five elements are interrelated principally in two ways: *trophism* (sheng 生) and *suppression* (ke 克). (See diagram.)

Trophism indicates sequential production and stimulation: thus, Wood produces Fire, Fire produces Earth, Earth produces Metal, Metal produces Water, and Water produces Wood. It is clear there are two aspects to this relationship for each element: each is stimulated by another and in turn stimulates another.

Suppression indicates sequential check and inhibition: Metal suppresses Wood, Wood suppresses Earth, Earth suppresses Water, Water suppresses Fire, and Fire suppresses Metal. Here too, there are two aspects to this relationship for each element: each is suppressed by another and in turn suppresses another.

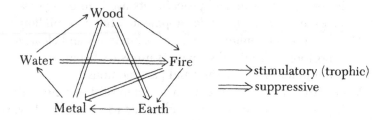

These two ways of interaction, however, are not separate and independent but are themselves intimately related, so that in trophism there is suppression and in suppression there is trophism. For example, Wood suppresses Earth, but Earth stimulates Metal, and Metal in turn suppresses Wood. This regulated interaction is a necessary mechanism for maintaining homeostasis, for stimulation without suppression makes the strong stronger, whereas suppression without stimulation makes the weak weaker. Within this regulatory system, there is also the abnormal phenomenon of an element turning around to suppress the element by which it is normally suppressed. For example, Water normally suppresses Fire, but under certain circumstances Fire can turn around and suppress Water. This is known as *disrespect* (wu 侮).

Whether it is trophism, suppression, or disrespect, there is one condition to be met: an element must be strong before it can stimulate or produce another. When an element is stronger than minimally adequate, it can suppress or show disrespect to its own suppressor. When it is too weak, not only does it fail to suppress, but it is now at risk of being actually suppressed by its natural suppressee.

As with Yin-Yang, the five elements must be balanced and in equilibrium. For example, when Wood is properly balanced, it spreads harmony; if it is deficient, there is male genital atrophy and impotence; if it is excessive, growth becomes unrestrained.

C. Diagnosis and Management

Symptoms are manifestations of the influence of the Improper Qi on the body, reflecting the nature of the disease "evil" and the strength of the body's normal functions. From the obvious to the minute, from the superficial to the deep, the symptoms reflect the cause of the abnormal processes and their progression or regression; the direction of development of these forces can be deduced from the disappearance or extension of the various symptoms.

The individual symptoms must be observed and analyzed. They are integrated into significant clinical patterns, because only in this way can the physician accurately assess the nature and status of the disease and not be misled by false clues. From the common symptoms, the physician can usually form a preliminary impression. For example, a patient may complain of a dry mouth and feeling hot inside, and may have in addition fever and headache. This is generally due to Heat. Closer observation may reveal that although thirsty, this patient does not desire liquids, which, if taken, produce a bloated feeling; or if he drinks at all, he prefers warm liquids. It is clear that here the thirst is a false clue, and the illness is not due to Heat.

Symptoms, then, may be simple or complicated. *Complicated* does not mean "confused" or "illogical," but the physician does need to understand the interrelationships among the various symptoms, and to analyze and integrate them to discover their cause and consequences. The appearance and disappearance of the symptoms reflect changes in the illness; sometimes the symptoms may seem to have changed only very slightly and yet the direction of progression of the illness has already changed. For example, fever is a common symptom; yet the following are only some of the questions that need to be clarified: Is there cold intolerance? Is there perspiration? How high is the fever? Following perspiration, is fever reduced and does cold intolerance disappear? As the temperature falls, does the pulse become calmer? Following perspiration, does cold intolerance disappear but the temperature actually rise, or does the temperature slowly fall but the perspiration continue unabated? Or do chills and fever alternate several times a day? Furthermore, does the sensorium remain clear? Is there thirst, real or apparent? Is there constipation or diarrhea? Are there the symptoms of headache, general aches, cough? As the temperature rises or falls, what happens to the appearance of the tongue?

Detailed understanding of such a simple and common symptom as fever is necessary because the diagnosis varies depending on the associated pattern, and therefore the treatment must also vary. Nor does diagnosis end here, for the struggle between the normal and abnormal forces frequently produces a very complicated natural course; and during this course of events, the patient's condition may suddenly change, depending on the interaction and balance between the opposing forces and with the various organs of the body, thereby forming the sequential phases of the illness. Diagnosis is as important at every step of the disease process as at the initial evaluation.

Management is determined by three aspects of the illness: the cause, the symptoms, and the location of the disease. For example, when the diagnostic process indicates that an illness is caused by retention of food, affecting the gastrointestinal tract and manifested by distention of the abdomen, management is then aimed at relieving the retention and eliminating the retained food by means of drugs that induce vomiting, elimination, or catharsis. Another example: if the cause is blood deficiency, manifested by dizziness, palpitation, and nervousness, the disease affecting the heart and the liver, then management is aimed at strengthening the heart and regulating the liver, supplemented by suppressing Yang and sedation. It can be seen from this that diagnosis and management are interrelated, the basic requirement being the flexible and proper application of principles and careful analysis of the facts.

D. The Total Approach

Yin-Yang and the five elements apply to the largest and smallest, pervading all nature. Hence, in Chinese medicine the viscera and the somatic body, the various organs and the various systems are recognized as intimately related and inseparable. Chinese medicine also recognizes that changes in the environment have a profound influence on the functions of the body in normal and in diseased states. In clinical practice, therefore, the physician must always consider all aspects of the problem at hand—the season, the weather, and the habitat; the patient's mood, emotions, and personal habits; and the diseased organ or region. This total approach is fundamental to the management of disease.

1. The Unity of the Body

Each of the twelve viscera recognized in Chinese medicine has its specific function; and the twelve viscera are grouped into two categories, the Zang (脏) and the Fu (腑) organs. The viscera do not function separately and independently. Each Zang organ is paired with a Fu organ, forming an interior-exterior dyad. Each organ is also reciprocally related to its respective system in the somatic body. Thus, the heart governs the pulse and the tongue; the liver governs the sinews and the eyes; and so forth. These exemplify the functions of the viscera and the relationship of the viscera to the somatic structures.

Even more important, the vasculature, through its superbly organized meridians with their afferent and efferent flow, serves as the connecting pathways that link the interior and exterior body and the various viscera, and in so doing promotes the functional unity of the body as a whole.

It is because of this unity that in the treatment of a disease of a visceral organ, attention is not restricted to this organ alone. Indeed, sometimes attention is not directed to the diseased organ at all, but instead to other organs, which then indirectly influence the diseased organ and effect a cure. For example, stomach ailments require treatment of the spleen as well; lung diseases can often be approached via the spleen and stomach, thereby secondarily enhancing the lung's resistance and recovery. Similarly, diseases of the somatic body frequently necessitate treatment directed at the viscera. For example, inflammation of the eye induced by Wind or Fire is best managed by cooling the liver; stasis necrosis (tissue death due to poor circulation) of a toe is prevented by stimulation of the circulation and warming the vasculature. Exterior diseases such as rashes, skin boils, and ulcers are usually treated with herbs taken by mouth to dissipate, to drain, or to close.

2. The Body and Climate

All biological processes are directly influenced by the environment. Chinese medicine greatly emphasizes this intimate relationship. Harmony with the natural environment must be established if the body is to remain free of disease and to achieve longevity.

Out of observations of the annual cycle, the special characteristics of the seasons have been recognized: spring warmth, summer heat, fall coolness, winter cold. Further, six types of changes of the seasons are defined: Wind, Cold, Heat, Dampness, Dryness, and Fire. It has further been recognized how by appropriate adaptation to the environment disease can be avoided, or how by contrary measures disease can be brought about. From the same principles have evolved the various techniques of diagnosis and treatment.

Thus, if the Qi (see chapter 2, section C) is appropriate but the hour is not, such as cold or heat instead of warmth in spring, then the Qi is improper; and such Improper Qi must be avoided promptly. Conversely, the regular progression of the four seasons produces Qi that is quite normal. This is called Proper Qi and is beneficial to the body. The normal cyclical changes of the four seasons are often used in the management of diseases.

3. The Body and Geographic Locale

Some habitats are severe, others mild. The higher altitudes are generally dry while (in China) the lowlands are generally humid. These different habitats require different living habits and can produce different illnesses. The choice of therapy and drugs, and their dosages, must frequently be modified according to the locale.

4. Other Factors

The strength or weakness of the constitution; the physique; the gaiety, depression, or nervousness of the mood; the excitement and stimulation of the mind; and so on—these are also emphasized in Chinese medicine and are recognized to play a very important role in the development and progression of disease. The physician must therefore consider them during therapy. For example, the strong of constitution can tolerate potent drugs, whereas the weak of body should be given small doses; the obese frequently have excessive Dampness and Phlegm, whereas the lean frequently lack Yin and have excessive Heat. Though these relationships are far from being constant, they nevertheless have much practical utility.

E. Preventive Management

The aim of preventive medicine is the maintenance of health—if necessary, after elimination of disease. These principles were recognized by the ancients and guided the early development of knowledge about personal and public hygiene, much of which was recorded in ancient texts.

The main features of Chinese preventive medicine are as follows:

1. Causation of disease, in addition to disturbance in the daily processes of living and nutrition, has intimate connection with the changes in nature and the weather, and particularly with the strength or weak-

ness of the body. To maintain health one must build up bodily vitality and avoid the invasion of external evils. To do so requires harmonizing with the four seasons and normal climatic progression to condition the body—for example, in spring and summer to conserve the Yang Qi, in fall and winter to conserve the Yin Qi.

2. Therapy is more effective if started promptly, before an illness has progressed. By the time an illness has reached the Zang viscera, it is usually very serious and difficult to cure.

3. The causation and natural course of diseases have their laws, and one must anticipate what is to come in order to grasp the status of an illness. For example, because liver diseases often extend to the spleen, if one pays special attention to the spleen while treating liver diseases, one can prevent damage to the spleen and thereby minimize the risk of extension of the liver disease, allowing a much easier recovery.

2

Bodily Functions

In this chapter, the functions of the internal organs, the circulation, and the various fluids and vital forces are described. It is important to realize that the functions ascribed to these organs and systems are not the same as those ascribed to them by modern Euro-American medicine. Indeed, the three sphincters (jiao 焦) do not correspond to any organ known to modern medicine.

A. The Viscera

The viscera are internal organs. There are five Zang (脏) viscera (heart, liver, spleen, lung, kidney) and six Fu (腑) viscera (gallbladder, stomach, small intestine, large intestine, bladder, and the three sphincters). The pericardium, a membrane that envelops the heart, is sometimes regarded as a sixth Zang organ, although in function it is a part of the heart. Although both groups are internal organs, the Zang organs store and preserve the vital forces and Qi and are Yin, whereas the Fu organs propel and digest and are Yang (within Yin). (See also table in chapter 1, section B.)

1. Heart

The heart belongs to the element Fire. It generates blood and stores Shen (神) (see below, section D). It governs the life and activities of the entire body. If the heart is weakened, disturbed by emotions, or invaded by external evils, the person may manifest fearfulness, anxiety, insomnia, forgetfulness, inappropriate gaiety, mental confusion, and so forth. When the heart is diseased, not only does it lose self-control, it can also affect the activities of the other viscera, causing dysfunction.

Heart diseases are most commonly due to deficiency: blood deficiency, Yin deficiency, Qi deficiency, and Yang deficiency of the heart. Of these, Yin blood deficiency is seen most often, although simultaneous deficiency of both Qi and blood is not uncommon.

2. Liver

While the heart generates blood, the liver stores it and governs thinking and deliberation. Belonging to the element Wood, liver has a strong and rigid nature, hence it is also known as "the general." When liver function is disturbed, it often leads to rage reactions, such as expanding or pounding types of headache, and sometimes even to backflow of the Fire Qi, causing vomiting of blood. In the female, the liver is inherently associated with reproductive capacity, so special attention must be paid to it in order to regulate menses and improve fertility.

Liver by nature tends to move and disperse, and to rise; hence most liver diseases are caused by the upstream rising of liver Yang. Blockage of liver Qi prevents its movement. Thus trapped, liver Qi builds up and often transforms into Fire; and if liver Yang is flourishing too, then liver Wind is generated and moves internally. Insufficiency of liver Yin, resulting for example from excessive passion, which allows the liver Yang to wax, can also lead to internal movement of liver Wind, especially when combined with trapping of liver Qi. Thus, liver Qi and liver Wind are intimately related; whether there is strength or deficiency must be determined on the basis of clinical findings.

3. Spleen

The spleen belongs to the element Earth. It commands the blood and governs transportation and is responsible for digestion of fluid and grains (shuigu 水谷) and the delivery of the extract from all foods to the entire body; and nutrition is the principal factor in maintaining life. Thus, the spleen is the basis of "postnatal acquisition." If spleen function is chronically insufficient, the person develops indigestion and bloating following eating. If this state is prolonged, muscle wasting and fatigue can develop. The spleen also governs the movement of fluids. Impedance of fluid movement causes such manifestations as tightness in the chest, vomiting or diarrhea, and edema.

Most spleen illnesses are due to deficiency Cold. Among the deficiency illnesses, deficiency of spleen Qi is fundamental. If there are cold intolerance and coldness of the limbs as well, then spleen Yang is deficient. Sinking of the Central Qi is a further development of insufficiency of spleen Qi. Spleen diseases are also intimately connected with Dampness: spleen deficiency can generate (internal) Dampness, while an excessively strong Dampness evil can confine the spleen, preventing its normal function.

4. Lung

The lung belongs to the element Metal. It governs Qi and is in charge of calm dignity. If lung Qi does not descend properly, cough and breathing difficulty readily develop. When the lung is weak, there is often inadequate respiration and difficult and weak speech. Although blood is governed by the heart, its circulation is also regulated by the lung. The lung is related to the heart as the chief minister is to the king.

The main symptoms of lung disease are cough, difficulty with breathing, and sputum production. The character of sputum permits analysis of Heat and Cold; the character of the cough and dyspnea (shortness of breath) permits analysis of strength and deficiency.

5. Kidney

The kidney belongs to the element Water. It stores Jing, the vital force (see below, section D), and governs vigor; it is therefore essential for the vitality and vigor of the body. Deficiency of the kidney leads to such symptoms as vertigo, tinnitus, loss of vision, flank pain, thigh weakness, and drowsiness and lassitude. In analogy with the liver for the female, the kidney is inherently associated with male reproductive capacity. Hence, loss of sexual desire, spontaneous seminal leak, and impotence and premature ejaculation are all treated via the kidney.

A major difference between the kidney and the other viscera is the fact that the kidney is a paired organ. The left is the kidney proper, and the right is the life gate (mingmen 命门); the left is Yin, and the right Yang; thus the kidney is sometimes called the water and fire organ (shuihuozhizang 水火之脏).

Most kidney illnesses are due to deficiency. Because both the Yin and the Yang of the kidney are essential for the entire body, illness arises whenever one or the other is deficient, leading to imbalance. The fundamental principle in the treatment of kidney disease is therefore to restore and support the weak rather than to attack the adequate.

6. Gallbladder

The gallbladder is the house of purity and governs judgment and decisiveness. The gallbladder and the liver are intimately related: the gallbladder is the external of the liver, whereas the liver is the internal of the gallbladder. Even strong liver Qi would be ineffectual without the gallbladder. It is when the liver and gallbladder function together harmoniously that courage and daring are born. Abnormal functioning of the gallbladder produces the symptoms of impatience, irascibility, head pressure, chest tightness, flank pain, bitter taste, and vomiting of bile.

7. Stomach

The stomach is the "sea of water and nutrients" (shuiguzhihai 水谷之海) and governs acceptance. It is the external counterpart of the spleen. The ancients assigned the function of acceptance (of food and drink) to the stomach and the function of digestion to the spleen. However, the basic functions of the stomach include both; indeed, without acceptance there can be no digestion.

The stomach Qi tends to sink. Only when the stomach Qi sinks can water and food move downward, permitting digestion, absorption, and excretion. If the stomach Qi rises instead, there are then eructation (burping), hiccough, nausea, and vomiting.

The stomach also prefers lubrication and dislikes dryness. It is easily injured by the Heat evil, which damages the stomach fluids and causes such symptoms as thirst and dryness of the mouth and tongue.

8. Small Intestine

The small intestine is an organ of reception and governs metabolism. It receives the digestive slurry from the stomach and further separates it into the clear and the impure, so that the nutrient essences are delivered to the Zang organs for storage, whereas the remains are delivered to other Fu organs for excretion. The water from the slurry is delivered to the bladder, and the residue from the slurry to the large intestine.

Most small-intestine diseases are related to the other organs. For example, Heat strength in the small intestine is usually due to descent of the heart Fire; Cold in the small intestine often relates to "deficiency Cold" (i.e., Cold due to deficiency) in the spleen and kidney.

9. Large Intestine

The large intestine is an organ of transportation, governing excretion. It receives the residue from the small intestine for excretion, performing the terminal step in the entire digestive process. Thus, cases of constipation, diarrhea, dysentery, and blood in the feces are generally approached by treating the large intestine.

The large intestine and the lung are related in an exterior–interior dyad. Therefore, in treating lung Heat strength one can, for example, use catharsis of the large intestine to facilitate movement of lung Qi.

10. Bladder

The bladder is the reservoir for fluids and controls Qi development. Blockage of Qi development causes urinary distention, whereas uncontrolled Qi development results in urinary incontinence. However, control of Qi development by the bladder is closely linked with kidney function—only when the Qi from the kidney is full can it develop and the bladder regulate its development. Thus, in treating oliguria (scanty urine) or polyuria (excessive urine), one must frequently warm the kidney.

11. The Three Sphincters (Sanjiao 三焦)

These sphincters—the upper, the middle, and the lower—together manage drainage and fluid movement. Thus, ascites (fluid accumulation in the abdomen) and edema (fluid accumulation under the skin) are often treated with drugs that open the sphincters.

12. Interactions among the Viscera

The organs do not function in isolation but are intimately linked through the meridians. Each viscus has its own principal function, but the functions of these organs proceed cooperatively and in an integrated manner.

Among the several Zang organs there is the relationship of governance (xiangzhu 相主) derived from the theory of the five elements (see chapter 1, section B). The concept of governance includes shades of control and of regulation. The kidney (Water) is the governor of the heart (Fire), the heart that of the lung (Metal), the lung that of the liver (Wood), the liver that of the spleen (Earth), and the spleen that of the kidney. In this way, the Zang organs restrain one another and maintain homeostasis. Similarly, they support one another, so that the kidney nurtures the liver, the liver nurtures the heart, the heart nurtures the spleen, the spleen nurtures the lung, and the lung nurtures the kidney.

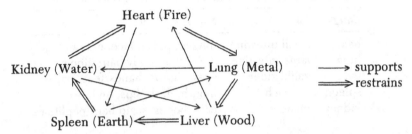

Between the Zang and the Fu organs there is also the relationship of complementation (xianghe 相合). The lung complements the large intestine, the heart the small intestine, the liver the gallbladder, the spleen the stomach, the kidney the bladder. This principle of complementation illustrates how the Zang organs form the substance and the Fu organs the exercise of their integrated functions. Also, the Zang organs are deeper and belong to Yin, whereas the Fu organs are closer to the exterior and belong to Yang, so that their mutually complementary relationship is also one of interior-exterior and Yin-Yang linkage.

The viscera are also intimately related in function with various structures of the somatic body. Consequently, observation of these somatic structures can reveal much of the state of the viscera. This principle is of great practical importance. Frequently used examples of this relationship include the following:

- The liver has its external opening in the eyes, its fulfillment in the sinews, and its blossoming in the hands and feet.
- The heart opens through the tongue, is fulfilled in the pulse, and blossoms in the face.
- The spleen opens through the mouth, is fulfilled in the flesh, and blossoms in the lips.
- The lung opens through the nose, is fulfilled in the skin, and blossoms in the body hair.

- The kidney opens through the ears, is fulfilled in the bones, and blossoms in the scalp hair.

Other examples:

- The limbs belong to the spleen.
- The elbow joints belong to the heart and lung.
- The axillae (armpits) belong to the liver.
- The thighs belong to the spleen.
- The popliteals (backs of knee joints) belong to the kidney.

CORRELATIONS BETWEEN VISCERA AND SOMATIC BODY

Zang	Fu	Somatic Body
heart	small intestine	tongue, pulse, face; elbow
lung	large intestine	nose, skin, body hair; elbow
liver	gallbladder	eyes, sinews, hands/feet; axillae
spleen	stomach	mouth, flesh, lips; limbs
kidney	bladder	ears, bones, scalp hair; popliteals

13. The Unclassified Viscera

In addition to the Zang and Fu organs, there are several viscera that are not classified by the usual scheme: the brain, the bones, the bone marrow, the vasculature, and the uterus. These organs are unclassified because in some ways they resemble both Zang and Fu organs, yet are different from them in structure and function. They are indispensable parts of the body, and like the other organs they are not isolated. For example, the brain is functionally connected with the heart and liver; further, because the brain is related to the bone marrow, and the marrow to bone, and bone to kidney, the brain is also functionally related to the kidney. Another example: the uterus is related to the liver; but because of its functions in menses and gestation, it is linked with blood, and thereby also linked with the heart and spleen.

B. Circulation (Jingmai 经脉)

The circulation determines the life and death of the organism, rules over the hundred diseases, and harmonizes the weak and the strong. Its functions are internally to service the viscera; externally to maintain the form of the somatic body; to move Qi and blood; and to modulate Yin and Yang. Thus the theory of the circulation constitutes one of the pillars of Chinese medicine.

The meridians are the structural pathways for the circulation of both Qi and blood. These longitudinal and transverse pathways form a network that subtends the entire body, interlinking all the various parts.

1. Circulation in General

Normal function of the body is principally determined by the viscera. The circulation, however, is indispensable in mediating the interactions between the exterior and interior, between the upper and lower body, and in the maintenance of homeostasis, so that the entire body functions as a whole. Because of the circulation, external influences can progress from the exterior to the interior. Similarly, illnesses caused by internal factors can be reflected externally.

The main branches of the vasculature are the twelve regular meridians (mai 脉). They course through the viscera, head, and limbs, and are grouped into the six Yin and the six Yang meridians. From these regular meridians branch the twelve collateral meridians. These branches form an interior linking network between the Yang and Yin meridians. There are also twelve (minor) superficial collateral meridians. These begin at the extremities of the limbs and course along the wrists, elbows, and axillae, or along the ankles, knees, and hips. They have a superficial course and provide superficial communication for the regular meridians. Apart from the function of interlinking the regular meridians, the collaterals are of minor importance.

In addition, there are eight irregular meridians. These are concerned with the regulation of the other meridians.

Each of the principal meridians has a series of points in well-defined positions along its course, which are not physically open but are nonetheless where the Qi of the Zang organs is transmitted to the somatic body and concentrated there. These are also the points for acupuncture. Altogether, there are more than 360 of these points distributed along the entire meridian network. In therapeutics, Chinese medicine groups the various drugs, depending on their actions and efficacy, to correspond to the twelve main meridians; and drugs are selected to treat illnesses of their corresponding meridians.

2. The Regular Meridians

Also called the proper meridians, the twelve regular meridians are subgrouped (each with its main corresponding viscus) as follows:

Hand Yin Meridians
a. hand Greater Yin (taiyin 太阴)—lung
b. hand Lesser Yin (shaoyin 少阴)—heart
c. hand Dark Yin (jueyin 厥阴)—pericardium

Foot Yin Meridians
d. foot Greater Yin—spleen
e. foot Lesser Yin—kidney
f. foot Dark Yin—liver

Hand Yang Meridians
g. hand Greater Yang (taiyang 太阳)—small intestine
h. hand Lesser Yang (shaoyang 少阳)—the sphincters
i. hand Bright Yang (yangming 阳明)—large intestine

Foot Yang Meridians
j. foot Greater Yang—bladder
k. foot Lesser Yang—gallbladder
l. foot Bright Yang—stomach

The Yin meridians link the Zang viscera to the somatic body, with the foot Yin meridians coursing from the foot to the viscera, and the hand Yin meridians coursing from the viscera to the hand. The hand Yang meridians pick up from the hand Yin meridians at the hand and course to the head; the foot Yang meridians then pick up at the head and course to the foot, where the foot Yin meridians take over. The cyclical sequence of the individual meridians is as follows:

hand Greater Yin (head to lung to hand)
hand Bright Yang (hand to large intestine to head)
foot Bright Yang (head to stomach to foot)
foot Greater Yin (foot to spleen to head)

hand Lesser Yin (head to heart to hand)
hand Greater Yang (hand to small intestine to head)
foot Greater Yang (head to bladder to foot)
foot Lesser Yin (foot to kidney to head)

hand Dark Yin (head to pericardium to hand)
hand Lesser Yang (hand to sphincters to head)
foot Lesser Yang (head to gallbladder to foot)
foot Dark Yin (foot to liver to head)

Hand Greater Yin then takes over. In this manner, the pathway leads endlessly from Yin into Yang and from Yang into Yin, from exterior to interior and from interior to exterior, from below to above and from above to below.

As the meridians course through the body, they very naturally organize the body into various regions and establish the interior-exterior relationship between the viscera and the somatic body. Consequently, from the symptoms in any given region one can deduce the diseased meridian or visceral organ and use appropriate treatment. Examples of symptoms of diseases of the regular meridians:

- hand Greater Yin: cough, pain above the clavicle, pain in the anterior and medial aspects of the elbow, heat in the palms
- hand Bright Yang: dental pain, throat numbness, upper arm pain, pain and dysfunction of the index finger
- foot Bright Yang: nosebleed, mouth sores, knee pain and swelling, pain from the breast along the outer buttocks down to the dorsum of the foot, dysfunction of the middle toe
- foot Greater Yin: thickening and hardening of the tongue, upper abdominal pain, cold swelling of the inner thigh, dysfunction of the big toe
- hand Lesser Yin: pain in the heart area, rib pain, pain and spasm in the inner and posterior elbow, heat in the palms
- hand Greater Yang: pain or difficulty in swallowing, swelling of the jaw, pain in the shoulder and elbow
- foot Greater Yang: headache, spastic stiff neck, lumbago, pain behind the knee and in the instep, little toe dysfunction
- foot Lesser Yin: throat inflammation, restlessness, pain and atrophy in the sacroiliac area, heat and pain in the sole
- hand Dark Yin: heat in the palm, spastic flexion of the elbow, axillary swelling, rib distention
- hand Lesser Yang: deafness, throat numbness, pain in the jaw, pain behind the ear, pain in the axillae and outer arm, dysfunction of the fourth finger
- foot Lesser Yang: headaches, pain around the outside corner of the eye, axillary swelling, pain along the side from the ribs to the ankle
- foot Dark Yin: throat dryness, chest distention, groin pain, urinary incontinence or scanty urine

3. Irregular Meridians

There are eight irregular meridians, which regulate the functions of the regular meridians. They are:

a. The Overseer (du 督) courses inside the spine and governs the Yang of the body.
b. The Official (ren 任) courses along the abdomen in front and governs the Yin of the body.
c. The Flood (chong 冲) arises in the perineum, courses inside the abdomen, and spreads out in the chest.
d. The Girdle (dai 带) courses around like a girdle just below the lowest ribs, uniting all the various meridians.
e. The Nimble Yang (yangjiao 阳蹻) courses along the outside of the limbs.
f. The Nimble Yin (yinjiao 阴蹻) courses along the inside of the limbs.
g. The Yang Connector (yangwei 阳维).
h. The Yin Connector (yinwei 阴维).

Of these, the most important are the overseer and the official—so much so that they are sometimes grouped with the twelve regular meridians.

C. Qi and Blood

Qi is a potential, a capacity to perform. It has many names, such as Original Qi (yuanqi 元气), Genuine Qi (zhenqi 真气), and Essential Qi (jingqi 精气); these reflect merely the different interactions of the one Qi with the various parts and functions of the body. There are also the Yang Qi and the Yin Qi, which are the two functional aspects of the Original Qi, one that protects the body and the other that preserves strength.

In Chinese medicine, abnormal Qi function often results from blockage of function of the various organs or to processes generated by indigestion. Common symptoms such as diaphragmatic impedance (strained respiration), chest distention and epigastric distress, and tendinitis and abdominal rumbling are interpreted using such terms as impedance, stagnation, hindrance, oppression, accumulation, gathering, and closure of Qi. Diseases that cause such symptoms are thus frequently named in accordance with what happens to Qi. Similarly, there are many methods of treatment dealing with Qi, such as to smooth its path, disperse it, blend it, regulate it, move it, dissipate it, facilitate it, bring it down, break it, and so forth.

Blood is generated by the heart, stored by the liver, and governed by the spleen. When the heart is weak or blood deficient, circulation becomes irregular, and the patient manifests palpitations, anxiety, and irregular pulses. When overexcitement affects the liver's function of storing blood, nosebleeds or vomiting of blood is common. When the spleen is diseased, so that its governance of blood is compromised, the patient may develop intestinal bleeding, excessive menses, or other vaginal bleeding. Prescriptions for harmonizing blood, generating blood, or inducing blood to return to its proper path are generally directed at the heart, liver, or spleen respectively.

Blood becomes like gel when exposed to Cold and courses wildly when exposed to Heat. This Heat or Cold includes external environmental influences, the characters of food and drink, and the effects of various diseases of the viscera.

Qi and blood are inseparable and of equal importance. Qi is essential for blood to perform its functions. If Qi is affected, whether by emotions or environmental factors, blood will also be affected. When Qi is impeded, so is blood. Stasis of blood is therefore often treated by facilitating the flow of Qi, and persistent bleeding by enhancing Qi to bring about hemostasis.

D. Jing, Qi, Shen (精气神)

These are called the three treasures, illustrating their importance to the body. Qi has already been discussed.

Jing, the "vital force," is the basic force underlying growth and fertility. It is the foundation of life and is the first thing formed when a person is conceived. It is housed in the kidney, and for this reason the kidney is called the organ of prenatal endowment. Jing has intimate effects on bodily strength. Thus, patients with frequent spontaneous seminal emission often have backache, weak flanks and legs, and staggering gait. In severe cases there are lethargy, generalized weakness, shortness of breath, dryness of the skin, ringing in the ears, and dull and shrunken eyeballs; this is known as extreme Jing depletion. Because the kidney stores Jing, these symptoms are generally due to failure of the kidney, and they are treated by strengthening the kidney.

The ancients also postulated a formless, nonmaterial force that directed each material organ in the performance of its functions. This force they called Shen, "spirit." Jing comes with conception, whereas Shen arises out of the interactions of Jing. The soul, the mind, thinking, anticipation of the future, and wisdom are all actions of Shen.

The viscera house these treasures: the liver houses the soul, the lung the mind, the heart Shen, the spleen intention and wisdom, the kidney Jing and will. The soul, mind, intention, and so on describe the functional manifestation of each organ; and though the names differ, they are basically all the same as Shen. Because the heart is chief among the viscera, the term *Shen* is generally used to encompass the other terms (soul, mind, intention, wisdom, will). If Shen is injured, the patient develops symptoms such as heaviness in the chest, inability to concentrate, weakness in the limbs, delirium, amnesia, atrophy of the external sexual organs, or pain and stiffness of the spine. In treating diseases of Shen, however, it is necessary to include methods that generate blood and supplement Qi.

Jing, Qi, and Shen are also closely connected. Qi arises out of Jing, and Jing transforms into Qi. When Jing and Qi are full, Shen becomes lively; conversely, if Shen weakens, then Jing and Qi also become deficient. Similarly, if Shen is overactive, Jing and Qi are also affected, so that the body weakens. Therefore, in both maintenance of health and treatment of disease, each attends to the others.

E. The Body Fluids

The body fluids pervade the body and are in equilibrium with the blood. Excessive flow opens the subcutaneous compartment and causes excessive perspiration; whereas loss causes withering, dehydration, weakness, ringing in the ears, joint dysfunction, and so forth.

Because the fluids and blood are in equilibrium, in Chinese medicine they are regarded as coming from the same source. Preservation of fluids is essentially the same as preservation of blood, and blood formation also produces fluid. In clinical practice, blood loss and fluid loss are often mentioned together; thus, a patient with blood loss must not be made to sweat, and every little part of fluid retained increases the chances of survival.

Nontraumatic blood loss can occur by four major processes: vomiting of blood, nosebleed, blood in the feces, and blood in the urine. Likewise, fluid loss can occur by four major processes: vomiting of fluids, perspiration, diarrhea, and excessive urine. These processes demonstrate significant parallel features: vomiting of blood resembles vomiting of fluid; nosebleed is also called red sweat, resembling perspiration; blood in the feces resembles diarrhea; and blood in the urine resembles excessive urine.

Fluids can also be transformed into sweat, tears, nasal secretion, and saliva. These are governed mainly by the kidney. However, persons with weak spleen and intestines may not be able to transport fluids, which can then accumulate as thick phlegm. The phlegm can block the internal upflow of fluids, leading to dryness of the mouth and refusal to eat or drink. Such conditions are often treated with warming drugs that mediate the block.

A common symptom of fluid deficiency is thirst, and this usually results from diseases of Heat. Mild cases may not need treatment; elimination of Heat may be sufficient to reverse the process. Severe cases, however, require methods that generate blood and enhance Yin.

3

Causes of Disease

The causes of disease are classified as (a) external evils that attack the body from the outside, (b) internal alterations that weaken the body or cause imbalance and loss of homeostasis from the inside, and (c) a small group of factors that are not readily classified as either external or internal. The first group is by far the most important, and its members are responsible for the majority of illnesses that afflict humankind.

A. External Causes

Of the external causes, the principal ones are the six evils (liuyin 六淫): Wind, Cold, Heat, Dampness, Dryness, and Fire. Except for Fire, these are all normal phenomena of the four seasons: spring Wind, summer Heat, midsummer Dampness, fall Dryness, and winter Cold. (The associations between the seasons and the external evils are clearly specific to China's geography. Historical China is a northern hemispheric, temperate zone country on the east coast of a continent—hence the association of Dampness with midsummer and Dryness with fall. A similar pattern can be seen on the East Coast of the United States. In areas on the West Coast, such as California, Oregon, and Washington state, a different pattern obtains.) These are normal climatic factors, but when present at the wrong time (season, or time of day) these influences become evil Qi. Disease occurs under their influence when the internal milieu of the body and the external environment are in disharmony.

Under special conditions these five influences, particularly extreme Heat, can all turn into Fire, and so Fire is included in this list. (Note that the term *Fire* is used both with reference to a disease and as one of the five elements. The context usually indicates which one it is.)

Wind, Heat, and Fire are Yang in nature and are also called the Yang evils. Dampness, Cold, and Dryness are Yin in nature and are also called the Yin evils.

1. Wind (Feng 风)

Wind by nature is active and changeable and wanders widely. It is frequently active between seasons or as weather conditions change. Wind also often combines with the other evils to form Wind-Heat, Wind-Dampness, Wind-Dryness, Wind-Fire, and so on. Thus, the ancients regarded Wind as the captain of all diseases.

In mild cases, Wind affects only the upper position (see chapter 4) or the exterior; this is Wind injury (shangfeng 伤风). Its symptoms are wind intolerance, fever, headache, nasal congestion, cough, and hoarseness. As Wind progresses into the meridians and the viscera, it causes Wind invasion (zhongfeng 中风), manifested by one-sided weakness of the facial and ocular muscles, difficulty with or loss of speech, paralysis of one side, and sudden collapse. In less severe cases, consciousness returns shortly; in the most severe cases coma persists.

This kind of illness results from attack by external Wind and is to be distinguished from illnesses resulting from internal causes. Internal Wind is usually caused by deficiency of Yin and blood; or excessive heat from Fire and Phlegm causing fainting, seizures, dizziness or vertigo, numbness, and spastic neck stiffness.

2. Cold (Han 寒)

Cold injury (shanghan 伤寒) results from the Cold evil in the exterior and manifests as cold intolerance, fever, headache, generalized aching, superficial and tight pulse, and white and greasy tongue coating. (See chapter 4 for description of pulses and so forth.) Treatment is directed at the symptoms. Cold injury can change into Heat, and this must be recognized to avoid stubborn adherence to inappropriate treatment of the Heat evil.

If damage extends to the internal organs, Cold invasion (zhonghan 中寒) is the result, and the patient vomits clear liquids and develops cramps and rumbling in the abdomen and diarrhea. More severe cases also involve coldness of the limbs and a hidden pulse. Treatment consists of warming the interior.

Cold invasion rarely transforms into Heat, but the virulent Cold evil can damage Yang effectively, and it frequently causes Yang to decline progressively. Weakening of Yang can manifest the symptoms of Cold, such as vomiting, abdominal pain, diarrhea, and cold limbs. Such coldness comes from inside and is called internal Cold. Because internal Cold arises from deficiency of Yang, its treatment is based on strengthening Yang and differs from that used for Cold invasion.

3. Heat (Shu 暑)

Heat is the principal Qi of summer. Diseases caused by the Heat evil mainly show high fever, thirst, restlessness, and spontaneous perspiration. Because Heat injures the body Qi and can affect the heart, the patient may develop rapid and sighing respiration and a tidal but deficient pulse.

A person who overexerts under the hot sun may develop Heat invasion (zhongshu 中暑), also called Heat exhaustion. The main symptoms are fever, thirst, headache, heavy respiration, a feeling of heaviness and weakness, lethargy, and scant and dark urine. As the body weakens and becomes exhausted, perspiration becomes profuse and the heart weak, causing dizziness, restlessness, and even fainting or coma.

Because Yang governs movements, such diseases as Heat invasion are also called Yang Heat. Conversely, even in the summer heat one can develop disease from being inactive—for instance, excessive exposure in a cool area, sleeping outside at night, or sitting undressed in the wind. These can result in cold intolerance, fever, headache, and loss of sweat. If there is overeating too, then abdominal pain and diarrhea occur in addition. Although called Yin Heat (yinshu 阴暑), it is actually a disease due to the Cold evil.

The Heat evil can easily injure Qi and Yin. If unresolved, it can exhaust the Yin fluids and cause lassitude and fatigue, even lethargy. This is known as Heat decay (shuji 暑瘵).

4. Dampness (Shi 湿)

As an external factor, dampness or moisture generally refers to fog, dew, rain, or humidity. Exposure also occurs through staying on damp ground, living in a moist area, working in water, or wearing damp clothing (from perspiration or otherwise). The Dampness evil is heavy, impure, sticky, viscous, and difficult to dissolve. The symptoms of damage by Dampness are mainly chills and fever, nasal congestion, bandlike pressure in the head, and joint pains. If Dampness has entered the meridians and muscles, there are edema and swelling of the tissues as well.

Internal Dampness arises when there is dysfunction of the spleen because of excessive indulgence in fats, grains, and spices, or in cold fruits, nuts, and sweet, sticky foods. If the internal Dampness is high in the body (upper position), the chest feels tight, with impeded respiration, and there is much sputum; if it is in the midsection (middle position), outflow from the stomach is blocked, with vomiting, anorexia, and indigestion; if it is low in the body (lower position), there is abdominal distention, diarrhea, and scant urine. Internal Dampness can also rise to the head and cause facial swelling, sink to the feet and cause edema there, or flow through the vasculature and cause aching and pain in the limbs.

Dampness is a Yin influence. Combined with Wind, it is Wind-Dampness; combined with Cold, it is Cold-Dampness. These conditions are relatively easy to cure. On the other hand, Dampness-Heat, which results when Dampness and Heat combine to cause disease, is slow to respond. Dampness and Heat are of quite different character, so that their joint diseases show variable, often inconsistent symptoms—for example, hot body but cold limbs, thirst but craving for warm liquids, or thick yellow and greasy tongue coating. There may also be tightness in the chest and excessive vomiting. In such illnesses, Dampness and Heat must be approached simultaneously.

5. Dryness (Zao 燥)

Dryness is the principal Qi of autumn. Diseases from external Dryness mostly affect the upper position and resemble Wind injury. The symptoms are mild chills and mild fever; headache; dry mouth, lip, nose, and throat; a cough that is nonproductive or productive of scant sputum, which is thick, mucoid, and sometimes blood-tinged; and large stools, sometimes leading to constipation.

Dryness is also a remnant of Fire, so that following recovery from Heat diseases there are often symptoms of Dryness. Dryness can also result from depletion of either blood or body fluids. This is internal Dryness and has a broader range of effects: on the body surface there are dry skin, dry and cracked lips, dryness of the eyes, and dry and hot nose; in the interior, thirst, frequent hunger, insufficient saliva for swallowing, hiccoughs, constipation, and dark yellow urine; in severe cases, weakness, spasticity, and chronic cough may occur.

Excessive ingestion of foods of Heat nature; excessively aggressive induction of perspiration, vomiting, or diarrhea; or diuresis can deplete the body fluids and lead to internal Dryness.

6. Fire (Huo 火)

As an external cause, Fire is a form of the Heat evil and results from the transformation of the other five evils. When Fire burns the three positions, the patient manifests throat inflammation, a hairy tongue, chest tightness, restlessness, thirst for cold liquids, abdominal distention, dark urine, sometimes skin eruptions, delirium, and rapid and wild pulse.

The viscera can also generate Fire. This is "strength Fire" (shihuo 实火); the most common is from the liver and gallbladder. The symptoms are eye redness, bitter taste, dizziness with expanding headache, facial flushing, ringing in the ears, restless sleep with nightmares, chest distention and tightness, and even nocturnal emission and cloudy urine.

When Yin is deficient and Heat comes from within, there is high fever, loss of perspiration, restlessness, insomnia, and denuded and red tongue. If Yang is deficient below, then Fire floats to the top, resulting in such symptoms as gum inflammation, agitation, perspiration on the head, and ringing in the ears. Such Fire is called deficiency Fire (xuhuo 虚火).

External Fire is treated by dissipation, strength Fire by reduction, and deficiency Fire by restoring Yin. Both strength Fire and deficiency Fire show signs of dehydration, but strength Fire begins with excess Fire and consequent loss of fluids and moves rapidly, whereas deficiency Fire begins with fluid loss and consequent increase in Fire and in general moves more slowly.

7. Other External Causes

Contagion refers to the process of communication from one person to another; the resultant disease is similar regardless of age. Pestilence refers to a type of virulent vapor in nature. It differs from ordinary evils and is most harmful to health. The pestilent vapor arises mostly from excessive rain, severe drought, the death of animals from the plague, or the decay of excreta. These diseases by their natures fall into two categories, the cold epidemics and the plague epidemics. Generally, the external factor enters by way of the mouth or nose and goes directly to the stomach and intestines. These diseases develop and progress rapidly.

8. General Considerations

a. Diseases externally caused by the six evils refer to those diseases induced when the six evils attack the somatic body (exterior) or invade the meridians and internal organs (interior). On the other hand, internal Wind, internal Cold, internal Dampness, the internal Dryness of fluid or blood deficiency, and the internal Fire of viscera, even though they all have names of the external evils, are of very different natures, and they must be carefully distinguished from their external counterparts. This is especially important in diseases caused by internal and external factors occurring simultaneously. In those conditions, the treatment differs significantly from that used when either an internal or an external factor is acting alone, and great care is needed in diagnosis.

b. Illnesses from the six evils do not necessarily become symptomatic promptly but may be delayed for a period of time. In this situation they are known as the hidden evils (fuxie 伏邪). For example, exposure to Cold in winter may cause symptoms of Heat disease in summer; exposure to Heat in summer may show up in winter. Hidden-evil illnesses are the obverse of newly acquired illnesses. Distinction can be made on the basis of the position (interior versus exterior) of the affected organ, the degree of severity, and the rapidity of progression. Consider Heat disease, as an example: in newly acquired Heat disease, the initial symptoms are those of the exterior; they are milder and progress slowly into the symptoms of Heat, going deeper only gradually. Hidden Heat disease, in contrast, has no exterior symptoms but starts with severe interior Heat and shows a strong tendency to injure Yin and to exhaust the body fluids. In the unusual case where a newly acquired illness activates the hidden evil, although at the outset there are exterior symptoms, the illness rapidly progresses to the more severe interior effects.

B. *Internal Causes*

The principal internal causes are the seven passions. Other important causes include Phlegm, food and drink, and parasites.

Although the causes of disease are classified into external and internal causes, they cannot be entirely isolated. Without internal influences at work, the external evils do not easily attack the body; similarly, internal causes often are induced or activated by external factors. At the same time, the physician must pay close attention to other factors, such as living habits, nutrition, home environment, and so forth, all of which have major bearing on susceptibility to and causation of disease.

1. The Seven Passions

Diseases of the passions are brought about when environmental factors excite the mind and cause undesirable changes. Because the environmental factors vary, the changes in the mind also vary.

The seven passions are anxiety, preoccupation (or melancholy), joy, rage, grief, fear, and fright (or terror). The basic effect in a disease of passion is a change in Qi. Thus rage makes Qi rise, joy makes it slow down, grief makes it shrink, fear makes it sink, and fright throws it into pandemonium; while preoccupation injures the spleen, anxiety injures the lung, and fear injures the kidney. Diseases caused by the passions are therefore best understood in terms of the vicissitudes of Qi.

Common examples of passion diseases are depression, unpredictable joy or rage, troubled and uncertain thought, a state of being apprehensive and suspicious (paranoia), insomnia with excessive dreaming, grief with incessant crying, anorexia (nervosa), and chest tightness with frequent sighing. More severe conditions are mental confusion, incoherence, and psychosis.

2. Phlegm (Dan 痰)

Phlegm is formed when the spleen and intestines are weak and fail to disperse water and moisture, which become collected and thickened. When there is Heat in the lung, the body fluids become thickened and heavy, and Phlegm is formed also. Of all the viscera, therefore, Phlegm is most closely connected with the lung and the spleen.

The principal symptom of disease caused by Phlegm is cough. If the smooth movement of air is hindered, there is heaviness of breath as well. If Phlegm escapes into the meridians, one finds numbness of the hands and feet, hardening and difficulty of movement of the tongue, scrofula, and carbuncles. If Phlegm combines with other causes, as in Cold-Phlegm, Heat-Phlegm, Dampness-Phlegm, Dryness-Phlegm, and Wind-Phlegm, the symptoms become complex. See chapter 9, "Common Symptoms of Disease."

Other diseases can also cause sputum production, simple examples being Wind injury and Cold injury. In Wind invasion, it is particularly important to eliminate Phlegm and clear clogged openings.

3. Food and Drink

Food and drink are the sources of nutrition, but if unregulated, the digestive and metabolic processes can be overwhelmed and disease may result—for example, epigastric pressure, abdominal distention, and vomiting of bile and acid; or, secondarily, chills and fever, headache, and diarrhea. These are together called food injury or indigestion. Indigestion often progresses to diseases of the stomach and intestines. If the person can eat but does not digest, then the stomach is strong but the spleen is weak (bloating after eating, loose and watery diarrhea). If there is hunger but inability to eat, then the spleen is strong and the stomach weak (vomiting).

4. Parasites

The common intestinal parasitic worms are roundworm (*Ascaris*), pinworm (*Oxyuris*), and whipworm (*Trichuris*). In most cases, they are the result of chronic Dampness and Heat, poor hygiene, and eating various raw vegetables, nuts, fruits, and excessively spicy foods.

C. Unclassified Causes

A number of causes of disease belong neither to external nor to internal factors.

1. Excessive sexual indulgence injures Jing and Qi. Not only does the body weaken, but susceptibility to the various other causes of disease is also increased. Common symptoms are haggard appearance, anxious and insecure demeanor, back and flank strain, cold limbs, nocturnal emissions, premature ejaculation, night sweats, and recurrent fever.

2. Injury by animals may involve various degrees of poisoning in addition to the physical damage.

3. Poisoning generally refers to poisoning by ingestion of foods or drugs, although contact with animals and plants can also be responsible. For example, excess salt damages the lung; raw alum damages the heart and liver.

4. Other causes, such as trauma and burns, are not discussed in this book.

4

Diagnosis

A. Physical Diagnosis

Once the physician has mastered the basic principles of Chinese medicine and has gained some familiarity with the symptoms caused by the various diseases, it is time to meet the patient and diagnose his or her illness. Physical diagnosis is the process by which a physician obtains all the relevant clinical information and, based on this information, deduces the cause of a patient's illness, its status, and its course. The most effective way to do so without leaving any gap is to approach it in a systematic manner. One time-honored approach is as follows: First, look at the patient (inspection); then listen and smell (auscultation and olfaction); then ask (history); and finally touch (palpation). Only the most basic and important aspects of physical diagnosis are indicated here. For details, consult chapter 9 on the common symptoms of disease.

1. Inspection
    a. Vigor and complexion
        (1) Look for indications of vigor, such as bright eyes, clear speech, orderly mentation, and easy and confident deportment. Observe the degree of activity (for example, whether passive, active, restless or agitated). Are the eyes bright or dull?
        (2) Inspect the complexion for its color. In Chinese medicine, five colors are recognized to be of clinical significance: green, pallid, yellow, red, and gray. Is the color superficial or deep? Observe also whether the complexion is bright and clear, light and faint, dense and deep, dry and flaccid, or heavy and murky.

(3) Note whether the patient is obese or emaciated, well coordinated or unsteady, has difficulty with movements, and if the activity seems purposeful or aimless.

b. Tongue and its coating (tai 苔)

(1) This is a very important part of inspection. The texture and color of the tongue reflect the deficiency or fullness of the Qi of the Zang viscera; the tongue coating reflects the clarity or murkiness of the stomach Qi and the nature of the external evil. Observation of changes in the texture, color, and coating of the tongue can reveal much about the character of the illness and the rise and fall of the Proper Qi and of the disease evil.

(2) The location of disease can often be recognized, as the different parts of the tongue are governed by the different viscera. Thus, the heart governs the tip, the kidney the root, the lung and stomach the body, and the liver and gallbladder the two edges of the tongue. In reference to the three positions, the tip belongs to the upper position, the middle to the middle position, and the root to the lower position.

(3) Does the tongue have a coating, or is it denuded? Note the color of the coating of the tongue (white, yellow, or gray), whether it is thin and smooth or thick and greasy, dry or moist. Are there blisters on the tongue?

(4) Assess the texture of the tongue, whether firm, dry, or supple. Is there fasciculation (twitching) or swelling? Is it smooth or "hairy"?

c. Teeth and gums

(1) Are the teeth stained black? Are they decayed? Are they chattering? Are they normal in shape, or misshapen?

(2) Are the gums pale, purple, or dark? Do they appear baked dry? Are they red and swollen? Is there purulent drainage?

d. Sputum. If there is sputum, is it thick, viscous, and lumpy, or thin, clear, and fluid? Does it appear foamy, purulent, or bloody? What is its color? Is the quantity large or small?

e. Feces. Are the feces watery, thick, or very dry? What is the color—light, dark, yellow, black, white, green, red, or gray like fish brain? Is there any blood or pus? Is there any undigested food? What is the quantity?

f. Urine. What is the color of the urine—yellow, red, very dark like soy sauce? Is it clear, cloudy, or bloody? Is it scanty in quantity or excessive?

g. Limbs
   (1) Do they appear well developed, or do they resemble a dry twig? Are they swollen? Do the knees resemble those of a stork? Are the fingers misshapen, or the joints enlarged?
   (2) Is there weakness in the limbs, or any contracture? Are there abnormal movements, especially rhythmic contractions? Is there any tremor?
   (3) Is there any painful inflammation?
   (4) Are the feet rotated abnormally?
   (5) Are the fingernails pitted, concave, or convex? Are the nails firm or soft? Are they pale, red, or green?
h. Skin
   (1) Does the skin appear swollen or dry? Is it peeling? Is it rough and cracked? Does the hair appear burned?
   (2) Observe the skin color. Is it yellow? Bright or dull? Does it appear grayish black, pallid, or red?
i. Abdomen. Is the abdomen distended? If so, is the skin thick with blue-gray color, or thin with bright color? Is the umbilicus protruding or sunken?

2. Auscultation and Olfaction
   a. Voice and speech. Is the voice loud but unclear? Soft but clear? Is it weak, whispering? Hoarse? Is the speech coherent? Is it repetitive?
   b. Respiration
      (1) Is respiration rapid? Is inspiration loud or quiet? Is expiration bubbly or hesitant? Is the breathing rattlelike, with wheeze, grunt, or moan?
      (2) Is respiration difficult, as if it would stop? Is it rapid with short inspiration and prolonged expiration? Are the breaths short and intermittent? Is there sufficient breath to permit speech? Does the patient appear to be straining?
   c. Cough. Is the cough dry, moist, productive? Is it weak, loud and forceful, silent, choking, or paroxysmal? Is the coughing associated with vomiting or blood?
   d. Odor. Does the patient have halitosis? A fruity odor, or sour and rotten gas? Is there a foul body odor? Is the sputum fishy and malodorous, or foul? Is the urine malodorous? Is the flatus foul?

3. History
   a. In diagnosing an illness, it is often essential for the physician to understand the patient's living habits and psychological temperament as well as the circumstances of the illness and its changes.

In general, the main subject of inquiry is the beginning and the course of the illness and the patient's subjective symptoms. One should also inquire into the past medical history and family medical history. In females of childbearing age, one should always ask about pregnancy and the menses. In taking the history, an orderly sequence should be followed.

b. Fever and chills. Ask about the timing and pattern of the fever, especially if it recurs, and where the fever is located. Ask also about associated symptoms, such as chills, perspiration, and aches and pains.

c. Perspiration. Note the amount and timing of perspiration, especially in relation to fever and chills and the day-night cycle. Note also whether the perspiration is generalized or localized.

d. Headache. Note the timing of the headache. The character of the headache can also be a very helpful clue, such as persistent and steady versus intermittent, or an expanding type. Ask also about associated symptoms, such as dizziness, blurring of vision, photophobia, and relationship to exertion. The location of the headache can also be a clue.

e. Cough and chest

(1) Cough may be paroxysmal or prolonged, and it may be associated with difficulty with breathing (especially on lying down) or disturbance of sleep. If the coughing brings up sputum, that should be examined as well.

(2) Pain in the chest may be stabbing or spastic, tight or distended in character, and may be located in specific regions or move from one location to another. It may also be associated with palpitations of the heart or a feeling of agitation or oppression.

f. Appetite, vomiting, and defecation

(1) Ask about anorexia, or the converse, excessive eating or drinking. There may be a feeling of bloating following eating. There may be an abnormal taste in the mouth—bitter, sweet, acid, or salty—or a lack of taste.

(2) Vomiting is a common symptom. Ascertain its relationship to eating and to time of day. Ask about associated symptoms, such as pain or tightness in the chest just prior to vomiting. The character of the vomitus may also provide valuable clues —for example, watery, acid, or bitter; containing sputum, blood, or undigested food.

(3) There may be diarrhea or constipation, and diarrhea may be

frequent, explosive, or recurrent. Ascertain the character of the feces: dry and hard, watery, light in color or dark or red or green, foul smelling, containing blood or pus or undigested food. Note any associated pain, vomiting, or anorexia.

g. Sleep and mental status

(1) Sleep may be excessive or frequently interrupted and restless. Note increased dreaming or night terrors. There may be insomnia.

(2) Note any forgetfulness, restlessness, or anxiety. Assess for abnormal mentation.

h. Urine and urination. Note whether urination occurs more or less frequently, and whether the urine dribbles out. Bed-wetting or incontinence should be noted. Ask about and observe whether the urine is clear or cloudy, light in color or dark, or containing mucus, blood, or gravel.

i. Male genitalia. There may be an itch, pain, or swelling. Ask about impotence, premature ejaculation, night emission, priapism, and scrotal atrophy.

j. Menses

(1) Absence of menses during childbearing age must always raise the possibility of pregnancy. A number of diseases can also cause loss of menstrual flow.

(2) Menses may be early or late, or irregular. The flow may be reduced or excessive, or it may contain clots.

(3) Vaginal bleeding not associated with menses may be sudden with gushing, or persistent with oozing. Ascertain the amount of flow, its color, whether there are clots, its odor, and such associated symptoms as flushed face, hot palms, restlessness, anorexia, pelvic pressure or pain, and abnormalities of complexion or the tongue coating.

k. Vaginal discharge. Note its color, amount, and odor, and any associated symptoms, such as pain or itch.

4. Palpation

a. Palpation of the pulse is one of the most important techniques in diagnosis. No Chinese physician can be successful without mastering this technique and the implications of its findings. The pulse configurations reflect the rise and fall of the external evil and the Proper Qi, the nature of the disease evil, and the location of the illness.

b. Basic technique. The pulse is taken near the head of the radius bone, which is the small bulge just behind (proximal to) the wrist on the thumb side. Apply the second, third, and fourth fingers, slightly inside the bone, using the digital pulp (the soft part of the fingertip opposite the nail). The position adjacent to the radial head is the gate (guan 关) position; just in front (distally) is the inch (cun 寸) position; and just behind (proximally) is the foot (chi 尺) position. These positions correlate with the viscera:

left inch	heart and pericardium
left gate	liver and gallbladder
left foot	kidney, bladder, small intestine
right inch	lung
right gate	spleen, stomach
right foot	kidney, large intestine

The correct way to take the pulse is as follows: Half stretch the patient's arm comfortably with the palm up. The wrist is supported to a height of just over one inch, relative to the elbow. The middle finger is applied first to determine the gate position, then the index finger for the inch, and finally the ring finger for the foot. For tall patients, slightly separate the fingers; for short patients, squeeze them together slightly; for infants, only one finger is used. First palpate lightly for superficial pulses, then deeply for deep pulses.

(1) If the patient has just engaged in physical exertion or has just left an extreme environment, or if the clothing is too tight, or if the position of sleep has put undue pressure on the pulse, or if the patient is influenced by passions or excessive food or drink, it is best if possible to postpone taking the pulse.

(2) For proper analysis, examine at least fifty beats.

(3) The patient's physique, height, age, sex, and overall condition also affect the pulse and its interpretation.

c. For each pulse configuration there are subtle variations, and sometimes differences between the two wrists or in the three pulse positions. The physician must therefore determine what constitutes the principal pulse. Most importantly, the pulse configuration must be correlated with the symptoms and the information gathered by the other methods.

d. The twenty-eight basic configurations

(1) These pulse configurations are grouped as shown in the diagram.

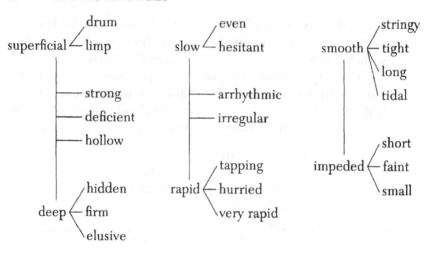

(2) Their descriptions are:

Superficial (fu 浮): palpated with light pressure
  Drum (ge 革): superficial and elastic, as if feeling a drum
  Limp (ru 濡): superficial, soft like loose cotton under
    water
  Strong (shi 实): forceful at every depth
  Deficient (xu 虚): weak at every depth, empty-feeling
  Hollow (kou 芤): superficial, large but empty
  Hidden (fu 伏): deep, palpated only when pressing on
    bone
  Firm (lao 牢): deep, hard and forceful
  Elusive (ruo 弱): deep, weak, palpable only gently
Deep (chen 沉): palpated only with heavy pressure

Slow (chi 迟): three beats or fewer per breath
  Even (huan 缓): four beats per breath, smooth and even
    to and fro
  Hesitant (jie 结): like even but stopping every now and then
  Arrhythmic (dai 代): now slow, now fast, overall rate even
  Irregular (san 散): rapid but frequent missed beats,
    irregular in rhythm
  Tapping (dong 动): rapid, no head and no tail to the beat
  Hurried (cu 促): rapid but missing occasional beats
  Very rapid (ji 疾): seven or eight beats per breath
Rapid (shu 数): five beats or more per breath

Smooth (hua 滑): unimpeded flow to and fro
   Stringy (xian 弦): smooth as if feeling a musical string
      instrument
   Tight (jin 紧): forceful to and fro, like a twisting rope
   Long (chang 长): neither large nor small, as if tracing a
      long pole
   Tidal (hong 洪): full and large coming, decayed and
      long going
   Short (duan 短): feels like a passing pea; as soon as it is
      felt, it is gone
   Faint (wei 微): impeded, small and soft, as if pressure
      would destroy it
   Small (xi 细): faint and small
Impeded (se 涩): impeded flow to and fro

(3) Most pulse configurations are double: for example, superficial
and tight; deep and stringy; slow and impeded; rapid and
tidal; smooth and strong. Sometimes they may be triple: for
example, superficial, tight, and rapid; superficial, smooth,
and rapid; deep, small and faint.

e. The seven strange configurations. In addition to these twenty-
eight configurations there are also seven strange configurations.
These all indicate an extremely exhausted heart, with death being
imminent. They are:

(1) Sparrow peck pulse (quezhuo 雀啄): like the pecks of a sparrow feeding, now there are several beats close together, now
there is none.

(2) Leaky roof pulse (wulou 屋漏): like the dripping of water
through a slow leak, a drop every now and then, with no
force in the splash.

(3) Rock tapping pulse (tanshi 弹石): like snapping at a rock with
a finger, the beat comes hard and hurried or comes late but
goes rapidly.

(4) Knot-untying pulse (jiesuo 解索): it comes in several beats,
then becomes dispersed and disorderly.

(5) Swimming fish pulse (yuxiang 鱼翔): the pulse has a steady
head but wavering tail, now floating, now drifting.

(6) Shrimp swim pulse (xiayou 虾游): like a shrimp swimming at
the water surface, suddenly it is gone; in a while it may be
back.

(7) Steaming kettle pulse (fufei 釜沸): only coming out, not going in; like boiling water, with no distinguishable separate beats.

B. Diagnosis by the Eight Fundamentals (Bagang 八纲)

Because most illnesses produce many symptoms, the number of deductions from them and their correlations with disease processes may become large and bewildering. A number of very useful approaches have been developed to make order out of this chaos.

An illness arises out of imbalance of the Yin and Yang Qi of the body or from the interaction of disease evils with the body's Proper Qi. The first step in the formulation of a diagnosis is thus to determine whether the illness belongs to Yin or to Yang. Only then should the physician determine the location of the disease (whether exterior or interior), the nature of the disease evil (whether Heat or Cold), and the relative ascendancy of the disease evil versus the Proper Qi (whether due to weakness of bodily functions or to strength of the disease evil). Thus, of the eight fundamentals, Yin-Yang are the chief, and these other six are really developments of Yin-Yang.

1. Analysis by Yin-Yang

Yin and Yang are key and serve to coordinate the other six fundamentals. Interior, Cold, and weakness belong to Yin; exterior, Heat, and strength belong to Yang. Hence, the Chinese physician analyzes the nature of an illness, its course, and its development in terms of Yin-Yang, saying that it is a Yin disease or a Yang disease, or that the disease is in Yin or in Yang.

a. Yin diseases. Patients with Yin diseases show fatigue and debility, a weak and low voice, a dull gray complexion, slow movements, and a cool body with cold intolerance. There is no thirst, and the urine is clear; the feces are watery; the tongue coating is white and smooth; and the pulse is deep and slow, with little force.

b. Yang diseases. Patients with Yang diseases show vigor and excitement, even agitation or delirium. The voice is loud and coarse; the face is flushed; fever and thirst are present; respiration is coarse; there is heat intolerance and preference for cold; the urine is scanty and dark; the tongue coating is yellow and dry; and the pulse is rapid, large, and full of force.

c. Yin destruction. There is a superficial resemblance to Yang diseases, but the fundamental defect is loss of Yin. The body is intolerant of heat and the hands and feet are warm, as are the muscles and sweat. There is a salty taste in the mouth; respiration is coarse; and the pulse is tidal and large, but rootless.

d. Yang destruction. The fundamental defect here is loss of Yang, with superficial resemblance to Yin diseases. There is much perspiration and yet cold intolerance; the hands and feet are cold, as are the muscles and sweat. The mouth is sticky and has no taste; the breath is shallow; and the pulse is superficial and rapid, but hollow.

Yang and Yin destruction are both very serious diseases. They usually appear under conditions of very hot and humid weather, with excessive perspiration, excessive vomiting or diarrhea, or prolonged blood loss.

Some essential considerations should be kept in mind.

Pay close attention to the natural course and changes in the status of the illness. As a result of the body's resistance and its changes, a Yang illness can transform into a Yin illness, and a Yin illness into a Yang illness. In general, a Yang illness transforming into a Yin illness indicates worsening; conversely, a Yin illness transforming into a Yang illness indicates improvement.

When Yang waxes too strong, Yin may be damaged, even destroyed; conversely, if the Yin fluids are exhausted by diaphoresis, not only Yin but also Yang is destroyed. Therefore pay close attention to the interaction and interrelationship between Yin and Yang.

Difficulties in diagnosing Yin-Yang most often arise in either prolonged illnesses or very severe illnesses. Carelessness at this stage can have dire consequences.

2. Analysis by Exterior-Interior (Biaoli 表里)

In the human body, exterior is the somatic body, including the skin and muscles; interior means the viscera, including the Zang and Fu organs, brain, and so on. When the external evils attack the body, they usually first injure the somatic body, causing exterior symptoms. The passions and other internal causes, in contrast, usually start internally, giving rise to interior symptoms.

a. Exterior symptoms. Typical exterior symptoms are cold or wind intolerance, perspiration, fever, headache, stiff neck, generalized aching, weakness of the limbs, thin and white tongue coating, and a superficial pulse.

      (1) Exterior Cold: cold intolerance, low-grade fever, superficial
        and tight pulse.
      (2) Exterior Heat: high fever, superficial and rapid pulse.
      (3) Combined exterior Heat and Cold: head and body aches,
        superficial pulse.
      (4) Exterior weakness: perspiration, superficial and even pulse.
      (5) Exterior strength: no perspiration, superficial and tight pulse.
      (6) Exterior strength and weakness combined: cold intolerance,
        fever, superficial pulse.
  b. Interior symptoms. Typical interior symptoms are high fever,
lightheadedness or drowsiness, incoherence, restlessness, thirst,
chest tightness, nausea and vomiting, diarrhea, abdominal distention or pain, blockage of intestinal or urinary excretion, thick and
yellow tongue coating, and a deep pulse.
      (1) Interior Cold: no thirst, nausea, vomiting, diarrhea, abdomi-
        nal pain, cold limbs, white tongue coating, deep and slow
        pulse.
      (2) Interior Heat: thirst, fever, restlessness, scanty and dark
        urine, red tongue with yellow coating, deep and rapid pulse.
      (3) Interior weakness: loss of appetite, fatigue with reluctance to
        talk, palpitation, dizziness, light or white tongue coating,
        deep and elusive pulse.
      (4) Interior strength: constipation, abdominal distention with
        tenderness and guarding, fever with diaphoresis, delirium,
        thick and yellow tongue coating; deep, strong, and forceful
        pulse.
  c. Exterior-interior transformations
    The exterior evils can and do proceed internally into the vis-
cera to produce interior symptoms. When the disease evil has
reached the meridians but not yet the viscera, the illness is said
to be half exterior, half interior. After internalizing, the exterior
may still be affected, in which case the illness is said to be simultaneously exterior and interior.
    As the external evils progress from the exterior toward the inte-
rior, the illness tends to become more severe or more complicated. The Cold evil is an example. When Cold injury first
begins, there are fever and chills, headache, and stiff neck; these
are exterior symptoms. If the fever does not break, and there are
symptoms such as bitter taste, persistent vomiting, tightness or
fullness of the heart and lung, or scanty and dark urine, these
symptoms indicate that the evil is tending toward the interior

(and is in the meridian). When high fever, thirst, agitated delirium, and abdominal cramping with constipation or diarrhea develop, the evil has reached the internal viscera.

Conversely, when an interior illness progresses outward, the illness is resolving. Thus, in the clinical analysis of exterior versus interior, of more importance is the determination of the direction of change.

Care should be taken to distinguish from these conditions those mixed illnesses that can result from a second illness developing during an unresolved illness—for example, exterior Heat-interior Cold; exterior Cold-interior Heat; exterior weakness-interior strength; and exterior strength-interior Heat.

3. Analysis by Heat-Cold (Rehan 热寒)

Analysis by Heat-Cold determines the basic nature of an illness. A Cold disease may come from the external Cold evil or arise out of the waning of the Qi or functions of the organs, whereas a Heat disease may come from the external Heat evil or arise out of excessive organ function or other causes.

a. Cold symptoms. The principal Cold symptoms are absence of thirst, preference for warm drinks, cold intolerance even without wind, cold limbs, copious clear urine, watery stools, pale complexion, white and smooth tongue coating, and slow pulse.

b. Heat symptoms. The principal Heat symptoms are fever; heat intolerance; thirst for cold drinks; flushed face; restlessness; dark and scanty urine; yellow, gluelike, and malodorous feces with rectal burning; coarse yellow tongue coating; and rapid pulse.

c. Location. Cold and Heat diseases sometimes do not affect the entire body. For example, dark and scanty urine may reflect total body Heat or Heat localized in the urinary bladder. Thus, one must further determine the location of the Cold or Heat.

(1) Upper Cold: acid regurgitation, vomiting of clear liquid, indigestion, cold feeling inside the chest.

(2) Upper Heat: head pressure, red eyes, throat inflammation, gum inflammation, dry mouth and preference for cold.

(3) Lower Cold: abdominal pain with guarding with the arms, watery stools or diarrhea, cold legs and feet.

(4) Lower Heat: constipation, cloudy yellow urine or scanty urine with painful urination.

(5) Exterior versus interior: See above, Section 2 (page 49).

These may occur in any combination. Sometimes even a single illness affecting the stomach and intestines may show Heat in the stomach but Cold in the intestines, or vice versa.

Genuine versus False Symptoms. In differentiating Heat and Cold, it is important to distinguish the genuine from the false. For example, if a patient is cold but has no desire to put on clothing, there is genuine Heat in the interior and false Cold in the exterior. Similarly, if a patient has a high fever yet wants to put on more clothing, there is genuine Cold in the interior and false Heat in the exterior.

4. Analysis by Deficiency-Strength (Xushi 虚实)

The Proper Qi may be weak or strong, and the evil Qi may be waxing or waning. In clinical practice, however, deficiency (or weakness) generally refers to the Proper Qi and strength to the evil Qi, because neither strong Proper Qi nor weak evil Qi have any abnormal consequence.

a. Symptoms of Qi deficiency. Weakness of Proper Qi causes weakening of vital functions and exhaustion from prolonged illness. The principal symptoms are loss of vitality or vigor, wasting of the body, fatigue, weakness, soft and weak voice, shortness of breath, dizziness, palpitations, impaired vision or hearing, spontaneous perspiration or loss of perspiration, flabby and swollen tongue, and small, faint, and elusive pulse.

b. Symptoms of strength. A strength disease occurs because of strong evil Qi, but the bodily functions and vigor are also strong. The principal symptoms are abdominal distention with guarding, much sputum causing blockage of the airway, chest tightness, difficulty with urination, large and dry feces or malodorous diarrhea, cold intolerance, firm tongue, and tidal smooth and large pulse.

c. Fluctuations of Qi

(1) If the body constitution is strong and the illness is recent, the illness is likely due to evil Qi strength. If the body constitution is weak and the illness chronic, it is mostly an illness of Proper Qi deficiency.

(2) Some diseases are pure deficiency or pure strength states, and these are relatively easy to recognize and treat. Other illnesses, however, are mixed, and we must attend to such variations as weakness in strength, strength in weakness, exterior strength and interior weakness, exterior weakness and interior strength, upper strength and lower weakness, and so on.

For example, in injury by Wind and Cold, the principal symptoms are cold intolerance, fever, and superficial and tight pulse; this is an exterior strength disease. If, following induction of sweating, the perspiration persists, the temperature falls rapidly, and cold intolerance intensifies, the illness shows changes toward a deficiency state; or if the cold intolerance disappears but fever heightens and thirst increases, the illness is internalizing.

(3) If a Heat disease shows a dry tongue, the patient's body fluids are already depleted; or if the tongue is denuded and dark red, Yin has been injured by the Heat evil, and therefore treatment cannot be restricted to removing the Heat.

(4) In general, if the Proper Qi is strong, then even though the evil is strong and the illness severe, the prognosis is good. If the Proper Qi is weak while the evil is strong, then even though the illness appears mild, it is still dangerous.

5. Combination Patterns

The combinations of exterior-interior, Cold-Heat, and deficiency-strength produce the eight basic patterns.

a. Exterior-Cold-strength

Cold and Wind attack the body exterior. Principal symptoms: cold intolerance, headache, body ache, superficial and tight pulse, with or without fever.

b. Exterior-Cold-deficiency

Resistance is low. Principal symptoms: intolerance of cold and wind, ready perspiration, increased cold intolerance upon perspiring.

c. Exterior-Heat-strength

Early injury from external Heat. Principal symptoms: wind may or may not be tolerated; fever, headache, perspiration may be spontaneous or absent.

d. Exterior-Heat-deficiency

This belongs in the category of Yin deficiency with Dampness and Heat. Principal symptoms: heat in the muscles after noon, warm palms, spontaneous perspiration.

e. Interior-Cold-strength

The Cold evil goes directly into the viscera. Principal symptoms: abdominal pains and diarrhea; if severe, cold and clammy extremities, deep and hidden pulse.

f. Interior-Cold-deficiency

This arises most commonly when the Yang of the spleen and kidney is deficient. Principal symptoms: loss of stamina, fatigue, the limbs cannot be warmed, feces remain loose, the pulse is faint and elusive, and the tongue is soft and large without inflammation.

g. Interior-Heat-strength

The external evil transforms into Heat and reaches the interior. Principal symptoms: thirst, restlessness, scanty urine that is dark; when severe, delirium with incoherence.

h. Interior-Heat-deficiency

This is mostly due to deficiency of the Yin of the liver and kidney. Principal symptoms: hot palms, lightheadedness, thirst, agitated insomnia. If there is Dampness and Heat also, see exterior-Heat-deficiency (5d above).

6. Synthesis

Looking at a single symptom has little meaning, because every symptom can appear from both sides. Thus, cold intolerance is seen in diseases of the exterior as well as those of the interior, in diseases of deficiency as well those of strength, in diseases of Cold as well as those of Heat. To decide which disease is causing this symptom, one must consider many symptoms, analyzing them and grouping them according to their nature.

Symptoms belong primarily to the surface, but some are hidden and misleading; this is known as false presentation. Cold-Heat is an example: true Cold should show a pulse that is deep and small or slow and elusive, with cold limbs, vomiting, abdominal pain, diarrhea, clear and frequent urine, and unwillingness to uncover even with fever. These symptoms indicate floating Heat on the surface and sinking Cold inside. True Heat causes rapid, smooth, large, and strong pulses, with restlessness, coarse respiration, chest tightness, thirst, abdominal distention, constipation, red and scanty urine, and no desire to cover up. False Cold manifests Cold on the surface but Heat internally: rapid pulses, being afraid of cold but not wanting to cover up, stool with a foul odor, or thirst with excessive drinking. This kind of cold intolerance is not a symptom of Cold but of Heat, and reflects what is known as extreme Heat generating Cold, or extreme Yang presenting as Yin. False Heat is the appearance of Heat affecting the surface but really Cold internally: the pulse is faint and elusive or deficient though rapid, superficial and large but unrooted; the body is hot but the person is comfortable and calm; speech is irrational yet the voice is weak and small, or it is ranting but easily stopped; or the skin shows fine and faintly red rash; or there is preference for cold liquids but not drinking much, or adequate urine flow, or absence of constipation. These symptoms are not truly of Heat but of Cold, reflecting extreme Cold generating Heat, or extreme Yin presenting as Yang.

In the case of deficiency-strength, extreme deficiency also can give the appearance of strength, that is, false strength; extreme strength also can give the appearance of deficiency, that is, false deficiency.

C. Diagnosis by the Six Regions (Liujing 六经)

Diagnosis by the eight fundamentals is relatively static. It reveals the patient's status, but it does not help much in understanding the course and progression of an illness. An alternate approach is needed that emphasizes the dynamic aspects of a disease. Two such approaches are commonly used in Chinese medicine: diagnosis by the six regions, described in this section, and diagnosis by the three positions and four levels, described in the following section.

Diagnosis by the six regions uses the properties and effects of Yin and Yang development to analyze diseases. These regions are given the same names used in describing the circulation and its vasculature. The three Yang regions are Greater Yang, Lesser Yang, and Bright Yang. The three Yin regions are Greater Yin, Lesser Yin, and Dark Yin.

Most illnesses start in Greater Yang, at which stage the disease evil is in the exterior. As the disease evil leaves the exterior, the illness shifts into the Lesser Yang region, and when it becomes stronger and reaches the interior, the illness is now in the Bright Yang region. If the patient fails to recover and his Proper Qi begins to decline, the illness enters the Greater Yin region. Thus, illnesses in the Yang regions are generally strength illnesses (that is, strength of the disease evil) and often show fever. Illnesses in the Yin regions are generally deficiency illnesses (that is, deficiency of the Proper Qi) and manifest symptoms of Cold rather than Heat. All illnesses in Lesser Yin are serious, and the physician must constantly watch for exhaustion of the body's Yin and Yang Qi. The Dark Yin represents the critical or terminal stage of an illness, with very grave prognosis.

By dividing the body into these six regions, this technique provides another way of systematically analyzing illnesses. It enables the physician to grasp the development and progression of diseases induced by external evils.

1. Analysis of Greater Yang

At the outset of an illness, the patient's Proper Qi is in general strong, and the appearance of the illness reflects vigorous struggle; such is a Yang disease. Greater Yang is the initial phase of such an externally caused disease. Although the symptoms are mostly those of the body exterior, the illness can internalize via the meridians into the Fu viscera.

    a. Principal symptoms: headache, cold intolerance and fever, superficial pulse.

    b. Greater Yang meridian illness
- (1) Exterior-deficiency: principal symptoms; and spontaneous perspiration, wind intolerance, even pulse.
- (2) Exterior-strength: principal symptoms; and body aches, no perspiration, tight pulse.

    c. Greater Yang Fu organ illness
- (1) Water accumulation: principal symptoms; and restlessness, thirst yet vomiting upon drinking, difficulty with urination.
- (2) Blood accumulation: besides fever, cold intolerance, and spastic arching backward of the head and spine (opisthotonos), the main symptoms are madness, pelvic spasm and cramps, urinary incontinence, deep and faint pulse.

    d. If other factors are discovered, they too must be analyzed. Thus, combined illnesses, simultaneous illnesses, illnesses in both interior and exterior, meridian symptoms not yet resolved, or complications due to erroneous treatment, and so forth, all need to be considered.

2. Analysis of Lesser Yang

Illness in the Lesser Yang results as the disease evil leaves the exterior of the Greater Yang but has not yet entered the interior of Bright Yang; it is thus in the stage between these two, and often manifests symptoms that are half exterior and half interior.

    a. Principal symptoms: bitter taste, dry throat, blurred vision, repeated chills and fever, chest tightness and distention, nausea, loss of appetite, palpitations, stringy pulse.

    b. In a Lesser Yang illness, it is important to clarify the direction of tendency of the illness, whether toward the exterior (improving) or toward the interior (worsening).

    c. Any illness that is half exterior and half interior can be regarded as a Lesser Yang illness.

3. Analysis of Bright Yang

Disease of the Bright Yang arises when disease in the Greater Yang fails to resolve, and the disease evil becomes stronger and progresses inward. Its symptoms are generally those of interior Heat and strength—of Heat when disease is located in the meridian, of strength when disease is located in the Fu organs. This is a stage of rapid rise or advance and often manifests severe or dangerous symptoms. Prompt diagnosis or treatment is essential.

    a. Principal symptoms: high fever, diaphoresis, heat intolerance, thirst, large pulse.

    b. Disease in the Bright Yang meridian manifests with high fever, diaphoresis, restlessness, excessive drinking, heat intolerance, large and tidal pulses.

    c. Disease in the Bright Yang Fu viscera manifests with repeated spiking fever in the afternoon, incoherence, diaphoresis, abdominal distention and pain with guarding, constipation; pulse is either deep and strong or smooth and rapid; tongue coating is yellow, dry, thick, and greasy.

    d. Bright Yang illnesses may be caused by combinations of disease evils, such as Heat and Dampness together, causing jaundice, blood accumulation in Bright Yang, or deficiency and Cold symptoms. It is thus important, in clinical practice, not to be constrained by the two categories of meridian and Fu viscera.

4. Analysis of Greater Yin

When in the course of an illness the patient's Proper Qi tends toward decline and the patient seems to have deteriorated, the illness has become one of Yin disease. In general, diseases of the three Yang all have fever, whereas diseases of the three Yin are mainly diseases of deficiency and therefore manifest symptoms of Cold rather than Heat.

    a. Greater Yin illness can be caused by two mechanisms: transformation of a Yang disease, and chronic deficiency of the stomach and spleen so that the external evil invades the Greater

Yin directly. These illnesses generally show symptoms of interior deficiency and Cold.

b. Principal symptoms: abdominal distention with vomiting or abdominal pain somewhat relieved by pressure, inability to eat, no thirst, severe diarrhea, warm hands and feet, smooth, white, and greasy tongue coating, even or elusive pulse.

c. Although illnesses of Greater Yin and Bright Yang affect the same locations, their natures are opposite. Caution is required in analyzing such similar symptoms to avoid error, particularly because illnesses of Greater Yin usually result from transformation of other illnesses and may be accompanied by some symptoms of the original illness. In a Greater Yin illness, the stool may become hard in several days, and the pulse may change from faint and impeded to long; the illness is then developing from Yin to Yang (that is, improving), and should be so recognized.

5. Analysis of Lesser Yin

An illness of Lesser Yin is one step more serious than illnesses of Greater Yin and reflects deficiency of Yang Qi. Lesser Yin governs Water and Fire, and deficiency of Yang transforms with Cold whereas deficiency of Yin transforms with Fire.

a. Principal symptoms: somnolence, faint and small pulse.
b. Types of Lesser Yin diseases
   (1) Deficiency-Cold: cold intolerance without fever, diarrhea with undigested food, paradoxically cold hands and feet, clear urine, deep and faint pulse.
   (2) Deficiency-Heat: restlessness with insomnia, dry mouth, sore throat, chest fullness, diarrhea, deep, small, and rapid pulse, bright-red tongue tip.
c. All illnesses of Lesser Yin are serious, particularly the deficiency-Cold type. Look carefully for indications of Yin exhaustion and Yang collapse. Many Lesser Yin illnesses are in fact untreatable.

6. Analysis of Dark Yin

Dark yin is the terminal stage in the course of disease caused by an external evil, where the Proper Qi puts up a final struggle against the disease evil. The symptoms are consequently mixed, with those of Yin and of Yang, of Cold and of Heat, being present simultaneously.

a. Principal symptoms: excessive urine with unquenchable thirst, Qi rising into the chest and against the heart with pain behind the breast bone, hunger without appetite, eating followed by vomiting, sometimes vomiting of *Ascaris* worms.

b. Although the symptoms are complex, there are only two main types.

   (1) Mixed chills and fever. Symptoms of upper Heat: persistent thirst, Qi rising against the chest, heart pain, fever. Symptoms of lower Cold: hunger without appetite, vomiting upon eating.

   (2) Cyclic fluctuations between heat and cold. Limbs may be cold and then warm up spontaneously, but they turn cold again; and so forth. If the cold stage lasts longer than the heat stage, or if the limbs fail to warm up again, then Yang is subsiding and Yin growing, and the illness has a grave prognosis. If the heat stage lasts longer than the cold, or warming returns, then the Proper Qi is recovering and the prognosis is better.

c. Dark Yin disease is a grave stage, and precise diagnosis is critical. The key is to analyze the direction and progression of the Proper Qi and of the disease evil, and to base the decision on this knowledge.

7. General Analysis

   a. The appearance of the symptoms of the six regions depends on the development of the disease evil. This phenomenon of progressing from one region to another is known as region transmission. Whether a particular illness will show region transmission depends on the struggle between the body's forces of resistance and the disease evil. If the disease evil is strong and the Proper Qi weak, the risk of transmission is high; conversely, if the Proper Qi is strong and the disease evil weak, the risk of transmission is small. Also, if the body resistance is strong, the transmission will be mostly limited to the three Yang regions; but when the body resistance is weak, the transmission easily encompasses the three Yin regions.

   b. Region transmission usually progresses in an orderly fashion, moving from Greater Yang to Lesser Yang to Bright Yang to Greater Yin to Lesser Yin to Dark Yin. Sometimes, however,

one or two regions may be skipped; this is known as skip transmission. The cause of skip transmission is usually the rise of disease evil at the time when the Proper Qi is deficient. Additionally,
illnesses of the three Yin regions do not necessarily begin in
any of the Yang regions but may begin directly in Greater Yin
or Lesser Yin, or even Dark Yin; this is known as direct invasion. This usually happens when the Proper Qi is already very
weak.

c. Each of the six regions has its characteristic symptoms and
characteristic pulse configurations. These symptoms, however,
can and often do appear simultaneously. When more than one
region is affected at the same time, not because of transmission,
it is known as simultaneous illness. If one region is affected by
transmission before the previous region has cleared of its symptoms, it is known as combined illness.

d. Analysis based on the six regions not only explains the develop-
mental course of illnesses induced by external evils but also clari-
fies how the six regions mutually interact to function as a unified
system. One can in this way look at the entire process of illnesses
induced by an external evil and apply the principles of treatment
effectively.

D. Diagnosis by the Three Positions and the Four Levels

Diagnosis by the three positions (sanjiao 三焦) and the four levels is
designed for analysis of diseases of Heat. The approach evolved from
that of the six regions. On one hand, an illness progresses from the
upper through the middle and to the lower positions; on the other
hand, it also proceeds from the superficial into the deeper levels. Analysis of position and analysis of level are usually combined.

1. The Three Positions

In an illness caused by the Heat evil, at the outset the evil is in the
upper position and the illness is shallow and mild; as it progresses to
the middle and lower positions, it becomes more severe.

a. Upper Position. The upper position encompasses two meridians:
the hand Greater Yin lung and the hand Dark Yin pericardium.
The lung governs Qi and regulates the skin and hair. When the
Heat evil first injures the lung, the symptoms are mild wind and

cold aversion, fever, spontaneous perspiration, headache, sometimes thirst, cough, superficial smooth and rapid pulse. The pericardium governs blood and enhances vitality. If the Heat evil
reaches the pericardium, the symptoms are restlessness, thirst,
depressed consciousness with incoherence, restless sleep, and
deep red tongue. Usually the Heat evil goes from lung to
stomach, that is, from the upper to the middle position. This is
known as orderly transmission (shunchuan 顺传). It can, however, go rapidly from the lung to the pericardium, that is, from
the pneuma to the blood level (see below); this is known as contrary transmission (nichuan 逆传).

b. Middle Position. The middle position encompasses two meridians: the foot Bright Yang stomach and the foot Greater Yin
spleen. Bright Yang governs Dryness. When the Heat evil progresses from the upper position into Bright Yang, the symptoms
are high fever and diaphoresis that worsen as the day wears on,
flushed face and red eyes, coarse respiration, constipation, dark
and scanty urine, thirst with excessive drinking, and coarse yellow or black and hairy tongue. Greater Yin governs Dampness.
When illness is transmitted into Greater Yin, the symptoms are
marked discomfort from heat that worsens in the afternoon,
head pressure, body heaviness, chest pressure, loss of appetite,
overflow of stomach contents with nausea, painful urination, and
white and viscous or light-yellow tongue coating. At this stage,
Heat becomes extreme, or Dampness and Heat cause evapora-
tion so that red or pale rashes appear on the skin, and there is
agitated delirium or semicoma.

c. Lower Position. The lower position encompasses two meridians:
the foot Lesser Yang kidney and the foot Dark Yin liver. The kidney governs the Yin Qi, while the liver governs blood. When the
Heat evil has reached this stage, often the illness proceeds from
depletion of body fluids to damage of blood and Yin Qi. In illness
in the kidney, the symptoms are relative quietness in the daytime
but restlessness at night, thirst but little drinking, throat inflammation or aphthous sores with loss of voice, diarrhea, and dark
and scanty urine. In illness in the liver, the symptoms are cyclic
fluctuations between cold and heat, pain and heat in the heart,
agitated protestations, frequent dry heaves, headaches with foaming at the mouth, and inability to eat. Above there is dry mouth
with maceration; below there is watery diarrhea. Or there are
seizures, scrotal atrophy, and abdominal pains.

2. The Four Levels

These are the guard (wei 卫), the pneuma (qi 气), the encampment (ying 营), and the blood (xue 血) levels, progressing from the most shallow to the deepest. The course of the disease evil through these levels is intimately related to its progression through the three positions.

a. The Guard Level. Early diseases in the upper position all belong to this level and are in the exterior. Symptoms: fever, mild aversion to wind and cold, nasal congestion, cough, headache, thin and white tongue coating, superficial and rapid pulse. The skin is injured, as is the lung internally.

b. The Pneuma Level. Diseases in the middle position and Bright Yang all belong at this level and are in the interior. Symptoms: high fever, disappearance of cold intolerance, thirst, yellow tongue coating, smooth and rapid or tidal and large pulse.

c. The Encampment Level. The disease evil is in the upper position but has arrived at the pericardium by contrary transmission, causing the symptoms of restlessness, incoherence, and depressed consciousness. Alternately, the evil is in the middle position, causing bumpy rashes and incoherence and depressed consciousness. At this stage, the most reliable diagnostic finding is the dark red tongue.

d. The Blood Level. The Heat evil has entered blood. Symptoms: agitation, incoherence and depressed consciousness, seizures; externally there are bumpy rashes, internally there are vomiting, nosebleeds, and bloody stools; the pulse is small and rapid or stringy and rapid, the tongue deep red with little saliva. These symptoms belong to the lower position.

3. Combined Analysis

Most illnesses begin in the upper position at the guard level and progress into the middle position at the pneuma level. These correspond to the three Yang regions. Further deterioration allows the disease evil to reach the encampment level, corresponding to the Greater Yin region. As the evil enters the blood level, first body fluids and then Yin become damaged and depleted; when Yin is depleted, the evil has entered the lower position. These correspond to the Lesser Yin and Dark Yin regions; and when the illness has progressed to this extent it becomes critical indeed. In a combined analysis, Heat diseases can be summarized as follows.

a. Stage of Cold Intolerance. This is the earliest stage of Heat diseases. The patient first feels a chill and aversion to wind. There is a low-grade fever that rises somewhat after noon, and in addition, headache, cough, and aching of the four limbs; there may be spontaneous perspiration and dryness of the mouth, and the tongue coating is thin and white.

This is thus an exterior illness, with the disease evil in the upper position and at the guard level. Treatment should be by dispersing the exterior evil. If the fever persists even when the chill and wind aversion have subsided, and there is no further development, it still belongs to the upper position at the guard level.

b. Stage of Heat transformation. Following clearing of aversion to cold and wind, the fever rises, followed by dry mouth, restlessness, dark and scanty urine, or worsening of cough. This is the beginning of Heat transformation, when in general the Heat is still in the upper position at the guard level. Thereafter, the body starts to burn, and the patient develops heat intolerance, diaphoresis, thirst with craving for cold liquids, a yellow tongue coating, and smooth and large pulse. The Heat evil has now progressed to the middle position and reached the pneuma level.

The middle position belongs to the stomach, and the stomach to Bright Yang. Treatment at this stage should be based on cooling to reach the evil, and constipation can be managed by catharsis.

c. Stage of entering the encampment level. Heat is trapped in the middle position and leaves the pneuma level for the encampment level. The tongue now turns deep red and sleep becomes restless. There are three characteristic findings: incoherence with depressed consciousness, bumpy rash, or bleeding from the mouth and nose.

Although the Heat evil is still in the middle position, it has reached the pericardium and thus the encampment level, and the situation begins to deteriorate. It is therefore a critical point. Treat by dispersion combined with drugs that cool the blood. There is still hope of repulsing the evil back to the pneuma level.

d. Stage of Yin injury. Any Heat disease, if prolonged, depletes the body fluids and damages Yin. Fluid depletion is mainly in the middle position and is relatively less serious, whereas Yin damage is mainly in the lower position and is most serious.

Damage to the kidney Yin and liver blood: the tongue is denuded and red, followed by wild movement of the Yang of deficiency, which precipitates seizures. This is also known as the stage of the evil entering the blood level. Treatment must be powerful, to nourish Yin and suppress Yang. Death from Heat disease occurs mostly in this stage.

5

Herbal Pharmacology

Pharmacology is the study of the properties of drugs, how they are collected and prepared, and how they are applied in the treatment of illnesses. About six thousand drugs are known in Chinese medicine. The vast majority of these are derived from plants; for this reason books about Chinese *materia medica* have traditionally been called herbals and Chinese drugs herbs. Less than 5 percent of the known drugs are used commonly.

Section A details the material aspects of Chinese drugs. Section B describes the properties that make them suitable for treating diseases. Section C lists the factors that influence dosage—how much of an herb to use. Section D discusses the interaction between different herbs and the principles that aid the physician in exploiting such interactions.

A. *Materia Medica*

1. Collection

In Chinese medicine, the locale where an herb grows and the time of its collection are of intimate importance to its effectiveness (see chapter 1). Indeed, many Chinese herbs are partially named according to their place of origin, and in some prescriptions the sources of certain ingredients are specified.

Because plants grow and mature according to their own schedules and each plant has different structural parts, the preservation of the herb's potency as a drug depends very much on the appropriateness of the season and manner of collection. Even the time of collection must be varied somewhat, because seasons can be early or late and the weather can change, affecting the growth and maturation of the plant.

a. Root. The root is used for its rising Qi. Collect before the shoot appears or after the herb has wilted, because the essence is then stored in the root.

b. Stalk. The stalk is the pathway for going up and down and is used for this property in mediation. Collect when the herb is most luxuriant.

c. Leaf. The leaf is used for its ability to disperse and dissipate. Collect when the plant is most luxuriant—but not when wet from rainfall, to avoid rotting.

d. Branch. The branch is used for its ability to go to all the limbs. Collect when the plant is most luxuriant.

e. Flower. The flower is used for its fragrance and its ability to dissipate and disperse. Collect when the bud is about to open or has just opened, when its Qi is strongest.

f. Fruit. The fruit is used for its descending Qi. Collect when it has just ripened.

g. Seed. The seed is used for its Qi, which has already descended. Collect when the fruit has overripened.

h. Kernel. The kernel is used for its ability to moisten and lubricate. Collect when the fruit has overripened.

i. Node. Nodes (the joints in a stalk) are used for their ability to loosen joints. Collect when the nodes are firm and strong.

j. Sprout. The sprout is used for its ability to scatter, to throw out. Sprouts can be grown by horticulture.

k. Thorn. The thorn is used for its ability to breach.

l. Peel. The peel is used for its ability to reach the skin.

m. Center. The center (of a stalk or branch) is used for its ability to move through the internal viscera.

n. Vein. The veins are used for their ability to enter the meridians. Collect veins when the herb is ripe.

o. Vine. The vine is used for its ability to reach the meridians and the limbs. Collect when it is luxuriant.

These rules apply only in general. The actual structure of a part makes a difference. For example, the root of *Pueraria* is firm and thus raises fluid but not Qi; the root of *Cimicifuga* is hollow and raises Qi but not fluid; the root of *Achyranthes* is solid and has a bitter taste, and it has no raising ability at all.

2. Preparation

Freshly collected herbs may be poisonous or too potent for direct use; or have an offensive odor or taste; or have an unsuitable part; or may require cooking to bring out their intended actions. Most herbs have to be prepared properly. For example, raw *Pinellia ternata* can irritate the throat, causing hoarseness, even poisoning, and should be treated with ginger juice before use. Raw *Rehmannia glutinosa* is of cold nature and can chill blood; if steamed first, its nature becomes warm, and it can nourish blood; if dry-stir-fried into ashes, it can stop bleeding.

   a. Basic techniques

     (1) To fire. The drug is placed directly in the flame or in a fire-proof container. This technique is most often used with minerals or shell-type drugs, such as the shell of the female oyster, *Ostrea rivularis*, and fossil bone.

     (2) To toast. The drug is placed in a dry and hot pan and rapidly stirred until the surface is burned yellow and has cracked (e.g., toasted *Zingiber officinale*, or ginger).

     (3) To roast. The drug is wrapped in paper or some other suitable material, then either buried in appropriate hot ashes or toasted in low fire until the wrapping material has burned black (e.g., roasted *Saussurea lappa*).

     (4) To dry-stir-fry. The drug is placed in a pan over a fire and stirred until cooked, browned, burned, or turned into ash (e.g., dry-stir-fried *Atractylodes macrocephala*, burned *Gardenia jasminoides*).

     (5) To moist-stir-fry. While stir-frying, add honey, butter, or another suitable material, until the drug is browned (e.g., moist-stir-fried *Glycyrrhiza uralensis*).

     (6) To heat-dry. The drug is dried over a low fire (e.g., the leech, *Hirudo nipponica*).

     (7) To warm-dry. The drug is simmered dry (e.g., *Chrysanthemum, Lonicera japonica* flowers).

     (8) To wash. The drug is washed clean of dirt, soil, and so on.

     (9) To soak. The drug is soaked in water as long as necessary, for instance to get rid of fishy or salty taste. This takes longer than washing and requires frequent changes of water (e.g., *Cistanche salsa, Laminaria japonica*).

    (10) To peel. The drug is put in clear water or boiling water in order to remove its peel (e.g., *Prunus armeniaca* kernel).

(11) To moisten. The drug is softened with water to facilitate cutting.

(12) To pulverize. The powdered drug is further ground with water to make it finer (e.g., talc, cinnabar).

(13) To steam. The drug is steam-cooked over boiling water (e.g., *Rheum palmatum*, *Polygonum multiflorum*).

(14) To boil. The drug is boiled in water or some other liquid until cooked (e.g., *Daphne genkwa*).

(15) To temper. The drug is heated red hot in the flame, then thrown into water or vinegar (e.g. lodestone, pyrite).

b. Liquids and other materials used

Sometimes liquids other than water, or other materials, may be used to prepare the herbal medicines, depending on treatment requirements.

(1) Wine: for its ability to lift up.

(2) Ginger juice: for its ability to disperse and dissipate.

(3) Salt water: for its ability to enter the kidney and soften what is solid.

(4) Vinegar: for its ability to go to the liver, and for its astringency.

(5) Child's urine: for its ability to cool Fire and descend.

(6) Rice water: for its ability to moisten dryness and mediate the interior.

(7) Milk water (milk diluted with water): for its ability to moisten severe dryness and generate blood.

(8) Honey: for the ability of its sweetness to restore the spleen.

(9) Earth: frying with earth for its ability to move into the middle position.

(10) Wheat husk: frying with wheat husk for its ability to strengthen the stomach and intestines.

(11) *Glycine max* (black bean) and *Glycyrrhiza uralensis* (licorice): for soaking with potentially poisonous herbs and peeling them to remove their poison.

(12) Goat curd or lard: for their ability to diffuse into bone.

c. Drug form

(1) Pill form. Grind the ingredient(s) into a fine powder; add water, honey, rice paste, or other sticky substance. Mix and roll into round shapes. The size depends on clinical needs.

Pills are digested and absorbed slowly, so the pill form is used in chronic diseases that require long-term treatment.

Diseases in the lower position are also frequently treated with drugs in pill form to keep the drugs from becoming active before they reach the intestines. Sometimes pills are used even for urgent or severe illnesses, as pills can conveniently be prepared ahead of time.

(2) Powder form. The drugs are simply ground into powder or flake form. In most cases the ingredients are ground together. They are ground individually if they are sticky, or are very potent, or are rare and expensive. The stepwise procedure, wherein ingredients and/or portions are added periodically, is used when the formula includes a small quantity of expensive ingredient or some ingredients that require separate individual grinding.

The powder form is usually taken by mouth, and its actions usually begin faster than those of the pill form. The powder form can also be snorted or externally applied as a plaster.

(3) Gel form. The herbs are soaked in water overnight and boiled. The liquid is filtered, and the residue is boiled again. The procedure is repeated two to four times. The filtrates are then combined and simmered until they form a gel so thick that it does not soak into paper. To use, dilute an appropriate quantity in boiling water, let cool, and drink.

The gel form is used mostly for restorative drugs.

A different procedure extracts the medicinal principles from the herbs with plant oil. This is intended for use as a topical ointment.

(4) Distillate form. This form is suitable mainly for medicinal minerals and is prepared by sublimation or melting. Occasionally herbs are mixed and prepared in this manner. The form varies; it can be a pill, a powder, or a cake. The distillate is used the same way as a pill or a powder.

(5) Alcohol extract. The herbs are extracted with white wine, hence the common term, *medicinal wine*. Extraction can be performed cold or hot. Cold extraction involves simply soaking the herbs in wine for a period of time. Hot extraction involves sealing a mixture of herbs and wine in a glazed pot, putting the entire pot in a vat of water, and warming it with slow fire to maintain an appropriate temperature (usually just below boiling); after three to seven days, the fire is stopped and the contents of the pot are allowed to cool.

Alcohol extracts are mostly used for rheumatism, taking advantage of the alcohol's ability to increase the circulation of Qi and blood, thus potentiating the drug's action.

(6) Decoction form. This form uses hot-water extraction by boiling the herbs. The liquid is poured out; this is the first extract. The herbs are boiled a second time to produce the second extract. Both extracts are used: in some cases, the two extracts are taken separately as two doses; in other cases, they are combined.

Decoction is the most widely used drug form in the practice of Chinese medicine. The drug is absorbed rapidly and has potent action, and the quantity can be readily controlled to suit the severity of the illness.

B. Drug Properties

1. Nature (qi 气)

The nature of drugs falls into four categories: hot, warm, cool, and cold. This categorization is derived from the body's reaction to the various drugs and provides an indication of the drug's action. Drugs of a cold nature are useful in diseases of Heat, and drugs of a warm nature are useful in diseases of Cold. Some authorities add a fifth category: neither warm nor cool.

Drugs of hot or warm nature are Yang drugs, and those of cool or cold nature are Yin drugs. Their application is governed by the principles of Yin-Yang.

2. Taste (Wei 味)

There are five categories of taste: acid, bitter, sweet, acrid, and salty. Some authorities add a sixth: bland. Acrid, sweet, and bland are Yang; acid, bitter, and salty are Yin.

a. Acrid
Acrid drugs can induce dispersion of external evils and movement of Qi, thereby also loosening of tightness or congestion in the lung. Acrid belongs to the Metal element and thus easily enters the lung. Excessive use of acrid drugs causes spasm of the sinews and wilting of the hands and feet. Acrid should be avoided in diseases of Qi.

b. Acid

Acid drugs can induce a pulling back and impedance of outflow, so that Yang is preserved and loss of Jing slowed. Acid belongs to the Wood element and thus can enter the liver. Excessive use of acid hardens the muscles. Avoid acid in diseases of the sinews.

c. Sweet

Sweet drugs can restore and nourish Yin and Qi and harmonize the interior. Sweet belongs to the Earth element and can enter the spleen. Excessive use of sweet drugs causes bone pain and hair loss. Avoid sweet drugs in diseases involving the flesh.

d. Bitter

Bitter drugs can induce firming, eliminate Fire by catharsis, dry Dampness, and eliminate Heat by catharsis and induction of defecation. Bitter belongs to the Fire element and can enter the heart. Excessive use of bitter drugs causes withering of the skin and hair. Bitter should not be used in bone diseases.

e. Salty

Salty drugs soften the firm and eliminate Phlegm and can lubricate the intestines and induce catharsis. Salty belongs to the Water element and can enter the kidney. Excessive use of salty drugs causes blood to stagnate and the pulse to become impeded. Salty should be avoided in diseases of blood.

3. Dispersion and Excretion, Rising and Sinking

In many cases, different drugs of the same nature and taste may nevertheless have different uses and actions, owing to the strength of the nature and taste.

- Drugs with strong nature tend to disperse.
- Drugs with strong taste tend to promote excretion.
- Drugs with weak taste tend to rise.
- Drugs with weak nature tend to sink.

To disperse, to excrete, to rise, to sink—these describe the tendencies of a drug's action. A drug that rises and disperses (strong nature, weak taste) generally rises upward and moves into the exterior and has the actions of raising Yang, inducing perspiration, and cooling the head and eyes. In contrast, a drug that sinks and excretes (weak nature, strong taste) generally lowers and moves internally. It has the actions of submerging Yang, reducing backward flow, and facilitating both urination and defecation.

It is clear that as diseases can affect the exterior or the interior, above or below, and can show upward or downward tendency, so must drugs be chosen that have the appropriate properties of nature, taste, and the tendency to rise, sink, disperse, or excrete. Furthermore, a drug's tendencies may often be altered by the technique of preparation. For example, preparing a drug with wine gives it a tendency to rise, with ginger juice a tendency to disperse, with vinegar a tendency to draw in, and with salt water a tendency to sink.

4. Nature, Taste and Tendency of Action

Every drug has nature and taste. Some drugs are similar in nature but differ in their taste, whereas others are similar in taste but differ in their nature. Some drugs have one nature but several tastes. These kinds of complex combinations of nature and taste reflect the wide variety of Chinese drugs.

The study of a drug's nature and taste and the tendency of its action is aimed at understanding the drug's application. To realize the full potential of Chinese drugs, all these aspects must be considered. For instance, *Pinellia ternata*, *Fritillaria cirrhosa*, and *Sargassum fusiforme* can all decrease sputum. But *Pinellia* is acrid, has warmth, and can decrease Dampness and Phlegm; whereas *Fritillaria* is bitter, has coolness, and can dissolve Heat and Phlegm; and *Sargassum* is bitter and salty, has cold, and can dissipate solidified Phlegm. Again, *Astragalus hoantchy*, *Dioscorea opposita*, and *Adenophora verticillata* are all restoratives. But *Astragalus* is sweet, has warmth, and is used to restore Qi; whereas *Dioscorea* is sweet, is neither warm nor cool, and is useful for spleen deficiency; and *Adenophora* is sweet and slightly bitter, has coolness, and is used to restore deficient lung Yin.

These drugs have seemingly similar actions, but their effects are quite different, largely because their natures are different.

5. Organ and Meridian Affinity

Through a large clinical experience, Chinese medicine recognizes that each drug has affinity for a particular organ or meridian. *Ephedra sinica*, for example, has affinity for the meridians of the lung and bladder, so that its acrid warmth is ideally suited to treat illnesses resulting from the Cold evil in the lung or bladder. Thus *Ephedra* is indicated for exterior Cold in the Greater Yang region.

In clinical application, the concept of affinity has major importance.

As pointed out earlier, drugs of cold nature can be used to treat Heat diseases, and drugs of warm nature can be used to treat Cold diseases. Yet the same Heat disease or Cold disease may be localized in different specific areas, such as the exterior or the interior, a Zang organ or a Fu organ. At the same time, certain cold drugs can cool exterior Heat but not necessarily interior Heat, or cool Heat in the lung (Zang organ) but not necessarily Heat in the stomach (Fu organ). For example, headache in the forehead belongs to Bright Yang and can be treated with *Pueraria lobata* root; headache in the occiput belongs to Greater Yang and can be treated with *Ephedra sinica*; headache in the temples belongs to Lesser Yang and can be treated with *Bupleurum chinense*. *Pueraria* is a drug with affinity for Bright Yang, *Ephedra* for Greater Yang, and *Bupleurum* for Lesser Yang.

The meridians are intimately linked with the viscera, and therefore these drugs also show affinity for the visceral organs. This affinity is related to the drug's nature and taste. For example, the bladder belongs to Water and Cold, and its meridian is Greater Yang. *Ephedra sinica* has multiple thin and long stalks that are hollow but go straight up, and is of cool and light nature and taste; hence it can facilitate the Yang Qi of the lower sphincter, conducting it to the skin to be dispersed as perspiration. It is thus an essential drug in treating Cold injury of the Greater Yang exterior. *Angelica sylvestris* can be used instead, also because of its deep root and straight stalk and its ability to conduct the bladder Yang to the meridian. Because of its somewhat stronger acrid taste, it is also able to mobilize Dampness, but it is not light and cooling like *Ephedra*. Hence *Ephedra* can lubricate the lung and facilitate urination, while *Angelica* can further treat pain in the body caused by Wind and Dampness.

C. Drug Dosage

The dosage of a drug is exceedingly important in achieving proper therapeutic results; indeed, inappropriate dosage may produce undesirable effects. The appropriateness of a compound prescription, for example, depends not only on the nature of the illness and the body's condition but also on whether the ingredient drugs are each properly selected and in the proper quantities. Such mastery comes only with experience.

Although there are standard doses for all the drugs, the following factors must be carefully weighed. Adjustment in dosages may be required according to these principles.

1. Nature of the drug. Drugs with a strong nature and taste and drastic action are used in smaller quantities, those with mild and bland taste and nature in larger quantities. Solid drugs are used in larger quantities, soft and light drugs in small quantities.

2. Nature of the illness. Severe illnesses require larger quantities, especially when rapid and aggressive therapy is needed. Milder illnesses and those requiring long-term treatment need lesser amounts.

3. Body constitution. If the patient's constitution is strong, it is permissible to use larger quantities; if weak, smaller quantities. In general, use larger amounts in the northwestern geographical areas (of China) than in the southeastern areas, the main reason being the difference in body constitution (for the Chinese).

4. Age of the patient. Use lesser amounts for children—in general, half the amount for adults. Infants need much smaller amounts.

5. Organization of the formula. The principal drug (see next section) is used in larger quantities, the supporting drugs in lesser amounts. Where there are many ingredients, use smaller amounts; where there are only a few ingredients, use larger amounts.

D. Drug Combinations

Each drug has its nature and actions. By combining several drugs into a compound, we can often enhance the intended therapeutic action or reduce the undesirable effects. Some combinations, however, can reduce therapeutic effectiveness or even produce severe undesirable effects.

1. Principal Types of Drug Interaction

   a. Mutual assistance: two or more drugs with similar actions helping one another to achieve their effect. For example, *Anemarrhena asphodeloides* combined with *Phellodendron amurense* mutually enhance each other's action to nourish Yin and reduce Fire.

   b. Mutual potentiation: two or more drugs with differing actions in combination achieve their therapeutic effects more readily and more directly than either alone (e.g., *Aconitum carmichaeli* and *Poria cocos*).

   c. Dislike: one drug is counteracted by another in such a way that the strength of its effects is reduced or eliminated. For instance, *Pinellia ternata* dislikes *Zingiber officinale*, so that *Zingiber* is used to control the effects of *Pinellia* whether in formulas of compound drugs or as treatment of overdose. Common examples of dislike:

(1) Sulfur, mirabilite
(2) Mercury, arsenolite
(3) *Stellera chamaejasme*, lead oxide
(4) *Croton tiglium, Pharbitis nil*
(5) *Syzygium aromaticum, Curcuma longa*
(6) Mirabilite, *Sparganium stoloniferum*
(7) *Aconitum carmichaeli*, rhinoceros horn
(8) *Panax ginseng, Pleropus pselaphon*
(9) *Cinnamomum cassia*, halloysite

d. Inhibition: two or more drugs reduce or neutralize one another's effectiveness. For example, *Scutellaria baicalensis* is of cold nature and can inhibit the warming action of *Zingiber*.

e. Antidote: one drug can eliminate another drug's poisonous effects. *Saposhnikovia divaricata*, for example, is antidotal to *Arsenolite*; *Phaseolus radiatus* is antidotal to *Croton tiglium*.

f. Mutual contrariness: several drugs in combination generate severe toxic effects. Common examples of mutual contrariness:

(1) *Aconitum carmichaeli* when combined with one of these: *Pinellia ternata, Tricosanthes kirilowii, Fritillaria* spp., *Ampelopsis japonica, Euonymus tengyuehensis*

(2) *Glycyrrhiza uralensis* when combined with one of these: *Sargassum fusiforme, Euphorbia pekinense* and *kansui, Daphne genkwa*

(3) *Veratrum nigrum* when combined with one of these: *Panax ginseng, Adenophora verticillata, Asarum heterotophoides, Paeonia lactiflora*

2. Ingredients

A compound drug is a prescription including two or more drugs designed for a broader range of effectiveness than can be expected from a single drug, or to reduce or eliminate the undesirable or poisonous effects of some of the ingredients. How to select and combine the ingredients is governed by established principles, including the types of drug interactions described above. The terms *king, minister, steward,* and *assistant* are used to distinguish the various ingredients, which are not of equal importance.

a. King. The king is the principal drug in a formula of a compound drug and is aimed at the basic cause of an illness or the principal symptom. There may be more than one king in a formula, and the king need not necessarily be a very potent drug. The important point is to determine the cause or principal symptom on the basis of the facts of the actual case.

b. Minister. The minister is to assist or potentiate the king's effectiveness. In any given formula there may be one or more ministers, particularly if there are two kings.

c. Steward. In addition to assisting the king to perform its function much as the minister does, the steward can also help overcome some of the lesser symptoms. For example, *Prunus armeniaca* kernel in formula 249 helps relieve the cough and soothe the lungs while the king, *Ephedra*, takes care of the diaphoresis. If the king has undesirable effects or is too powerful, the steward can also be used to ameliorate that.

d. Assistant. The assistant assists the minister just as the steward and minister assist the king. In pharmacological terms, its function is to reduce and direct the power of the compound drug to the site of the illness; thus it is also called the inducer.

3. The Seven Categories (Fang 方)

Because of the differences in the number of ingredients, their nature, and their rapidity of action, compound formulas are classified into seven categories.

a. The Powerful Formula (dafang 大方). When the disease evil is in full power, it cannot be overcome except by strong power, and a powerful formula is essential. When using a powerful formula, first consider whether the Proper Qi can withstand its effects. A powerful purgative can damage Yin, and a powerful diaphoretic can destroy Yang, and so on.

b. The Mild Formula (xiaofang 小方). When the disease evil is mild or weak, a gentle drug is adequate—either a milder drug, or a powerful formula in a reduced dosage.

c. The Slow Formula (huanfang 缓方). Most chronic diseases, especially those due to deficiency and weakness, cannot be resolved rapidly. They should be treated on a long-term basis using drugs with slow and gentle action.

d. The Urgent Formula (jifang 急方). These compound drugs are used in urgent situations when the illness is critical. An urgent formula should have concentrated action and is used in high doses, hence it is often used in combination with a powerful formula.

e. The Single-Action Formula (jifang 奇方). If there is only one cause of an illness, it is appropriate to use a single king to treat, so that the action of the compound drug is concentrated. A single-action formula need not be restricted to only a single ingredient.

f. The Double-Action Formula (oufang 偶方). This type of compound drug is designed to attack two causes simultaneously and thus generally contains two kings. It is used for such purposes as combined diaphoresis and catharsis, or simultaneous attack and restoration, and so on.

g. The complex formula (fufang 复方). Complex illnesses with several causes or many symptoms require complex treatment. Formula 41 contains formulas 249, 175, 76, 7, and so on, using one complex formula to eliminate Wind, Cold, Phlegm, and Dampness, and to dissolve accumulations and stagnation. Another use of a complex formula is when other, simpler drugs have not been effective.

6

Approaches to Treatment

Having examined the patient and made the diagnosis, the physician must now devise appropriate treatment. Like all other aspects of Chinese medicine, treatment is based on an understanding of Yin-Yang and the five elements.

Because illnesses can arise from Proper Qi deficiency or disease-evil strength, the usual approach is to treat the cause by providing what the patient lacks. Only in unusual circumstances would a Chinese physician be mainly concerned with treating the symptoms. In determining what treatment to select, the physician should keep the following considerations in mind in addition to factors relating to the specific illness:

- Weather. As the weather warms, use warming and drying drugs with caution to avoid damaging the body fluids. Similarly, as the weather cools, use cooling drugs with caution to avoid injuring the Yang Qi.
- Geographic locale
- Age
- Sex
- Constitution
- Emotion and personality
- Occupation

A. Standard versus Contrary Treatment

In Chinese medicine, the course of an illness is regarded as the struggle between the Proper Qi of the body and the evil Qi of the disease-causing agent. If the Proper Qi wins, the illness resolves; if the disease evil wins, the illness worsens, and the patient may die. The approach is thus to restore and strengthen the Proper Qi, or to eliminate the disease evil and its ravages, or both. There are numerous methods within this framework, but only one aim, to bring about recovery of health and well-being.

1. Standard Treatment (Zhenzhi 正治)

The standard treatment meets the cause head on. Thus, if the illness is due to Heat, treatment is with drugs that cool; if due to Cold, with drugs that warm; if due to deficiency, with drugs that restore; if due to strength (of disease evil), with drugs that eliminate this evil. This is the usual approach.

2. Contrary Treatment (Fanzhi 反治)

The contrary treatment seemingly uses drugs of similar nature to the symptoms—for instance, cooling drugs in the presence of Cold symptoms. On deeper analysis, however, the treatment still basically opposes the cause of the illness. For example, in deficiency states with abdominal distention due to inefficient digestive function, a restorative drug is used rather than a cathartic. The illness arises out of deficiency, so that it is not possible to bring about resolution of the symptom of abdominal distention unless the deficiency is first remedied. Another example: in diarrhea caused by internal blockage resulting from accumulation, a cathartic is used instead of a drug that stops diarrhea and solidifies, again because the symptom of diarrhea cannot be controlled unless the accumulation is eliminated.

Furthermore, in severe illnesses there may arise so-called false manifestations. For example, extreme (internal) Cold may repel Yang to the exterior, giving rise to the symptom of restlessness; using a cooling drug to treat the restlessness aggravates the basic disease process. However, a strong heat-generating drug may not be tolerated by the body. Here it is appropriate to administer a heat-producing drug together with a mild cooling drug. Such an approach also falls in the category of contrary treatment. Another example: in an illness of the Lesser Yin meridian with diarrhea and cold limbs, no cold intolerance but fever and face flushing, and so forth, the Cold is true while the Heat is false, and therefore the treatment requires warming and Yang drugs.

Contrary treatment has fewer uses than standard treatment.

B. Treatment of Root versus Treatment of Appearance

The analysis of root (ben 本) and appearance (biao 标) is intended
for sorting out the cause and the symptoms of an illness, the degree of
severity, the need for speed, and the order of importance of the various
factors.

1. Root versus Appearance

From the holistic viewpoint, the body is the root while the illness is the
appearance. The aim of treatment is to restore the root and eliminate
the appearance. From the viewpoint of the disease process, the cause
is the root and the symptoms are the appearance. The importance of
this distinction is underscored by the fact that different sets of symptoms may be due to different diseases of different causes. In complicated illnesses, the original symptoms are the root and the subsequent
symptoms are the appearance. When a patient has two diseases simultaneously, the first disease is the root and the second the appearance.

Because the terms *root* and *appearance* mean different things, depending on the specific situations, the treatment must be adjusted
accordingly.

2. Treatment of Root

Root is the basis, the cause. In general, Chinese medicine uses treatment of the root as standard practice. For example, in cough and fever
due to Yin deficiency, the fever and the cough are appearance, while
the Yin deficiency is root; treatment is therefore directed at nourishing
Yin, and when that is accomplished, the fever and the cough will disappear. Another example: a patient has a kidney disease that causes
absence of urine and total body swelling, along with subsequent damage to the lung with cough and shortness of breath; treatment is aimed
at inducing urine flow to reduce swelling. When the kidney disease has
improved, the symptoms of lung disease (cough, shortness of breath)
will naturally improve.

3. Treatment of Appearance

If symptoms are recognizably serious and severe, it may be necessary to
treat appearance first. In accumulation of fluid in the abdomen due to
liver or spleen disease, for example, the liver or spleen disease is root,

while the abdominal fluid is appearance. Yet when the abdominal distention has reached the point of causing severe respiratory difficulties and compromise of defecation and urination, one does not aim treatment at the liver or spleen but rather at prompt and rapid induction of urine flow, postponing treatment of the root until the appearance has improved considerably. Another example: when a patient with asthma develops critical air blockage, it is permissible to relieve the blockage before paying attention to the asthma. The ancients said, "When urgent, treat the appearance."

We must recognize, however, that treatment of appearance is really a temporizing approach. Sooner or later, one must come to the definitive treatment of root.

4. Simultaneous Treatment

When the root and the appearance are both urgent, one must treat both at the same time. Even when the appearance is not urgent, it is sometimes reasonable and advisable to treat the appearance at the same time as the root. Example: in an illness caused by Wind and Cold, there are symptoms such as fever, headache, and body aches. Wind and Cold are the cause and are thus root, while the fever and so forth are the symptoms and are thus appearance. The fever is a principal symptom, because the degree of fever may influence the severity of the other symptoms. In this case, use diaphoresis to dissipate the Wind and Cold as the principal treatment, but add some cooling drug to reduce fever and thereby relieve the other symptoms as well.

C. Treatment by Yin-Yang and by the Five Elements

1. Strengthen Water to Control Yang

Useful in such conditions as insufficiency of the Genuine Yin (as opposed to excessively strong Yang) in the kidney, this treatment uses rapid restoration of the kidney Genuine Yin to relieve the symptoms of rising Yang due to deficiency Yin's inability to control Yang—symptoms such as faintness, blurred vision, dry and painful throat, dental pain, pain in the heel with heat in the sole, and deep, small, and rapid pulse.

2. Enrich Fire to Dissipate Yin

Useful in such conditions as insufficiency of the Genuine Yang (as opposed to excessively strong Yin) in the kidney, this treatment uses rapid restoration of the kidney Yang to relieve the symptoms of Yin gelation resulting from deficient kidney Yang's inability to warm and melt—symptoms such as flank pain, weak limbs, cold below the waist, and spasm above the pubis.

3. If Deficient, Enrich Its Mother

By the principle of trophism (of the five elements), when the Qi of a particular visceral organ is deficient, it is possible to restore it by enriching its mother—that is, the visceral organ that bears the trophic relationship to it. For example, Earth produces Metal, thus spleen (Earth) is the mother of lung (Metal) and lung the son of spleen. If the lung Qi is insufficient, this may affect its mother organ, so that chronic lung deficiency with chronic cough, for example, sometimes induces dysfunction of the spleen and stomach, with loss of appetite, watery diarrhea, and so on. For treatment, one can use the technique of enriching the mother by strengthening the spleen, improving appetite and stopping diarrhea so the lung now receives nutrition and the cough is also relieved.

4. If Strong, Purge Its Son

The trophism principle also applies to excessive strength. If an organ is diseased because of excessive activity of its son, it can be treated by purging the son organ's excesses. Example: Water produces Wood; if liver (Wood) Fire is excessively strong, it may affect the ability of the kidney (Water) to hold and store, causing nocturnal emission and bedwetting; in this case, treatment should be directed at cooling and eliminating liver Fire.

5. Other Treatment by the Five Elements

Metal (lung) suppresses Wood (liver), and Wood suppresses Earth (spleen). If the lung is deficient and is unable to suppress the liver, the liver may show disrespect for the lung, causing such symptoms as rib pain, bitter taste, cough, and coughing up of blood. Furthermore, because the liver, being unsuppressed, is overactive, it may now affect the spleen's function, causing the symptoms of rib pain, acid regurgitation, loss of appetite, abdominal distention, diarrhea, and so on. In this example, treatment is directed at restoring and enriching the spleen, because by enriching the spleen (Earth) one can strengthen the lung (produce Metal), and a strong lung can then suppress the liver.

This sort of treatment is mostly used in very complicated illnesses. The ancients called this the technique of skipping one (or skipping two).

D. The Eight Methods (Bafa 八法)

To apply the principles just described, eight methods of treatment have been devised in the course of the years. The eight methods are diaphoresis, emesis, catharsis, mediation, cooling, warming, dissipation, and restoration. These methods can be applied singly or in combination, depending on the requirements of the patient.

For specific applications of these methods, see the Compendium (chapter 10) on Therapeutics.

1. Diaphoresis (han 汗)
   a. Synonyms: dispersion of the exterior, dispersion of the muscles, or simply dispersion.
   b. Purpose and indications
      This method is intended to dissipate external evils from the body exterior by sweating. It is indicated in the early stages of diseases caused by external evils, in the early stages of edema or skin ulcers and abscesses, and in measles when the rash is about to appear. Diaphoresis treatment includes soothing the lung, as applied in Wind injury with nasal congestion, cough, and hoarseness.
   c. Basic types
      (1) Acrid-warming diaphoresis is suitable for exterior Cold diseases with low-grade fever but marked cold intolerance, especially those due to external Wind and Cold.
      (2) Acrid-cooling diaphoresis is suitable for exterior Heat diseases with high fever and mild cold aversion, especially those due to external Wind and Heat.
      (3) Acrid-even diaphoresis is suitable when neither Heat nor Cold symptoms are prominent.
   d. Other types
      (1) Yin-nourishing diaphoresis is suitable for use in disease induced by external evil in a patient with preexisting Yin deficiency.
      (2) Yang-aiding diaphoresis is suitable for use in disease induced by external evil in a patient with preexisting Yang deficiency.

(3) Diaphoresis with elimination of water and Phlegm is suitable for use in disease induced by external evil in a patient with chronic water and Phlegm accumulation.

(4) Diaphoresis can also be combined with the other methods.

e. Precautions and contraindications

(1) Diaphoresis should be used only with great caution in such conditions as blood deficiency, severe vomiting and diarrhea, weak heart, or carbuncles, to avoid such complications as tetany or even collapse. Where diaphoresis is needed in these conditions, use in conjunction with Qi enrichment, blood generation, or other treatments.

(2) Diaphoresis can deplete the body fluids, so the treatment should not be used any more than absolutely essential. Pay attention also to the weather, the location, the patient's constitution, and the selection of drugs and dosages.

(3) Most exterior illnesses show fever and cold intolerance as the principal symptoms. If after diaphoresis the fever and cold intolerance both persist, the external evil has not been dispersed from the exterior, and further use of diaphoresis is appropriate so long as the body fluids are not damaged. If, however, the cold intolerance is gone but the fever persists, or the fever rises instead, the disease evil is showing a tendency to internalize; here, diaphoresis should not be used again.

(4) When using diaphoresis, the patient should be advised to avoid exposure to Wind and Cold and not to eat heavy, fatty or oily, or spicy foods.

2. Emesis (tu 吐)

a. Emesis is aimed at removing external disease evil or injurious materials by vomiting. It is an emergency procedure. When used appropriately, it is very effective. If used inappropriately, it can easily damage the Proper Qi.

b. Indications

(1) Emesis is suitable treatment when accumulated Phlegm causes overflow or blockage of the throat or chest, when retained food blocks the stomach and pylorus, and when ingested poisons are still in the stomach.

(2) Emesis can sometimes be used in favorable circumstances in place of the uplifting treatment—for example, in such conditions as certain types of difficulty with urination or frequent

lower abdominal pain during pregnancy. The inexperienced physician should avoid the use of emesis.

(3) Emesis is frequently applied in severe or urgent illnesses in which the accumulated evil must be vomited promptly.

c. Technique

Emesis is usually induced with emetics. Sometimes other drugs are given as indicated, and vomiting is then induced with a chicken feather or a finger stimulating the throat. This procedure is called gag-induced emesis.

d. Basic types

(1) Cooling emesis is suitable for illnesses in which the Heat evil is trapped above.

(2) Warming emesis is suitable for illnesses in which the Cold evil is trapped above.

(3) Fast-acting emesis is suitable for illnesses in which the evil is strong above and the condition is urgent.

(4) Slow-acting emesis is suitable for illnesses in which the evil is strong and the Proper Qi weak, the disease is located in the upper position, and emesis is a necessary part of the treatment.

e. Precautions and contraindications

(1) Emesis is contraindicated in the following conditions:

(a) Critical illnesses, especially in the aged, the weak, and those with markedly deficient Qi

(b) Massive blood loss

(c) Asthma

(d) Beriberi

(e) Pregnancy, or immediately following delivery (see paragraph 2.b.(2) above)

(2) In general, emesis should be used only once, not repeatedly.

(3) When undergoing treatment with emesis, the patient should be warned to avoid solid foods but to use soups, porridges, or gruels for nutrition; to avoid excessive passion; to avoid sexual activity; and to avoid exposure to Wind or Cold.

3. Catharsis (xia 下).

a. Catharsis is aimed at removing interior accumulations and sludges and at facilitating defecation. Catharsis may be precipitous or slow.

(1) Precipitous catharsis (or purgation) is used when the condition is urgent but the patient's constitution is still strong—

mostly when the Heat wanton shows a tendency to deplete body fluids and destroy Yin (called rapid purgation to preserve Yin).

(2) Slow or gentle catharsis is used when the illness is mild or when the patient's constitution is weak.

b. Indications

Catharsis is best suited for illnesses resulting from external evil in the interior, particularly in the stomach and intestines. Catharsis is also appropriate for external evil–induced constipation or fecal retention. Catharsis can also be applied in cases of water or Phlegm accumulation or parasitism.

c. Basic types

(1) Cooling catharsis is suitable for constipation due to Heat or interior or strength diseases; severe constipation, with or without leakage of liquid feces; and severe painful straining. This is the most commonly applied type of catharsis. It uses mainly drugs that are of bitter taste and cold nature.

(2) Warming catharsis is suitable for Cold-induced intestinal blockage or Cold-induced chest tightness. Warming catharsis uses mainly drugs of acrid taste and hot nature.

(3) Water elimination is suitable for water retention due to Yang Heat, with swelling in the upper body, fever, thirst, dark urine, and constipation.

(4) Moistening catharsis is suitable for constipation due to insufficiency of body fluids, Yin deficiency, or blood depletion.

(5) Mobilization of stagnation is suitable for illnesses due to stasis or stagnation of blood (hematoma, ecchymosis).

(6) Phlegm dissolution is suitable for illnesses due to accumulation and gelation of Phlegm.

(7) Expulsion of parasites is suitable for more severe cases of parasitism.

d. Precautions and contraindications

Inappropriate catharsis can lead to serious complications, and due caution is essential.

(1) If the disease evil is in the exterior, do not use catharsis.

(2) If the illness is half interior, half exterior, do not use catharsis.

(3) In Bright Yang disease, if the evil has not reached the Fu organs, do not use catharsis.

(4) In the aged with insufficient body fluids and constipation, or the constitutionally weak, or those with chronic insufficiency

of Yang Qi, or in women with blood deficiency following delivery, do not use precipitous catharsis.

(5) Use catharsis only with great caution in pregnancy or during menstruation.

(6) Do not overuse catharsis.

4. Mediation (he 和)

a. Indications and applications

Mediation has wide applicability. In general, it is suitable for illnesses that are half exterior, half interior, in which neither diaphoresis for the exterior nor catharsis for the interior would be
appropriate. For conditions in which the illness is not severe and
the Proper Qi only mildly decreased, mediation can also be used.
Thus, besides illnesses in the Lesser Yang, such illnesses as disharmony of liver and stomach, menstrual disturbances due to
trapping of liver Qi, and disharmony of liver and spleen can all
be treated by mediation.

b. Combined types

(1) Mediation with diaphoresis is suitable for illnesses that lean toward the exterior but require mediation.

(2) Mediation with catharsis is suitable for illnesses that show features leaning toward the interior but require mediation.

(3) Mediation with cooling is suitable for illnesses that show features of Heat but require mediation.

(4) Mediation with warming is suitable for illnesses that show features of Cold but require mediation.

(5) Mediation with dissipation is suitable for illnesses with accu-mulations but that require mediation.

(6) Mediation with restoration is suitable in illnesses with de-ficiency of Proper Qi but that require mediation.

c. Precautions and contraindications

Although mediation is gentle, if used inappropriately it can nonetheless aid the disease evil or damage the Proper Qi. It should not
be regarded as generally applicable to all illnesses; it is contraindicated in the following situations:

(1) The disease evil is in the exterior and has not entered Lesser Yang.

(2) The disease evil has entered the interior.

(3) Cold disease exists in the three Yin regions.

5. Cooling (qing 清)

a. Indications and applications

Cooling as treatment is designed to reduce fever and suppress Fire. It also includes protecting the body fluids, quenching thirst, and inducing sedation to eliminate restlessness. Cooling thus has wide application, being useful in Heat diseases at the pneuma, encampment, and blood levels, so long as the disease evil has left the exterior.

  b. Basic types

    (1) Acrid-cool cooling is suitable for Heat at the pneuma level with damage of the body fluids.

    (2) Bitter-cold cooling is suitable for Heat strength at the pneuma level.

    (3) Encampment-penetrating cooling is suitable for Heat at the encampment level.

    (4) Salty-cold cooling is suitable for Heat at the blood level.

    (5) Yin-generating cooling is suitable for damage of Yin by Heat so that Water is unable to control Fire.

    (6) Cooling to open conduits is suitable for persistent high fever with dull sensorium.

    (7) Other types include cooling heart Fire, cooling liver Fire, cooling lung Fire, cooling stomach Fire, and the like.

  c. Precautions and contraindications

    (1) Do not use cooling when the exterior evil is unresolved and the fever is due to trapped Yang Qi.

    (2) Do not use cooling if the constitution is chronically weak or the viscera already cold.

    (3) Do not use cooling in deficiency Heat due to Qi or blood deficiency.

    (4) Do not use cooling in illnesses of genuine Cold and false Heat, such as those due to waxing Yin attacking Yang, or kidney Fire deficiency.

    (5) Be cautious also concerning the location and depth of the Heat to avoid guiding the evil deeper.

6. Warming (wen 温)

  a. Indications and applications

Warming treatment is designed for elimination of Cold and protection and strengthening of the Original Yang. It is applicable to illnesses caused by the Cold evil entering directly the three Yin regions, or Cold diseases transformed from Heat diseases. Warming treatment also includes stimulation in such illnesses of Yang deficiency as spontaneous perspiration with cold body, indigestion, shortness of breath with weak voice, weak limbs with lassitude, urinary incontinence, and decline of sexual desire.

b. Main types

(1) Yang rescue is suitable in acute illnesses due to insufficiency of true Yang allowing the Cold evil to invade directly the three Yin regions, or due to Heat disease with perspiration and excessive use of cooling so that the disease evil enters the three Yin regions. This type aims principally at supporting Yang.

(2) Warming centrally to repel Cold is suitable in slower illnesses of chronic Yang deficiency allowing Cold invasion. This type aims at driving out Cold.

c. Precautions and contraindications

(1) Heat hidden internally with false symptoms of exterior Cold.

(2) Interior Heat causing vomiting of blood, blood in the urine, or blood in feces.

(3) Fever with diarrhea, semicoma, marked dehydration with gray complexion, or near exhaustion of body fluids.

(4) Chronic Yin deficiency with red tongue and dry throat.

(5) In pregnancy, avoid potent warming drugs.

7. Dissipation (xiao 消)

a. Definition, indications, and applications

Dissipation is designed for use in illnesses resulting from slow accumulation, gelation, or solidification of Qi, blood, foods, Phlegm, and even water. Parasitism and carbuncles can also be treated with this technique. Dissipation thus includes features of elimination and of dissolution and bears some resemblance to catharsis. However, dissipation is a much slower process and does not emphasize purgation.

b. Major types

(1) Dissolution and grinding of solids is suitable for abdominal masses.

(2) Mobilization of Qi and release of stagnation is suitable for illnesses due to gelation of Qi and stagnation of blood.

(3) Promotion of digestion and movement is suitable for dietary indiscretion and for dysfunction of spleen and stomach causing food retention and stoppage.

(4) Dissipation of accumulated Phlegm and water.

(5) Elimination of water and relief of swelling.

(6) Combinations. The accumulative and solidifying processes show different stages of evolvement. In accordance with the

status of the Proper Qi, dissipation should be combined with other treatments, such as mediation and restoration.
  c. Contraindications
    (1) Qi impedance causing interior distention.
    (2) Weakness of Earth (spleen) causing inability to control Water (kidney) leading to fluid swelling in the abdomen and limbs.
    (3) Deficiency Heat with thirst and loss of appetite, or spleen deficiency causing distention, diarrhea, and indigestion.
    (4) Phlegm generated by spleen deficiency or kidney deficiency with water overflow.
    (5) Blood depletion in women and consequent loss of menses.
8. Restoration (bu 补)
  a. Synonyms: nourishment, nurture, strengthening.
  b. Definition, indications, and applications
    (1) Restoration treatment is designed to strengthen the weakened Yin, Yang, Qi, blood, or function of specific organs, and to restore it to normal equilibrium. In conditions where the weakened Proper Qi is unable to eliminate the residual disease evil, using restoration treatment not only helps Proper Qi recover but also helps eradicate disease evil.
    (2) Because of variability in the severity of illnesses, restoration may be rapid or slow. Rapid restoration is often needed for patients near exhaustion or for resuscitating a patient in collapse. Slow restoration is indicated when the body is so weak it cannot withstand too rapid restoration, or when there is deficiency but only mild symptoms of Cold or Heat.
  c. Major types
    (1) Restoration of Qi is used in deficiency of spleen and lung Qi, fatigue and weakness, lethargy, shortness of breath, spontaneous perspiration, and large but deficient pulse—for example, falling of Central Qi; rectal prolapse; hernia; prolapse of the uterus; and Wind invasion with collapse. In patients with substantial blood loss, first restore Qi or use strong doses of restorative drugs, because restoration of Qi can generate blood.
    (2) Restoration of blood is suitable in blood deficiency or blood loss, with sallow complexion, pallor, light-headedness, ringing in the ears, confusion and nervousness, delayed and light menses, or even loss of menses. When restoring blood, look also for the presence of Heat or Cold, which must be treated also.

(3) Restoration of Yin is suitable in illnesses caused by deficiency of Yin or body fluids—for example, emaciation, dry mouth and throat, dry and wilted skin and sinews, blurred vision and ringing in the ears, nervousness and fearfulness, restlessness and insomnia, night sweats and night emissions of semen, bloody paroxysmal cough, or diabetes.

(4) Restoration of Yang is suitable in deficiency of the spleen and stomach Yang—for example, cold, pain and dysfunction of the waist and below the knee, weakness of the lower limbs, difficulty with walking, recurrent lower abdominal pain, diarrhea, urinary frequency, impotence, or premature ejaculation.

d. Precautions and contraindications

(1) When using restoration, first pay close attention to the spleen and stomach, because most restoratives are thick, viscous, and hard to digest. Patients with weak spleen and stomach function are unable to absorb and utilize these drugs and may indeed suffer further compromise of their digestive processes.

(2) Do not use restoration in the false deficiency of severe strength disease.

(3) When the disease evil is strong, even though there are symptoms of deficiency, do not use pure restoration, in order to avoid leaving behind disease evil. That would be like closing the door with the thief still inside.

(4) In general, it is recommended to add to restoratives some drugs that mobilize, in order to avoid Qi impedance that can result from an inability to utilize the restorative because of deficiency of function.

E. Combinations of the Eight Methods

1. General Considerations

Each of the eight methods has its characteristic properties and uses, but in clinical practice the physician must respond appropriately and flexibly to the diverse causes and symptoms of disease, and not be confined to the use of a single therapy.

a. The eight methods have been devised on the basis of the three categories of causes and of the eight fundamentals of diagnosis. Every illness has its cause and location, yet of the eight methods, four are more concerned with location than with cause (diaphoresis, catharsis, emesis, mediation), while the other four are more concerned with cause than location (warming, cooling, dissipation, restoration). Furthermore, the same cause in different locations can bring about different symptoms.

  b. In a sense, several of the methods form pairs of opposites.

  (1) Diaphoresis is aimed at illnesses of the exterior, while catharsis is aimed at illnesses of the interior.

  (2) Catharsis is aimed at driving out the disease evil, while restoration is aimed at supporting the Proper Qi.

  (3) Cooling drives out Heat and sedates, while warming drives out Cold and stimulates.

  c. Although opposites in this sense, these methods can be and often are used in combination. In using combined methods, however, it is important to determine carefully the appropriate ratio of the individual methods.

2. Diaphoresis and Catharsis

In combined exterior and interior disease (not half exterior, half interior), the usual procedure is to clear the exterior before treating the interior. When the exterior and interior symptoms are both urgent, however, the standard procedure may not be appropriate. Diaphoresis and catharsis may need to be used together. This is called double dispersion of exterior and interior.

3. Cooling and Warming

When an illness has symptoms of both Heat and Cold, using cooling or warming alone may cause further imbalance and complication. Such illnesses are common in clinical practice: upper Heat with lower Cold; Dampness and Heat; water accumulation and Heat; and so forth.

4. Attack and Restoration

In a patient with weak constitution, injury by external evil or unresolved internal disease evil can create a situation of evil strength and Proper Qi deficiency. Driving out the evil, used alone, may leave the Proper Qi still weak and unable to stand on its own, whereas restoring Qi alone may yet allow the disease evil to consolidate. Simultaneous application of the two methods may be the only way in this situation, so long as each method is applied to the correct degree.

5. Dissipation and Restoration

This combination is used as for attack and restoration, except that here the disease evil is slow acting and chronic (e.g., Phlegm), or the patient may not be strong enough to endure a method of vigorous attack.

PART TWO

Compendia

7

Common Diseases, by Cause

To practice Chinese medicine, the physician needs to know the manifestations of the common diseases in some detail. This compendium lists the major symptoms of these common diseases from the point of view of the various causes of disease. The next compendium, in chapter 8, provides a similar list organized according to the visceral organs.

A. *Diseases of Wind*

1. General Considerations
   Wind is mobile and flamboyant. Its diseases tend to develop rapidly and to resolve rapidly, with a short and variable course. Its symptoms tend to be changeable or active, such as shivering, contractions, seizures, and vertigo and fainting.
      There are two major categories of Wind diseases: external Wind diseases are generally caused by the Wind evil, whereas internal Wind diseases arise in the course of certain processes of internal damage. These should be distinguished. In analyzing Wind symptoms, note especially the location of the evil and the severity of the symptoms. Note also symptoms of combined diseases.
2. External Wind
   a. Wind injury. The evil is in the exterior, with disharmony at the guard and encampment levels. Principal symptoms: wind intolerance, perspiration, headache, nasal congestion, throat itch, cough with much sputum, fever, superficial pulse.

b. Wind invasion. The evil has reached the viscera or the meridians. Mild cases: dizziness or fainting, unresponsiveness of the tongue, inability to speak, numbness of the skin, aching of the limbs. Severe cases: sudden loss of consciousness, loss of speech, gurgling of sputum, seizure, weakness or paralysis on one side (hemiplegia).

3. Internal Wind
Principal symptoms: vertigo, fainting, shaking, numbness and paresthesia, asymmetry of mouth and eyes; when severe, spastic neck stiffness, coma, seizures, hemiplegia.
   a. Due to blood deficiency. In addition to the principal symptoms: palpitations, anxiety, lightheadedness, and symptoms of interior Heat or Dryness.
   b. Due to extreme Heat. Additional symptoms of high fever, drowsiness, tremor, or jitteriness.
   c. Due to kidney Yin deficiency: see chapter 8, section E.
   d. Due to rise of liver Yang or penting up of liver Qi: see chapter 8, section A.

4. Combined Wind Diseases
   a. Wind and Cold. In addition to the symptoms of Wind injury: cold intolerance, joint pain, shortness of breath, tight pulse.
   b. Wind and Heat. Headache, red eyes, thick yellow rhinorrhea, throat pain, inflammation of the tonsils, thirst, restlessness, yellow urine, tidal and rapid pulse. In severe cases, coma or delirium, rashes, dark-red tongue.
   c. Wind and Dampness
      (1) In the skin: rashes with itch, or water blisters.
      (2) In the exterior: pain and heaviness in the head, migratory joint pain, perspiration, wind intolerance, shortness of breath, fever, scanty urine.
      (3) In the interior: rumbling abdominal noises (borborygmi), abdominal pain, diarrhea.
   d. Wind and Water. Body edema, especially face and neck; cough; wind intolerance; persistent perspiration; superficial pulse.
   e. Wind and Dryness. Constipation, diabetes, dry and wrinkled skin, dry nails.

B. Diseases of Cold

1. General Considerations
The nature of Cold is to contract and to congeal. Thus it can readily

cause such effects as muscular contractions and stagnation of the blood or Qi.

Cold is a Yin evil and can easily damage the body's Yang Qi. Conversely, Yang deficiency often generates internal Cold.

All Cold diseases show cold intolerance and preference for warmth, but the converse is not necessarily the case (not all patients with cold intolerance or preference for warmth have a Cold disease).

2. External Cold
   a. Cold injury. The Cold evil is in the exterior. Principal symptoms: cold intolerance, fever, no perspiration, headache, body ache, joint pain, thin white tongue coat, superficial and tight pulse.
   b. Cold rheumatism. Nonmigratory joint pain that is alleviated by heat but aggravated by cold; or spasm, sometimes even contracture, of joints and muscles.
   c. Cold invasion. The Cold evil reaches the interior directly; this is more severe than Cold injury. Principal symptoms: sudden shivering; green complexion; vomiting of clear fluids; diarrhea; abdominal pain; cold body and limbs; spasm and pain in the limbs; lying motionless in a curled posture, even coma with icy extremities and stiffness; smooth white tongue; deep, small, slow pulse.

3. Internal Cold
   The Cold here arises internally out of Yang deficiency, especially of the kidney and spleen. It differs from Cold invasion in its slower onset and progression and its occurrence in a patient who is weak from prolonged illness.

   Principal symptoms: cold intolerance with preference for warmth, pallid complexion, limbs cold and cannot be warmed, vomiting of clear fluids, watery diarrhea, abdominal cramps, excessive urine, swelling, deep and slow pulse.

C. Diseases of Heat

1. General Considerations
   Heat has a broader and narrower meaning here. In the narrow sense of the Heat evil, it is the principal Qi of summer and is often accompanied by Dampness. In the broader sense, it includes the Heat evil and also the Heat that can be transformed from Wind, Cold, Dampness, and Dryness. In internal Yin deficiency, Heat can also arise.

   Heat can damage the body fluids and cause depletion. Heat also causes disease rapidly, and Heat diseases progress rapidly.

2. Heat Evil Diseases
   a. Heat injury. This is Heat in the exterior. Principal symptoms: chills and fever, heat intolerance, perspiration, restlessness, vomiting and diarrhea, dry lips and throat, rapid breathing, limb weakness, white and greasy tongue coating, rapid pulse that is either superficial and smooth or tidal.
   b. Heat invasion. This is Heat in the interior. Principal symptoms: sudden fainting, clouded sensorium, fever and restlessness, coarse respiration, cold or no perspiration, tidal and large pulse that is either forceless or hidden.
3. Symptoms of Heat per se
   Symptoms of Heat per se include fever, heat intolerance, preference for cold liquids, nasal flaring, parched lips, flushed face and eyes, restlessness, yellow sputum, scanty and dark urine, constipation, red tongue with yellow coating, rapid pulse, rashes, fainting, and agitated delirium.

   Internally generated Heat produces similar symptoms: flushed cheeks, exhaustion with recurrent fever, night sweats, anxiety, insomnia, parched mouth and tongue, sore throat, blood-streaked sputum, hot palms and soles, constipation, dark-red or smooth red tongue without a coating, and small, rapid, and forceless pulse.

D. Diseases of Dampness

1. General Considerations
   Dampness tends to become viscous and stagnant, and its diseases frequently become chronic. Its nature is heavy and impure, so its symptoms often show these characteristics—for example, heaviness in the limbs, head, or chest; foul vaginal discharge.

   Dampness is frequently combined with other causes of disease. It is also commonly localized to one organ.
2. External Dampness
   Body aches and joint pains, with heaviness in the body and difficulty of movement, joints moving only with difficulty, perspiration on the head, damp skin, persistent pain that tends to become localized, white tongue coating, limp but even pulse.
3. Internal Dampness
   a. In the upper position. Distention and heaviness in the head, distention and tightness in the chest, loss of taste, sometimes

stickiness with a sweet taste, anorexia, decreased drinking with preference for warm liquids, scanty urine, thick, white, and greasy tongue coating.

    b. In the middle position. Abdominal fullness or distention, food remaining undigested, eructation, watery diarrhea, limb weakness, spontaneous perspiration, scanty urine, thick, white, and greasy tongue coating.

    c. In the lower position. Dribbling of urine, diarrhea, vaginal discharge.

4. Combined Diseases of Dampness

    a. Wind and Dampness: See section A.

    b. Cold and Dampness. Generalized pain, especially joint pain; difficulty of movement; no perspiration; swelling of the limbs; scanty but clear urine; loose stools; white and greasy tongue coating; slow pulse.

    c. Dampness and Heat. Fever, restlessness, thirst, spontaneous perspiration, joint inflammation, chest fullness, jaundice, scanty and dark urine, yellow and greasy tongue coating, smooth and rapid pulse.

      (1) Variant: headache, cold intolerance, body heaviness and aching, anorexia with chest tightness, fever after noon, white tongue without dryness, pale yellow complexion, stringy, small, and limp pulse.

      (2) Variant: vomiting and diarrhea, fever with perspiration, chest and abdominal tightness, anorexia, smooth white tongue coating, deficient and limp or deficient and impeded pulse.

E. Diseases of Dryness

Dryness tends to damage the body fluids, so symptoms of fluid depletion are common. The Dryness evil has special affinity for the lung, whereas internal Dryness is more generalized.

1. External Dryness

    a. Cool Dryness. Headache, nasal congestion, cold intolerance more than fever, no perspiration, dry lips, dry throat, shortness of breath, superficial but impeded pulse.

    b. Warm Dryness. Fever with perspiration, thirst, sore throat, hiccough, chest pain, blood-streaked sputum, dry nose, white and thin tongue coating that is dry, red tongue, superficial and rapid or stringy and impeded pulse.

2. Internal Dryness

Internal Dryness is mostly caused by (a) excessive use of drugs that warm and dry; (b) excessive vomiting, diarrhea, diaphoresis, or blood loss; or (c) high and prolonged fever or chronic illnesses damaging or exhausting body Yin and fluids. Symptoms are those of exterior Dryness and interior Heat.

F. Diseases of Fire

1. General Considerations

Although Fire is one of the external evils, it is in clinical practice seldom considered in this manner. Instead, it is recognized as the extreme of Heat and can arise in many ways—by transformation from the other external evils, from overactivity of the passions, arising out of the viscera, and so on. Regardless of the cause, Fire easily damages the body fluids, blood, and Yin, and can progress rapidly.

Fire is subgrouped into strength Fire and deficiency Fire. Strength Fire shows obvious symptoms of Fire but not of Yin damage; deficiency Fire shows symptoms of Yin damage as well as those of interior Heat.

2. Strength Fire
   a. Principal Symptoms

   High fever; flushed face; inflamed eyes; dry lips, mouth, and throat with thirst and bitter taste; halitosis; inflamed throat and gingivae, sometimes gingival bleeding; nosebleed; occasional vomiting of blood; deafness or ringing in the ears; restlessness, even delirium; constipation, scanty dark urine; dark-red and dry tongue that is sometimes hairy; yellow or dark tongue coating; smooth, rapid, and strong pulse.

   b. Location of Fire
      (1) Upper position: head distention, vociferous complaining, throat swelling and pain.
      (2) Middle position: thirst, desire for cold drinks, tightness in the chest, restlessness.
      (3) Lower position: scanty dark urine with impeded flow, constipation.

   c. Fire of the viscera
      (1) Heart: palpitations, hot palms, maceration of tongue and buccal membrane.
      (2) Lung: bloody sputum, dry throat and nose.

(3) Liver: head distention, irascibility.

(4) Spleen: good appetite, loud and confused speech, inflammation of the lips.

(5) Kidney: bone weakness, dark urine with pain on urination, night emission.

3. Deficiency Fire

  a. Due to Yin deficiency. Recurrent fever, night sweats, restlessness, emaciation, dry throat and mouth, red tongue without coating, small, rapid pulse.

  b. Due to Qi deficiency. Fever before noon, cold and wind intolerance alleviated by warmth, fatigue and weakness, shortness of breath and disinterest in speaking, spontaneous perspiration, watery diarrhea, large but hollow pulse.

G. Epidemic Diseases

Epidemic diseases generally progress rapidly and spread from person to person rapidly. For each disease, the course of illness tends to be similar in all affected patients, regardless of age and other differences. Most do not follow the meridians, and although sometimes exterior and interior can be distinguished, they tend to accumulate in the middle position.

1. Pestilence Expressed in the Jaws (Mumps)

In mumps, both jaws below the ears are firmly swollen and painful, the swelling extending to the cheeks; inflamed throat; high fever with thirst; often inflammation of the testes; sometimes even depressed sensorium; drowsiness or nervousness; rapid and large pulse; thick yellow tongue coating.

2. Virulent Epidemic (Malaria)

The symptoms of malaria are cyclic chills and fever; when the fever is high, there is no perspiration; generalized body and head pain; chest tightness and vomiting; thirst with no desire to drink or unquenchable thirst; inflamed eyes; dark urine; sometimes lying as if dead with air blockage and coma; upon perspiration the patient awakens, or has tetany and incoherence; there may be a skin eruption; pulse is rapid and either large or hidden; tongue is red and dry with dry yellow coating.

3. Epidemic Dysentery

Epidemic dysentery progresses rapidly: fever with cold intolerance, body ache, thirst, restlessness or vomiting, severe abdominal cramps,

foul-smelling, red or clear diarrhea dozens of times a day, burning in the anus; if the poison is strong, then delirium, incoherence, tetany or convulsions; sometimes skin rashes; tongue coating is thick, greasy, and white; pulse may be limp, rapid, slow, faint, hidden, or irregular.
4. Epidemic Pharyngitis with Exanthem (Diphtheria)
   The symptoms of diphtheria are high fever, restlessness, thirst, marked sore throat with inflammation and necrosis, tiny rash on the neck and body, red tongue with yellow or viscous and greasy coating, rapid pulse.

H. Diseases Caused by the Passions

The passions mainly affect Qi but may progress to blood. They can also directly damage the viscera.
1. Principal Symptoms
   The principal symptoms of the passions are depression, unpredictable joy or rage, troubled and confused thought, apprehension with suspiciousness, insomnia with excessive dreaming, grief with incessant crying, chest tightness with sighing or hyperventilation, choking lump in the throat, abdominal fullness with loss of appetite, epigastric or gastric pain with acid regurgitation and eructation, movable abdominal mass; if more severe: mental confusion, incoherence, psychosis.
2. Passions and the Viscera
   a. Excessive anxiety. Lung damage; anxiety impedes Qi, causing depression. If prolonged, spleen is also damaged, and anorexia results.
   b. Excessive preoccupation. Spleen damage, with anorexia and fitful sleep; preoccupation causes Qi to knot up, so that excessive preoccupation or melancholy affects the mind and causes mental confusion.
   c. Excessive joy. Heart injury, with restlessness and nervousness; joy slows Qi down, causing its dispersion.
   d. Excessive rage. Liver damage, with pallid and green complexion; decreased eating with difficulty in swallowing; rage causes Qi to flow against stream.
   e. Excessive grief. Lung injury, making Qi diminish.
   f. Excessive fear. Kidney damage, with deficiency of kidney Qi; insufficiency of Qi and blood causes timidity and fearfulness.
   g. Excessive fright. Fright causes confusion of Qi and thereby disturbance of the heart and Shen, resulting in mental disquiet.

I. Diseases of Phlegm

Phlegm arises when the flow of body fluids in any area becomes impeded, allowing gelation to take place. Of the viscera, Phlegm is most closely associated with the spleen, the lung, and the kidney.

1. Principal Symptoms
   a. Main characteristics of Phlegm diseases
      (1) Productive cough and gurgling with respiration.
      (2) Symptoms of spleen deficiency (indigestion, loss of appetite, abdominal distention).
      (3) Greasy tongue coating and smooth pulse.
      (4) Most patients are obese and prefer inactivity.
   b. Phlegm is usually localized, causing characteristic symptoms in each location. Examples:
      (1) Stomach: nausea, vomiting.
      (2) Heart: palpitations, faintness, delirium.
      (3) Head: vertigo, fainting.
      (4) Skin: numbness, nodules under the skin.
      (5) Air passage: air blockage in the throat.
2. Combined Phlegm Diseases
   a. Wind and Phlegm. Vertigo or syncope, nausea, numbness of the four limbs, copious sputum with foaming, gurgling in the throat, tetany or tremor, superficial and smooth pulse.
   b. Heat and Phlegm. Yellow sputum that is thick and lumpy and sometimes blood-streaked, flushed face, dry lips and throat with frequent drinking, yellow tongue coating, tidal and smooth pulse.
   c. Cold and Phlegm. Thin and clear sputum, white and moist tongue coating, joint pain, cold intolerance, gray complexion and cold feet, deep and slow pulse.
   d. Dampness and Phlegm. Copious thin and clear sputum that comes up easily, sallow complexion, loss of appetite, abdominal distention, lassitude, thick and greasy tongue coating, even pulse.
   e. Dryness and Phlegm. Cough and shortness of breath, thick viscous sputum that comes up only with great difficulty and sometimes blood-streaked, dry and irritated throat, chills and fever, scanty dark urine, dry tongue coating, impeded pulse.
   f. Phlegm and Fire. Similar to Heat and Phlegm, but more prominent symptoms.

J. Diseases Caused by Food and Drink

1. General Considerations
   Dietary indiscretion may be the result of excess or deficiency. Over-
   indulgence causes indigestion. In starvation, occasional large meals
   may also cause indigestion; this is due to deficiency.
       Indigestion is closely related to stomach and spleen function. If
   the digestive function is chronically weak, so that the patient cannot
   eat much and has bloating following eating, ingestion of oils or fats
   frequently causes diarrhea; this is spleen deficiency. If the patient is
   able to eat but not digest, the stomach is strong but the spleen weak;
   if there is hunger but inability to eat, the spleen is strong but the
   stomach weak.
2. Symptoms of Indigestion
   In general, in indigestion the tongue coating is thick and greasy or
   yellow; the pulse is smooth and rapid or deep and strong.
   a. Damage in the stomach. Gastric pain, poor appetite, food aver-
      sion, chest and epigastric fullness, acid regurgitation and eructa-
      tion, thick tongue coating, smooth and forceful pulse.
   b. Damage in the intestines. Abdominal cramps and diarrhea.

K. Diseases of Water Accumulation

Water accumulation is closely related to Dampness and Phlegm and is
similarly closely tied to the function of the lung, the spleen, and the
kidney.
1. Principal Symptoms
   a. Water in the stomach and intestines. Cough, palpitations, aver-
      sion to drinking, water sounds in the abdomen, vomiting of clear
      liquids, chest and abdominal distention, emaciation, stringy and
      smooth pulse.
   b. Water under the axillae. Cough with pain, epigastric mass, fever
      with perspiration, deep or stringy pulse.
   c. Water in the somatic body. No perspiration when there should
      be, body heaviness with pain. Cold type: cold intolerance, no
      thirst, heavy respiration even without perspiration, white tongue
      coating, slow pulse. Heat type: fever, heavy respiration with per-
      spiration, yellow tongue coating, superficial and rapid pulse.
   d. Water above the diaphragm. Cough with air blockage, faintness,

shortness of breath on lying down that is relieved on sitting up, mild body edema, deep and tight pulse.

L. Diseases Caused by Parasites

The parasites generally reside in the intestines. They arise usually out of chronic Dampness and Heat, poor food hygiene, and dietary indiscretion.

1. Principal Symptoms

   The main symptoms of parasites are sallow face, emaciation, dark discoloration under the eyes and nose, itch in the nostrils and anus, grain-sized white cysts inside the lips, loss of appetite or excessive eating, sometimes craving for raw rice or tea leaves, abdominal cramps, and changes in complexion. Small children especially can develop malnutrition, with full and firm abdominal distention.

2. Differentiation of the Common Parasites

   a. The phthisis worm. The phthisis worm causes consumption (also known as the phthisis communicated from corpses) in the lung. Symptoms: cough, bloody sputum, hoarseness, rapid respirations, exhaustion with internal Heat, night sweats, pale and glossy complexion but red cheeks as if rouged. This disease causes severe damage.

   b. Roundworm. Facial freckles, periumbilical pain, vomiting of worms, worms in feces.

   c. Pinworm. Rectal itch disturbing sleep, worms in feces.

   d. Tapeworm. Hunger and increased appetite, nasal itch, irritability, worm segments in feces.

   e. Hookworm. Itchy skin eruptions, jaundice, and swelling.

8

Common Diseases, by Organ

As discussed in chapter 2, the Zang and the Fu viscera are intimately interrelated with each other; they are also closely linked with various parts of the somatic body. In evaluating actual patients, it is essential to observe and analyze the whole picture rather than any specific element in isolation, particularly because a disease often may manifest transmission from one organ to another and from one region to another. Nonetheless, it is often helpful to have a compendium of symptoms of the specific organs.

A. *Diseases of the Liver*

1. Cold in the Liver
   Firm flank swelling, abdominal distention with inability to eat, sinew atrophy, scrotal pain, distention and pain just above the pubis, vomiting of clear saliva, deep, stringy, and slow pulse, pale tongue with smooth white coating.
2. Heat in the Liver
   Head pressure, restlessness, inflamed eyes, flank pain, deafness, convulsion, restless and fearful sleep, cloudy dysuria, hematuria, stringy and rapid pulse, red tongue.
3. Liver Deficiency
   Dizziness, faintness, ringing in the ears, blurred vision, dry eyes, night blindness, convulsions, numbness and tingling sensation, hand and nail atrophy, urinary incontinence, quick anger and fear, agita-

tion, sometimes even recurrent chills and fever resembling malaria, stringy, small, and elusive pulse, red and denuded tongue.

4. Liver Strength

   Heat and pain inside the head, blurry vision with vertigo, ringing in the ears, impatience, irascibility, vomiting of acid fluids, chest and flank fullness with pain and guarding, shortness of breath, difficulty with turning and moving about, inability to urinate, stringy pulse, purple tongue with yellow and greasy coating.

5. Disease in the Liver Meridian

   Headache in the vertex, axillary swelling and pain, red eyes, green complexion, deafness, swelling of the forehead, dry throat, muscle spasm, testes that are drawn up, inflamed testes, leakage of urine or inability to urinate; in females, also inflammation of the vulvar area.

6. Liver Yang Rising against Stream

   a. Fire strength in liver meridian: headache, blurred vision with vertigo, flushed complexion and red eyes, irascibility, light-headedness, numb fingers, muscle twitching, ringing in the ears, bitter taste, excessive dreaming, bleeding from the gums and nose, constipation, urine dribbling, hard, stringy, and long pulse, red tongue with yellow coating.

   b. Pent-up Fire in liver meridian: head pressure, cyclic chills and fever, vomiting of acid fluids, distention and pain in flank and ribs, feverish and red face or scrofula, red tongue that is sometimes hairy, stringy and rapid pulse.

   c. Internal movement of liver Wind: Sudden collapse, asymmetric eyelids and mouth, paralysis on one side and loss of speech, usually stringy, long, and forceful pulse; the patient may gradually recover with residual weakness on one side, or die in coma.

7. Disequilibrium of Liver Qi

   Headache, blurred vision, spastic pain in the flank and ribs, flushed forehead and bitter taste, depression, loss of appetite, drowsiness, pelvic heaviness, irregular menses, stringy and large but deficient pulse.

8. Combined Liver Diseases

   a. Liver Fire invading lung: rapid and difficult breathing, cough with thick sputum, chest pain; in severe cases, vomiting of blood or blood-streaked sputum.

   b. Liver Qi invading heart: spastic and curled tongue, coma, snoring while awake, upward empty gaze, green complexion with red eyes.

c. Liver Qi invading stomach: chest tightness with diaphragmatic pressure, pain in the axillae, gastric pain, undigested food, eructation or vomiting of acid material, abdominal enlargement, irregular defecation, stringy pulse, thin and yellow tongue coating.

d. Disharmony of liver and spleen: wilted and yellow complexion, drowsiness, thirst without desire to drink, hunger without desire to eat, abdominal distention and pain, rumbling of the abdomen, watery diarrhea, stringy but even pulse, white and greasy tongue coating.

e. Disquiet of liver and gallbladder: restlessness with insomnia or nightmares with restless sleep, nervousness and easy fright, shortness of breath and weakness, blurred vision, bitter taste, vomiting of bitter fluids.

f. Yin deficiency in liver and kidney: wan and haggard face, cheeks red as if rouged, vertigo with dry eyes, pain above the eyes, pain in the axillae, sore and weak waist, night pains and drying of the throat, night sweats, hot palms and soles, night emission in males and pelvic pain in females, irregular menses, profuse vaginal discharge, impeded and difficult urinary and fecal excretion, small pulse, red tongue without coating.

g. Kidney Yin deficient, liver Yang rising: faintness with blurred vision, decreased sleep with increased dreaming, heat and restlessness with red cheeks, fearfulness and irascibility, heavy head with light feet, deafness with ringing in the ears, weak limbs, flank aches and night emission, red and glossy tongue, stringy, small, and rapid pulse.

B. Diseases of the Heart

1. Cold in Heart
   Palpitations of the heart, mental disorientation, sudden severe heart pain, cold limbs, slow pulse.

2. Heat in Heart
   Red face, dry throat, thirst with desire to drink, restlessness and insomnia, delirious and incoherent speech, uncontrollable frivolity, heat and tightness in the chest with stabbing pain, rapid pulse, red and dry tongue tip or swelling under the tongue, swollen and stiff tongue.

3. Deficiency in Heart
   Fearfulness, nervousness, forgetfulness, insomnia, restlessness, ex-

cessive dreaming, easy startling, spontaneous perspiration and night sweats, hot palms, small and elusive pulse, pale red tongue.

4. Strength in Heart
Agitation, uncontrollable frivolity, rage, blockage by Phlegm, faintness, red tongue tip, strong and large pulse.

5. Disease in Heart Meridian
Yellow eyes, dry throat, pain in the heart and ribs, thirst with desire to drink, pain in the inner and posterior aspects of the elbow or paradoxical cold, heat and pain in the palms.

6. Combined Heart Diseases
   a. Heart and spleen both deficient: sallow complexion, decreased intake and fatigue, poor stamina and timidity, forgetfulness, nervousness, loss of sleep, night sweats, irregular menses, small, weak, and forceless pulse, pale tongue with white coating.
   b. Heart and gallbladder both deficient: fearfulness, excessive dreaming, restlessness with insomnia, bitter taste, palpitations and nausea, stringy, small, and forceless pulse, pale tongue.
   c. Heart and kidney disconnected: nervousness, forgetfulness, restlessness with insomnia, night emissions, cyclical fever, night sweats, ringing in the ears with deafness, flank pain and weak legs, excessive urination at night, easy flushing of face, deficient and rapid pulse, red and coatless tongue.

C. Diseases of the Spleen

1. Cold in Spleen
Food not digested, persistent abdominal cramps, vomiting with diarrhea or constipation, cool limbs, dull and yellowish skin with smoked appearance or edema, deep and slow pulse, thin and white tongue coating.

2. Heat in Spleen
Red lips with sores, mouth sweet with stickiness, able to eat, bright yellow body, dark yellow urine, thin and yellow tongue coating, rapid pulse.

3. Deficiency in Spleen
Sallow complexion, weakness with loss of stamina, drowsiness, decreased appetite and undigested food, abdominal pain alleviated by pressure, cold limbs, muscle atrophy or swelling, even vomiting and watery diarrhea, deficient but even pulse, pale tongue with white and smooth coating.

4. Strength in Spleen
   Diaphragmatic discomfort, abdominal distention and pain, easy hunger at times, total body swelling, retention of urine and feces, rapid and strong or deep and smooth pulse, dry yellow tongue coating.
5. Diseases in Spleen Meridian
   Pain in the root of the tongue; body unable to move; food fails to go down; restlessness; painful spasm below the heart; very loose feces or cholera, or water retention inside, or generalized jaundice; restless sleep; swelling and cold in the inner thighs upon standing; inability to move the big toe.
6. Combined Spleen Diseases
   a. Yang deficiency in spleen and stomach. Abdominal pain alleviated by pressure, preference for warmth, increased clear saliva, belching and vomiting, loss of appetite with bloating upon eating, prolonged diarrhea, weakness and tiredness, cold limbs; sometimes scanty urine and swelling, copious clear white vaginal discharge; pale tongue and white coating, deep, small, and forceful pulse.
   b. Yang deficiency in spleen and kidney. Fearfulness, nervousness, cough, swelling, self-regulated feces, excessive but clear urine; in severe cases, abdominal fullness, diarrhea at dawn, gassy abdominal bloating, even and elusive or slow and small pulse, pale and dull tongue.
   c. Spleen and lung both deficient. Cough producing sputum, shortness of breath, stomach unable to receive food, emaciation, cold body, deficient but rapid pulse, white and dry tongue coating.
   d. Heart and spleen both deficient: see section B.6.a.

D. Diseases of the Lung

1. Cold in Lung
   Pale complexion, fever with cold intolerance, cough, thin and clear sputum, difficult breathing especially on lying down, clear nasal drainage, no thirst, superficial and stringy pulse, white and smooth tongue coating.
2. Heat in Lung
   Cough with thick yellow sputum, burning in nose with inflammation, shortness of breath with perspiration, thirst, inflamed throat, nosebleed, smooth and rapid pulse, dark red tongue; or, coughing up blood, dry throat and hoarseness, rapid pulse, red tongue.

3. Dryness in Lung

   Dry nonproductive cough, sometimes with scanty sputum; dry nose and throat; chest pain from coughing; red tongue tip with thin yellow coating; rapid pulse.

4. Lung Deficiency

   Glossy white complexion, soft voice and timorousness, shortness of breath, cold intolerance, easy perspiration, dry skin, brittle hair; or, red cheeks with night sweats, emaciation, cyclic fever with restlessness, cough and loss of voice, deficient and small or small, rapid, and forceless pulse, red or pale tongue.

   a. Lung Yin deficiency. Recurrent fever with night sweats, dry throat with thirst, dry cough with loss of voice and production of foul sputum; or, coughing up of blood, red cheeks, loss of voice, rapid and difficult breathing, generally small and rapid pulse.

   b. Lung Qi deficiency. Wilted white complexion, timidity with lassitude, cough productive of clear thin sputum, decreased food and drink, deep and faint pulse.

5. Strength in Lung

   Blocked air passage with rapid breathing, difficulty with breathing on lying down, loud and bubbly respiration, cough, distention and tightness in chest; or, purulent and foul-smelling sputum, smooth and strong pulse, thick greasy tongue coating.

   a. Water retention. Dry heaving, shortness of breath, anxiety, difficult breathing on lying down, foamy sputum, retractions and rib pain, deep and small pulse, white and slightly thickened tongue coating.

   b. Stasis of Phlegm and Dampness. Cold intolerance, fever, cough with rise of air bubbles, vomiting of porridgelike pus, even bloody pus in severe cases, fishy and foul sputum, full and painful chest especially on coughing, pressure over the area of pain aggravates the difficulty in breathing, smooth and strong or superficial large and forceful pulse, yellow and greasy tongue coating.

6. Disease in Lung Meridian

   Distended lung with cough and difficult breathing, pain above the clavicles, thirst, restlessness, chest tightness, pain in the front and inner side of the upper arm, or paradoxical cold, or heat in the palms.

7. Combined Lung Diseases

   a. Liver Fire invading lung: see section A.8.a.

   b. Spleen and lung both deficient: see section C.6.c.

   c. Deficiency in both lung and kidney. Difficult and rapid breathing, choking cough with blood-tinged sputum, sometimes even cough-ing up gross blood, scratchy throat, recurrent fever with night sweats, pallid face but red cheeks, restless insomnia, dark and scanty urine or urinary incontinence, red tongue with decreased fluid, thin tongue coating, rapid and either small or stringy pulse.

E. Diseases of the Kidney

1. Deficiency of Kidney Yin
   Dizziness and blurred vision, dry and inflamed throat, ringing in the ears with deafness, dry cough or spitting of blood, night sweats, cyclic exhaustion and fever, flank aching and limb weakness, in females loss of menses, in males scanty ejaculate, excessive drinking and urine, deficient, small, and rapid pulse, red tongue with scanty coating.

2. Deficiency of Kidney Yang
   Pain and ache in lumbar back, cold knees, weakness with decreased strength, loss of sexual desire, impotence and premature ejacula-tion, or decreased urine with edema, or loss of appetite with watery diarrhea.
   a. Insufficiency of kidney Yang. In addition, cold limbs, pale com-plexion that is glossy or dull, pale tongue that is soft and swol-len, thin white coating, deep and small pulse.
   b. Kidney deficiency with water retention. In addition, edema particularly below the waist, scanty urine; in severe cases, abdominal fluid accumulation, edema in the scrota, sometimes palpitations and shortness of breath, difficulty of breathing on lying down, pale tongue that is soft and swollen, thin and white or thick and greasy coating, deep and small pulse.
   c. Kidney deficiency with diarrhea. In addition, undigested food, prolonged diarrhea especially at or just before dawn, abdominal cramps before defecation and relieved by defecation, worsening when the abdomen is exposed to cold, pale tongue that is soft and swollen, deep, small, and elusive pulse.
   d. Kidney unable to receive Qi. In addition, wheezing (decreased inspiration, prolonged expiration) worsened by activity, cold sweats, or urinary incontinence during coughing, pale and swol-len tongue with thin white coating, deep and small pulse.
   e. Kidney Qi insecure. In addition, premature ejaculation or sponta-neous emission, urinary incontinence or frequency of urination,

    dribbling following urination, need to urinate during the night or
    bed-wetting, soft and swollen tongue with tooth markings, thin
    white coating, deep and small pulse.
3. Disease in Kidney Meridian
    The heart feels as if hungry and suspended in midair, palpitations
    and fearfulness, hot mouth with dry tongue, throat swelling, restless-
    ness, low-back pain, cold and atrophy of the buttocks, drowsiness,
    heat and pain in the soles.
4. Combined Kidney Diseases
    a. Yin deficiency in liver and kidney: see section A.8.f.
    b. Kidney Yin deficiency, liver Yang rising: see section A.8.g.
    c. Heart and kidney disconnected: see section B.6.c.
    d. Yang deficiency of spleen and kidney: see section C.6.b.
    e. Deficiency in both lung and kidney: see section D.7.c.

F. Diseases of the Gallbladder

1. Cold in Gallbladder Deficiency
    Face slightly dusty, dizziness and drowsiness, timidity and fear-
    fulness, frequent sighing, indistinct vision, depleted adipose (fat)
    tissue, stringy, small, and slow pulse, thin and smooth tongue
    coating.
2. Heat Strength in Gallbladder
    Pain in the temples and orbits, blurred vision, ringing in the ears,
    bitter taste, vomiting of bitter fluids, chest tightness and rib pain,
    chills and fever, irascibility, restless sleep or excessive sleep, stringy,
    rapid, and strong pulse, red tongue with yellow coating.
3. Disease of Gallbladder Meridian
    Headache, swollen chin, pain in the outer palpebral angle, painful
    swelling above the collarbones, nodules in the neck and the axillae,
    generalized aching, inability to use the toes.

G. Diseases of the Stomach

1. Cold in Stomach
    Persistent gastric distention and pain, preference for warmth and
    pressure and for warm foods and drinks; vomiting of clear liquids,
    feeding at dawn but vomiting at dusk, hiccoughs, cool limbs, deep
    and slow pulse, white and smooth tongue coating.

2. Heat in Stomach

Thirst with craving for cold drinks, good digestion with easy hunger, noisy vomiting upon eating, halitosis, gingival decay inflammation or bleeding; perspiration with nasal drainage or nosebleed; smooth and rapid pulse, red tongue with dry yellow coating.

3. Stomach Deficiency

No desire for food or drink, and the little food eaten is not digested well; fullness and pressure in the chest; regurgitation and vomiting of acid liquids; pale lips; soft and elusive pulse; pale tongue with scanty coating.

   a. Deficiency of stomach Yang. Gastric blockage and pressure, undigested food, frequent eructation, white and smooth tongue coating, deep and slow pulse.

   b. Deficiency of stomach Yin. Dry mouth and tongue or aphthous sores and gingival swelling, dry constipation, undigested food, sometimes even globus hystericus (a lump in the throat or choking sensation) and regurgitation, red tongue with scanty coating, small rapid and forceless pulse.

4. Strength in Stomach

Distention of the abdomen with guarding, regurgitation of acid, constipation, yellow urine, or abdominal fluid accumulation, strong and large pulse, thick yellow tongue coating.

5. Disease in Stomach Meridian

Asymmetry of the mouth, lip sores, pain along the front and side from the groin to the top of the foot, inability to use the middle toe.

H. Diseases of the Small Intestine

1. Cold in Small Intestine

Excessive clear urine or urinary frequency with dribbling; pain and heaviness just above the pubic area alleviated by pressure, or diarrhea with abdominal rumbling, or blood following defecation; small, elusive pulse, thin white tongue coating.

2. Heat Strength in Small Intestine

Sore throat, deafness, restlessness, tongue sores, groin pain extending to the lumbar back and tugging on the testes, fullness around the umbilicus, dark and dribbly urine with penile pain, smooth and rapid pulse, red tongue with yellow coating.

3. Disease in Small Intestine Meridian

Dry throat, jaw swelling with limitation in neck turning, pulling-like shoulder pain, elbow pain as if broken, deafness, pain along the meridian from the side of the neck and chin down the shoulder and arm to the elbow.

K. Diseases of the Large Intestine

1. Cold in Large Intestine
   Abdominal cramps and rumbling abdominal noises, diarrhea, excessive clear urine, cold hands and feet, slow pulse, smooth white tongue coating.
2. Heat in Large Intestine
   Dry mouth and parched lips, inflamed throat, constipation or foul watery diarrhea or blood in feces, burning in the anus with inflammation, dark and scanty urine, rapid pulse, dry yellow tongue coating.
3. Large Intestine Deficiency
   Chronic diarrhea, rectal prolapse, chills with shivering and cold limbs, small and faint pulse, thin smooth tongue coating.
4. Strength in Large Intestine
   Abdominal distention and pain with guarding, or pain in a fixed position with guarding; cold intolerance and fever; or no fever, right leg flexed—these are symptoms of intestinal abscess. Frequent urination; constipation or diarrhea with pus and blood, or urgency to defecate but inability to do so; deep and strong or smooth and rapid pulse; yellow and greasy tongue coating.
5. Disease in Large Intestine Meridian
   Dental pain with neck swelling, scleral jaundice, dry mouth, nosebleed or clear drainage, inflamed throat, pain in the front shoulder and inside arm, pain and inability to use the index finger.

J. Diseases of the Bladder

1. Cold in Bladder Deficiency
   Clear urine with frequency, dribbling, bed-wetting or incontinence, edema.
2. Heat Strength in Bladder
   Pain above the pubis and distention, painful urination with urgency, dark urine that is cloudy or urine with pus or blood, or gravel in the urine, or urinary blockage.

3. Disease of Bladder Meridian
   a. Qi rises improperly causing headache, eyes feel as if falling out, headache in the vertex as if being pulled, low-back pain as if broken, limited motion of the hip joints, frozen knees, back of the leg feels as if split.
   b. In addition, hemorrhoids, malaria, psychosis, yellow eyes with tearing, nasal drainage or nosebleed; pain from the head down the back, waist, buttocks, and behind the knees to the heel and foot; inability to use the fifth toe.

K. Diseases of the Three Sphincters

Indistinct hearing, inflamed throat with blockage, perspiration, pain in the outer palpebral angle, jaw swelling; pain behind the ears and in the shoulder, outer arms, and elbows; inability to use the fifth finger.

9

Common Symptoms of Disease

A. *Vigor*

1. When the Proper Qi is full, the patient is vigorous; the eyes are bright, speech clear, mentation orderly, respiration calm and easy. A vigorous patient has confidence and little worry and is able to withstand pain and suffering.
2. Conversely, if the Proper Qi is deficient, there is no vigor; the eyes are dull, the voice weak and hesitant, mentation incoherent, respiration short and rapid; even if the illness seems mild, be alert for complications.
3. Calm and inactive: Yin disease.
4. Lively: Yang disease.
5. Wandering mind, alternately clear or cloudy sensorium, blurred vision: most commonly fluid depletion or weakness of the heart or blood.
6. Restlessness: Heat disease, or exhaustion of Shen and Qi.
7. Fatigue: physical exhaustion, kidney deficiency, stomach weakness.
8. Agitated delirium: the Heat or Fire evil has reached the pericardium.

B. *Color and Its Appearance*

1. Color
   The complexion can show one of five colors: green, red, yellow, pallid, and gray. According to the theory of the five elements, these colors separately belong to the five Zang viscera. Furthermore, the Zang viscera are expressed in different locations on the face. Thus,

consider the color red, which reflects Heat. Heat in the liver causes reddening that starts in the left jaw; in the lung, reddening first in the right jaw; in the heart, first in the forehead; in the kidney, first in the cheeks; in the spleen, first in the nose. These correlations are often accurate but are not always constant.

a. Green. Usually caused by infantile convulsion or marked difficulty with breathing due to Phlegm. Green and gray: usually due to Cold and pain.

b. Pallid. Deficiency-induced Cold, depletion of blood and Qi, or depletion of body fluids. If there are white spots on the face also, there may be intestinal parasites.

c. Yellow. May reflect Dampness, Heat, or deficiency. Bright yellow is due to Heat; gray-yellow implies Dampness as well; light or wilted yellow reflects internal injury to the spleen and stomach; dry and wrinkled yellow means Fire in the stomach. If associated with yellowing of the sclerae of the eyes, it is due to jaundice. In prolonged illness, when the complexion changes to clear and smooth yellow, the illness is turning towards resolution.

d. Red. If the whole face is red, it is due to upstream rise of liver Fire, or to the Heat evil in Bright Yang; but if only the cheeks are red, the rising of Fire is due to Yin deficiency. Red resembling that in alcoholic intoxication reflects Heat in the stomach. Delicate red resembling cosmetic rouge with some pallor reflects abnormal rise of Yang.

e. Gray. Due to water Qi; in the female it reflects chronic jaundice; dark circles around the eyes in the female are associated with vaginal discharge.

2. Appearance
While observing color, also analyze its appearance.

a. Color in epidermis: superficial, indicating exterior illness.
b. Color deep in dermis: interior illness.
c. Bright, clear color: Yang disease.
d. Heavy, murky color: Yin disease.
e. Color is light, faint: illness is mild.
f. Color is dense, deep: illness is severe.
g. Color becomes sparse and dispersed: recovery is imminent.
h. Color is collected and concentrated: persistence of illness.
i. Fresh, bright, glossy appearance: good prognosis.
j. Dry, wilted appearance: grave prognosis.
k. In liver diseases causing pain and pressure in the axillae and ribs or infantile convulsion, a greenish-yellow color with glossy appearance is favorable, whereas pure white is unfavorable.

l. In lung and kidney deficiency causing cough and shortness of breath, night sweats and spontaneous emission, or exhaustion with internal Heat, a pallid yellow color is favorable, whereas pure red is unfavorable.

C. *Activity and Posture*

1. Obese: often deficiency of Qi, which also circulates poorly, so that Dampness often accumulates and causes Phlegm; Wind invasion is also common.
2. Thin or gaunt: usually Yin deficiency, with deficiency of blood and fluids; liver Fire rises readily, chronic cough is common.
3. Unsteadiness: common in deficiency of both Qi and blood, or following diaphoresis.
4. Weakness or paralysis of one side: usually due to Wind invasion.
5. Spastic arching back of the neck (opisthotonus): diseases in the Greater Yang meridian; when associated with involuntary rhythmic muscular contractions: epilepsy or infantile convulsion.
6. Decreased mobility of the knees with a hunched-over gait: disease in the ligaments and sinews; inability to stand for a prolonged period of time and unsteady gait: disease in the bone.
7. While lying down, body is light and able to turn over: illness is in Yang; if body is heavy and unable to turn over: illness is in Yin; frequent flexing of one leg or all curled up: usually due to abdominal pain.
8. Humped back resembling that of a tortoise: deficiency in the overseer meridian, or to the Wind evil having entered the marrow of the spine.
9. Chicken (pigeon) breast: bodily weakness or abnormal growth.
10. Constant aimless activity, such as absently smoothing clothing, touching the bed, grasping or scooping air, straightening threads: confusion of the mind.

D. *Voice and Speech*

1. Loud but unclear voice: disease of excess.
2. Soft but clear: deficiency disease.
3. Weak and whispering: internal injury and deficiency.
4. Sudden loss of voice: strength disease, mostly due to Wind and Cold with secondary Heat.

5. Prolonged hoarseness: deficiency disease, mostly due to internal damage to Jing and Qi.
6. Talkativeness: Heat disease.
7. Loud, incoherent speech: extreme Heat causing mental confusion.
8. Repetitive speech of minutiae: lack of concentration.
9. Loud abusive speech: delirium.

E. Respiration

1. Rapid, loud inspiration and bubbly expiration: strength disease.
2. Rapid, quiet inspiration and hesitant expiration: deficiency disease.
3. Difficult, as if breathing would stop and wishing for one deep breath: kidney is deficient and unable to accept Qi.
4. Rattle-like breathing, resembling a wheeze, but less air is expired, with sputum accumulating in the throat, and the air causes a moaning sound as it passes: internal blockage by Phlegm with external exposure to Wind and Cold, or excessive intake of salt or sugar.
5. Rapid breathing with short inspiration and prolonged expiration: internal blockage by Phlegm causing pressure on the diaphragm, or Yin deficiency allowing strong Fire.
6. Short breaths and intermittent respiration, resembling wheezing, but the shoulders are not lifted during breathing: interior strength disease, or fluid retention, or lung weakness.
7. Insufficient breath so that speech is intermittent and difficult: a sign of the weakness of prolonged severe illness.
8. Coarse breathing: Heat steaming the lung.
9. Rapid breathing with flaring of the nose: lung obstruction (an acute and dangerous condition).
10. Snoring with respiration that sounds like sawing: often seen in coma from Wind invasion.
11. Nasal congestion: external Heat disease.
12. Frequent sighing: usually sadness.
13. Tightness in chest and diaphragm: often seen in depression.

F. Chest, Cough, Sputum

1. Chest
   a. Side pain: liver depression, Fire in the liver, liver deficiency, and Phlegm accumulation can all cause this.

    b. Stabbing pain in the sides of the chest: usually Qi impedance and blood stasis.

    c. Spastic pain in the sides of the chest: impedance in the flow of liver Qi.

    d. Distention, fullness or tightness in the chest: liver depression, Qi impedance, or disease in the Lesser Yang meridian.

    e. Palpitations: palpitations aggravated by activity are due to insufficiency of the heart Yin or unbalanced rise of the heart Yang; intermittent palpitations are due to the water Qi oppressing the heart.

    f. Feeling of oppression, confusion, and disquiet in the heart: generally a manifestation of deficiency-induced Heat.

    g. Troubled and restless heart: Heat in the interior.

    h. Chest pain shooting into the back, and back pain shooting into the heart: chest wall disease.

2. Cough

    a. Dry cough: Heat injury of lung, consumption.

    b. Moist cough: external evil, internal Phlegm and Dampness.

    c. Productive cough: Wind and Cold residing in the lung, pent-up Phlegm and Dampness, or sputum accumulation.

    d. Weak cough: internal injury.

    e. Paroxysmal cough: often seen in whooping cough.

    f. Choking cough, sometimes with vomiting: whooping cough, sometimes coughing up of blood.

    g. Silent cough: mostly due to combined interior-exterior diseases.

3. Cough and Difficult Breathing

    a. Paroxysmal cough disturbing sleep: lung distention or internal water retention.

    b. Prolonged cough disturbing sleep, with persistently rapid respiration and diaphoresis: usually indicates impending demise of the lung Qi.

    c. Difficulty with breathing on lying down: Phlegm causing internal block, or the kidney refusing to accept Qi.

    d. Shortness of breath: seen in interior strength, fluid retention, lung deficiency, and so forth.

4. Sputum

    a. Appearance

        (1) Thick, viscous, and lumpy: due to Heat.

        (2) Thin, clear, and fluid: due to Cold.

        (3) Foamy: due to Wind.

        (4) Purulent: lung abscess.

        (5) Bloody: Heat injuring the lung meridian.

b. Color
   (1) Yellow: Heat.
   (2) Yellow and thick: Heat and Dryness.
   (3) White: Cold.
   (4) White and thin: Dampness, fluid accumulation.
   (5) Red and white with blood: Heat damaging the lung meridian.
c. Quantity
   (1) Large amounts, whether yellow or white: evil strength diseases.
   (2) Small amounts: deficiency diseases.

G. *Hiccough*

1. Loud and forceful hiccough: Heat strength.
2. Soft and hesitant hiccough: deficiency state.
3. Persistent hiccough: Heat strength.
4. In prolonged illness, infrequently intermittent hiccough: stomach Qi is about to disintegrate.

H. *Odor*

1. Halitosis: Dampness and Heat in stomach, or gum ulcers.
2. Acid, rotten odor in eructed gas: retained food in the stomach.
3. Fruity odor in the mouth: diabetes.
4. Fishy and malodorous sputum: Heat in the lung.
5. Foul sputum: lung abscess.
6. Foul and liquid diarrheal feces: Heat induced.
7. Malodorous urine: Dampness and Heat in the bladder.
8. Foul flatus: indigestion.
9. A patient may have a peculiar acidic and foul odor, particularly in seasonal (epidemic) diseases, Heat diseases, and those due to pestilences. A person with diminished resistance exposed to this odor may easily contract the illness.

I. *Fever and Chills*

In general, illnesses with fever and chills are exterior diseases caused by external factors, whereas those without fever are mostly interior dis-

eases caused by internal or miscellaneous factors. Cold intolerance with
fever is usually due to Yang disease; cold intolerance without fever is
usually due to Yin diseases.

1. Time of Fever
   a. Random: mostly externally caused Heat diseases.
   b. Fever in the morning: mostly Qi deficiency.
   c. Fever in the afternoon: mostly seasonal evil, but sometimes Yin
      deficiency or exhaustion.
   d. Fever at night: deficiency of Yin or of blood; sometimes indiges-
      tion.
   e. Cyclic fever (every second or third day): malaria.

2. Character of Fever
   a. Recurrent fever and chills: disease is half exterior and half inte-
      rior; also malaria.
   b. Fever without chills: strong Yang.
   c. Chills without fever: Yang deficiency.
   d. More fever than chills: Yin stronger than Yang.
   e. Fever with perspiration: deficiency in the exterior.
   f. Fever without perspiration: strength in the exterior.
   g. Fever with restlessness: interior Heat.
   h. High fever: mostly Heat evil in the interior.
   i. Persistent fever: mostly Yin deficiency.
   j. Fever and chills with aching of head and body: Greater Yang
      disease.
   k. Recurrent fever and chills with bitter taste, dry throat, and
      blurred vision: Lesser Yang disease.

3. Location of Fever
   a. Cold hands and feet: insufficiency of Yang Qi, or deep Heat
      locked in.
   b. Hot palms and soles: upstream Heat; also seen in some Heat
      diseases.
   c. Cold back: Cold in Greater Yang.
   d. Hot chest and abdomen: accumulated Heat internally.
   e. Cold chest and abdomen: Cold sunk in internally.
   f. Fever in the face: Heat evil in Bright Yang.

J. Perspiration

1. Character of Perspiration
   a. Perspiration is intimately connected with chills and fever. Thus,

externally caused fever without perspiration is Cold injury; with perspiration it is Wind injury; if fever subsides following perspiration, then the illness is resolving; but if fever increases despite perspiration, then the illness is tending inward.

   b. In Yin deficiency with night sweats, perspiration is followed by fatigue; in deficiency of Yang, spontaneous perspiration is followed by a cold feeling.
   c. Persistent perspiration in an exterior illness with lowering of fever by crisis and yet cold intolerance worsens: this is Yang depletion, and there is risk of collapse.
   d. Perspiration coming as if in collapse but the patient sleeps comfortably and the pulse is even: this is called battle sweat and is a sign that the illness is turning the corner.
   e. If the perspiration comes in droplets or is oily, the limbs are cold, and the pulse is hidden: this is a sign of imminent death and is called terminal sweat.

2. Location of Perspiration
   a. Head: deficiency in the exterior, Heat in the stomach, or Heat and Dampness evaporating upward; in addition, rising of the Yang Qi can also cause perspiration in the head.
   b. Chest: insufficiency of the heart Yin.
   c. One-sided perspiration: this generally comes before one-sided weakness with atrophy: a manifestation of one-sided deficiency of Qi and blood.
   d. Perspiration in the extremities: often seen in strength diseases in Bright Yang, or Dampness and Heat in the spleen and stomach, or bodily weakness.

K. Hair, Skin

1. Quantity of Hair
   Quantity of hair reflects fullness of circulation and Qi.
   a. Sparse hair: blood deficiency.
   b. Hair loss: deficiency of Jing and blood.
   c. Hair forming strands spontaneously: blood weakness, childhood malabsorption, or intestinal parasites.
   d. Wilted hair: blood and Qi are already exhausted, and the prognosis is very grave.
   e. Glossy hair: prognosis is good.
   f. Burned hair: severe lung damage or terminal lung disease.

2. Skin Appearance
   a. Swollen: mostly water, Wind, Heat poison, or blocked Qi.
   b. Dry: insufficiency of Qi and blood; waning of the Greater Yang Qi.
   c. Peeling: mostly following resolution of rashes.
   d. Ichthyosis: skin feels like cork, rough and prickly: lung wilts inside and skin dries outside.
   e. Ichthyosis associated with a dark countenance and dull gray eyes: terminal stage of dry blood exhaustion (chronic exhaustion with Heat accumulation, damaging Yin, and causing extreme depletion of blood).
   f. Ichthyosis associated with severe abdominal pain: intestinal ulcers.
3. Skin Color
   a. Yellow: a principal sign of jaundice.
   b. Yellow and bright: Heat and Dampness.
   c. Yellow and dull: Cold and Dampness.
   d. Black: congealing due to deep Cold, water accumulation, or fright and anxiety; in females, chronic gallbladder disease also.
   e. Pallid: insufficiency of Qi and blood.
   f. Red: acute Heat disease or Heat in blood; erysipelas.

L. *Head, Eyes, Nose, Ears, Throat*

1. Headache
   a. Time of headache
      (1) Before noon: mostly Qi deficiency.
      (2) After noon: mostly blood deficiency.
      (3) During the daytime: Yang deficiency.
      (4) During the night: Yin deficiency.
   b. Character of headache
      (1) Persistent and steady: usually external evil, particularly if associated with fever and chills.
      (2) Intermittent: usually internal or miscellaneous causes, especially if associated with dizziness and pressure.
      (3) Severe headache with facial pallor: liver Cold.
      (4) Expanding type of headache with hot feeling in the head: liver Fire.
      (5) Heavy head with dizziness, and humming: brain deficiency.
      (6) Blurred vision, dizziness and avoidance of strong light: liver

Yang excessive. Dampness and Phlegm blocked internally can also cause dizziness and blurred vision, but there is usually a greasy tongue and nausea as well.

(7) Headache aggravated by exertion: usually Qi deficiency.

(8) Dizziness only: deficiency of liver and kidney Yin, Wind and Cold, Wind and Heat, or excessive Phlegm accumulation.

c. Location of headache

(1) In the temples: Lesser Yang meridian.

(2) In the front: Bright Yang meridian.

(3) In the back: Greater Yang meridian.

(4) On top: Greater Yang or Dark Yin meridian.

(5) All over: the Wind and Cold evils reaching all three Yang meridians.

2. Face

a. Facial itch: Wind, Dampness, or Heat.

b. Facial pain: usually due to impedance of Qi and blood.

c. Facial numbness: insufficiency of Qi and blood so that the face is not adequately supplied with either, or invasion by Wind.

3. Eyes

a. Bright eyes: full Shen and Qi; conversely, dull eyes reflect weakness and deficiency of Shen and Qi.

b. Color

(1) Yellow in the sclerae: jaundice.

(2) Redness and swelling: Heat in the liver and lung.

(3) Green: liver disease.

c. External appearance

(1) Facial swelling: spleen Fire or deficiency.

(2) Excessive tearing: Heat in the liver.

(3) Swelling of eyelids: Qi deficiency; early water poisoning.

(4) Eyes closed and unable to open: Wind invasion with liver damage; belongs to Yin.

(5) Sleeping with eyes open: spleen deficiency.

(6) Spontaneous upward gaze: Wind in the liver.

(7) Fixed gaze: if transient, mostly due to obstruction by Phlegm; if permanent, mostly due to incurable illnesses.

(8) Widely dilated pupils: insufficiency of kidney water; Wind invasion.

(9) Dull appearance of the eyes: Heat disease; conversely, clear appearance reflects Cold disease.

(10) Drawn to one or the other side: convulsion.

    d. Eye pain: if red and swollen, mostly due to Heat strength.

    e. Eye itch: usually Wind or Heat.

    f. Dry eyes: usually insufficiency of liver, blood, or kidney Yin.

    g. Fear of bright light: if the eyes appear inflamed, disease of strength; if the eyes appear normal, usually insufficiency of kidney Yin.

    h. Blurred vision: usually insufficiency of Yin blood.

    i. Double vision: deficiency of both liver and kidney.

    j. Infant sleeping with eyes open: spleen weakness or chronic seizure disorder.

4. Nose

    a. Color

        (1) Green: abdominal pain; if associated with cold intolerance, the illness is severe.

        (2) Yellow: constipation.

        (3) Black like charcoal: excess Yang with deep Heat.

        (4) Bright red: Wind and Heat.

        (5) Pallid: deficiency of Qi or blood.

        (6) Gray: exertion; gray tinge suggests water.

        (7) Bright and clear: fluid accumulation.

    b. Shape and appearance

        (1) Nasal congestion: external Heat disease.

        (2) Copious (clear) nasal drainage: external Wind and Cold.

        (3) Thick nasal drainage: external Wind and Heat.

        (4) Nosebleed: liver Fire invading the lung, stomach Fire rising upstream, Cold injury with excessive perspiration, or congestion with Heat poison, Heat injury of the Yang meridians.

        (5) Dry nose: mostly excess Heat in the lung and stomach.

        (6) Swollen nose: evil Qi is waxing.

        (7) Inflamed nose: extreme Heat in lung.

        (8) Rosacea (a chronic condition with redness, papules, and pustules, leading later to coarsening and thickening of the skin): Cold concentration.

        (9) Shrunken nose: weakness of Proper Qi, pestilence, syphilis.

    c. Foul nasal odor: generally Wind and Dampness, with Heat; or sores in the nostrils.

    d. Pain in the nose: generally Fire in the lung.

    e. Nasal itch: Wind, Heat, or intestinal parasites.

5. Ears

    a. Color

      (1) Yellow-red: Heat, Wind.

      (2) Pale green: deficiency-induced Cold.

      (3) Gray: deficiency of kidney water.

  b. Helix

      (1) Dryness: diarrhea.

      (2) Geographical appearance: intestinal pus.

      (3) Dull and dry, whether yellow or pallid or green or gray: danger sign.

      (4) Red and glossy: favorable sign.

      (5) Thin and white, or thin and gray: kidney failure.

  c. Swelling of the ear: evil Qi is strong; waxing of Qi of the Lesser Yang.

  d. Sudden loss of hearing: usually due to evil strength, particularly the Fire of liver and gallbladder rising against stream; chronic deafness reflects deficiency and is caused by internal depletion of the liver and kidney Yin.

  e. Qi deficiency and disease in the Lesser Yang meridian can also cause deafness.

  f. At the beginning of hearing loss, there often is ringing in the ears. If the ringing resembles wind or tide sounds, it is due to Wind and Heat, particularly in the Lesser Yang meridian; if it resembles crickets singing, it is due to deficiency of Yin.

  g. Drainage of pus: inflammation with pus on the ear, with abscess or perforation, is mostly due to Wind and Heat invading during blood weakness in the three sphincters and the foot-Dark Yin-liver meridian, or liver Fire induced by anger.

  h. Sometimes there is drainage of pus and pressure with intermittent humming and hearing loss: this is Dampness and Heat in the liver meridian.

  i. Ear blockage: exhaustion of blood and Qi, allowing Heat to enter the foot-Lesser Yin meridian, so that as Heat accumulates, pus forms.

  j. Ear perforation: caused by ear blockage; also can result from Dampness and Heat in the liver and gallbladder.

6. Mouth and Lips

  a. Taste and odor

      (1) Slightly salty taste: generally deficiency or Cold diseases.

      (2) Sweet taste: generally Heat with Dampness in the spleen.

      (3) Bitter taste: Heat strength disease.

      (4) Acid taste: indigestion.

      (5) Fragrant taste: severe stage of diabetes.

(6) Halitosis: Heat in stomach.

(7) Increased salivation: Cold in the upper position or in the spleen.

(8) Dry mouth: depletion of Yin, or insufficiency of stomach fluids, or internal Heat rising.

(9) Sticky mouth: mostly Dampness and Heat.

b. Color

(1) Pallid: disease in the lung; blood depletion.

(2) Gray: disease in the kidney or extreme Cold.

(3) Red: disease of the heart, or Heat.

(4) Purple: extreme Heat; stasis or clotting of blood.

(5) Green: disease in the liver; extreme Cold.

c. Appearance

(1) Dry: blood deficiency.

(2) Baked dry: Heat in the spleen; retention of food (with intestinal blockage).

(3) Moist: blood is full.

(4) Inability to open mouth: tetany, Wind invasion.

(5) Mouth breathing with shallow breaths and foaming: lung weakness.

(6) Mouth breathing with dryness of the outer gums and teeth: interior Heat.

(7) Convulsion with staring eyes and open mouth and coma: dangerous (see Wind diseases).

(8) Pinched mouth: in an infant with inability to nurse, mouth pinched like a bag: this is a common manifestation of Wind in the umbilicus, due mostly to Heat in the womb.

(9) Mouth with pulplike mucous membrane: mostly due to Heat in the heart and bladder translocating to the small intestine.

(10) Swollen lips: Heat disease, particularly in the spleen, or full Wind and Dampness blocked in.

(11) Aphthous sores: Heat accumulation in the heart and spleen.

(12) Shrunken and curled lips: exhaustion of the Qi of the foot-Greater Yin meridian.

(13) Cystic lips, the cysts beginning as pea-sized nodules that develop into cocoonlike cysts that are firm and painful, making eating and drinking difficult: mostly due to chronic accumulation of Fire in the stomach and spleen, forming poison that is expressed in the lips.

(14) Asymmetric mouth: Wind invasion.

(15) Goose mouth (infants): mouth full of white patches resembling snowflakes, with throat swelling in severe cases, making suckling difficult: generally a result of Heat poison in the womb, subsequently collecting in the heart and spleen.

(16) Lip tremor: persistent tremor of the lips is usually caused by Wind or spleen deficiency.

(17) Peeling lips: mostly Cold diseases or excessive intake of acid foods.

(18) Cracked lips: diseases of Dryness.

(19) Harelips: generally congenital or a result of trauma.

7. Teeth and Gums

   a. Color

   (1) Black teeth: Heat in the kidney.

   (2) Teeth like decayed bone: kidney Yin exhausted.

   (3) Pale gums: chronic illness with blood deficiency or excessive blood loss.

   (4) Purple or dark gums: extreme Heat.

   b. Hydration

   (1) Gums baked dry: Yin and the body fluids damaged.

   (2) Teeth dry and stained: kidney deficiency with strong Fire but stomach fluids not yet exhausted; if no stain, stomach fluids already exhausted.

   (3) Dryness of front teeth: extreme Heat in Bright Yang, or Heat invasion.

   (4) Dryness of upper gums: extreme Heat in the stomach meridians.

   (5) Dryness of lower gums: extreme Heat in the intestinal meridians.

   c. Appearance

   (1) Chattering: Wind and Phlegm blocking meridians, causing Heat to transform into muscular contractions; also seen in stomach Heat, intestinal parasitic infestation, stomach deficiency, and Yin deficiency.

   (2) Gingivitis (gum inflammation): Heat in the stomach and intestines.

   (3) Pyorrhea: initially the gum is inflamed and painful, especially on exposure to Wind; later it rots and perforates, often draining foul-smelling pus, ending in exposing the dental roots: mostly due to Wind and Heat in Bright Yang, or in infantile ulceration.

   (4) Teeth shaped like the new moon: syphilis.

8. Throat
   a. Bright or dark red: evil strength or Heat.
   b. Pale or light red: deficiency or Cold.
   c. Inflamed and tight swelling: Heat evil.
   d. Mild and loose swelling: Cold and deficiency.
   e. Enlarged tonsils: interior Fire and Heat accumulation.
   f. White pseudomembrane: diphtheria.

M. Tongue and Its Coating

Examination of the tongue is a very important part of inspection. The texture and color of the tongue reflect the deficiency or fullness of the Qi of the Zang viscera; the tongue coating reflects the clarity or murkiness of the stomach Qi and the nature of the external evil. Observation of the changes in the texture, color, and coating of the tongue can reveal much about the character of the illness and the rise and fall of the Proper Qi and of the disease evil.

The location of disease can often be recognized in the tongue, as the different parts of the tongue are governed by the different viscera. Thus, the heart governs the tip, the kidney the root, the lung and stomach the body, the liver and gallbladder the two edges of the tongue. In reference to the three positions, the tip belongs to the upper position, the middle to the middle position, and the root to the lower position.

1. Tongue Color
   a. Pale
      A pale tongue reflects Cold in deficiency disease, or having lost massive amounts of blood.
   b. Red
      (1) Pale red with no coating: chronic deficiency of blood and Qi in the heart and spleen.
      (2) Fresh red: in externally caused illness it indicates extreme Heat; in deficiency and exhaustion induced internally it indicates Yin deficiency with complicating bright Fire.
      (3) Red tip only: strong Heat in the upper position, or rising of the heart Fire.
      (4) Red edges only: Heat in the liver.
      (5) Dry tongue with dull color: depletion of both fluids and Qi of the stomach, so that no fluid is available to moisten.
      (6) Tongue denuded and dry, but red and smooth, like a mirror: excessive perspiration causing depletion of the body fluids.

(7) Red tongue with bleeding: Heat injuring the pericardium.

(8) Tongue red with purple spots: the illness is about to break out in a rash.

c. Dark red

(1) Dark red: Heat reaches the encampment level.

(2) Dark red with yellowish coating: Heat has just reached the encampment level but has not yet dissipated from the pneuma level.

(3) Pure dark-red tongue that is well hydrated: evil in the pericardium.

(4) Dark red with central drying: burning Fire in the heart and stomach, destroying fluids.

(5) Dark red, looking dry, but well hydrated on palpation: fluids depleted, but Dampness and Heat bake and steam, so that Phlegm is formed and is on the verge of blocking the opening of the heart.

(6) Dark red with greasy dirt: the interior has impure Qi.

(7) Dark red with spotty yellow coating: the illness is about to progress to exhaustion.

(8) Dark red with large red spots: Heat poison reaching the heart.

(9) Dark red tongue that is smooth and glossy: stomach Yin has perished.

(10) Dark red tongue that is dried and shriveled: kidney Yin has dried up.

d. Purple

(1) Purple and swollen: alcohol poison has invaded the heart.

(2) Dull and gray-purple: blood flow is sluggish; there may be clotting.

(3) Purple with white smooth coating in the middle: Cold injury during alcoholic intoxication.

(4) Greenish-purple tongue that is smooth and moist: Cold directly invading the liver and kidney because of Yin deficiency.

(5) Purple with dry yellow coating: prolonged Heat in the viscera, particularly the spleen and stomach.

e. Blue

(1) Blue tongue with coating: visceral damage potentially curable.

(2) Faint blue with partial coating: unresolved Dampness and Heat, or Dampness and Phlegm, or Phlegm accumulation and blockage.

    (3) Full greasy coating with blue in it: Yin evil transforming into Heat.

    (4) Blue and smooth without coating: Cold in Yin deficiency. Danger signal.

    (5) Blue and dry: stagnant Heat. Danger signal.

2. Tongue Coating: Color

  a. White coating

    (1) Thin and smooth: beginning of externally induced disease.

    (2) Smooth and viscous: Dampness and Phlegm internally.

    (3) Thick and greasy: severe Dampness and murkiness.

    (4) Powdery: Heat pestilence with severe impurities.

    (5) Greasy and salty: indigestion with trapped Dampness and murkiness.

    (6) Note: a white coating in externally caused diseases is mainly an exterior symptom.

  b. Yellow coating

    (1) Light yellow and not dry: evil has reached the interior.

    (2) Greasy: Dampness and Heat.

    (3) Dirty greasy: Dampness is full in Heat.

    (4) Burned yellow: Heat is full in Dampness.

  c. Gray coating

    (1) Thin, greasy, and smooth: inability to drink, or direct invasion by Cold in Yin deficiency.

    (2) Black and dry: Fire has damaged the body fluids.

    (3) Black, smooth, and moist: Yin is deficient while Cold is strong, so that the Water element overcomes the Fire element.

  d. Stained tongue

  Food and drink can affect coating color. After drinking milk, for example, the coating is often white and greasy; orange juice makes it light yellow; soy pickle makes it gray or black. This sort of color is called stained tongue and has no diagnostic significance.

3. Tongue Coating: Denudation

  a. A completely denuded tongue generally reflects Yin deficiency; if it looks like a pork kidney stripped of its membrane, the Yin of the liver and kidney are severely damaged. (This is not to be confused with the congenitally denuded tongue, which is not associated with any illness.)

  b. If only a central area is denuded and red, there is Heat in Yin deficiency; if the coating is patchy, then Yin has been injured by Dampness and Heat.

  c. A "geographical tongue," or dry and cracked tongue coating, is

caused by damaged body fluids, and if there are red spots or spi-
cules, then internal Heat is severe.

    d. If the tongue develops white blisters that are tender on eating or
drinking, there is Heat in the stomach.

    e. A white coating that looks like curd and gradually expands is seen
mostly in diseases of Yin damage with persistent Heat.

4. Tongue Texture

    a. A firm tongue indicates a disease of strength, a soft tongue one of
deficiency; a dry tongue suggests depletion of body fluids; a supple tongue means that Qi and the fluids are self-generating.

    b. Twitching (fasciculation) and tremor are due to Wind in the liver;
if the repeated contractions cause difficulty with speech, there is
deficiency of the heart and spleen Qi; flaccidity (limpness) indicates that the Proper Qi is weak and deficient.

    c. Swelling of the tongue reflects excess water or Phlegm, or the
rising of Dampness and Heat; atrophy (shrinkage) suggests weakness of the heart or insufficiency of blood, or interior Heat causing loss of flesh.

    d. A hairy tongue means well-established chronic Heat; a heavy
tongue with a lump under it, unclear speech, and difficulty with
swallowing result from excessively strong Fire in the heart.

    e. Protruding and elongated tongue

        (1) Leaning to one side: Wind invasion.

        (2) Very weak: Qi deficiency.

        (3) Patient has a frequent desire to protrude the tongue beyond
the lips: interior Heat; this often precedes a convulsion.

5. Synthesis

After observing the changes in the tongue and its coating, a synthesis
of the information is necessary. For example, a deep-red tongue
indicates that the Heat evil has entered the encampment level, and
if the coat is yellowish white, then the pneuma level has not been
entirely cleared; a white coating on a red body means Dampness
has resolved but Heat has become submerged and hidden and cannot be treated solely by clearing the encampment. Or, again, a solid
tongue reflects Dampness, whereas yellow reflects transformation
into Heat in the stomach, and if it is thick, solid, and yellow and
the tongue itself is not red, it is still essential to dissipate Dampness; conversely, if the tongue is solid but not moist and already
showing red, then it is necessary to prevent transformation into
Heat and damage to the body fluids.

N. Food, Drink, Vomiting

1. Food
   The stomach governs reception, and the spleen governs digestion.
   a. Able to eat and develop hunger easily: strong stomach.
   b. Able to eat but slow to digest: weak spleen.
   c. Loss of appetite: stomach and intestinal obstruction.
   d. Hunger without appetite: Phlegm and Fire closing off the interior.
   e. Frequent eating but still hungry: Heat in the stomach, or interior dissipation.
   f. Bloating following eating: impeded Qi and retained food.
   g. Craving for unnatural foods: usually intestinal parasites.
   h. Children who overeat but have abdominal pain and are emaciated: also usually parasites.
   i. Pregnant women may develop nausea at the sight of food; this is normal.
2. Taste in the Mouth
   a. Bitter taste: Fire in the liver and gallbladder.
   b. Sweet taste: Dampness and Heat in the spleen.
   c. Acid taste: the liver and the stomach are not harmonious.
   d. Salty taste: deficiency in the kidney and water accumulation.
   e. Tastelessness with increased saliva: Cold in the stomach.
3. Drink
   a. Thirsty yet increased urine: diabetes, or Heat disease.
   b. No desire to drink: generally interior Cold, or Dampness trapped internally.
   c. Thirsty yet no desire to drink: Yin deficiency, blood stagnation, or water retention.
   d. Restless thirst: interior Heat.
   e. Preference for cold drinks: interior Heat.
   f. Preference for hot drinks: interior Cold.
4. Vomiting
   a. Vomiting immediately following eating: Heat disease.
   b. Eating at dawn and vomiting at dusk: Cold invading a deficient stomach.
   c. Vomiting of food with acid: food retention.
   d. Vomiting of water: water retention.
   e. Vomiting of acid liquids: pent-up liver invading stomach.

f. Vomiting of bitter liquids: the liver and gallbladder Qi flow upstream.

g. Vomiting of sputum: internal Phlegm accumulation.

h. Vomiting of blood: anger damaging liver, Heat accumulation in the stomach, or excessive worry damaging the spleen.

i. Nausea without vomiting: mostly due to "dry cholera."

j. Tightness in the chest leading to vomiting: stomach deficiency resulting in indigestion, or the evil Qi trapped above.

k. Thirst after vomiting: obstruction has been relieved, or body fluids injured from the vomiting.

O. *Abdomen, Anus and Rectum, Feces*

1. Abdomen
   a. Abdominal pain
      (1) Epigastric distention with stabbing pain: Qi impedance.
      (2) Burning epigastric pain: Heat in the stomach. If the pain is alleviated by food or by pressure: deficiency disease. If it is aggravated: strength disease.
      (3) In diseases of the Bright Yang meridian caused by (evil) strength, there is abdominal distention accompanied by intolerance for abdominal pressure, preference for the cold, and constipation.
      (4) In dysfunction of the spleen, abdominal pain is accompanied by preference for abdominal pressure and for warmth, and watery diarrhea.
      (5) Enlarged spleen: usually due to stasis and clotting of blood and Qi impedance.
      (6) Crampy pain: mostly internal carbuncle.
      (7) Intermittent pain: mostly Cold arising out of deficiency.
      (8) Pain above the pubis and in the groin: hernia, disease of the liver meridians, or (in women) menstrual cramps.
      (9) Pain around the umbilicus: (evil) strength in the Fu organs that belong to the Bright Yang meridian, intestinal parasites, or Cold in deficiency.
      (10) Rumbling abdominal noise with pain: usually water accumulation, but also diseases of Dampness and Heat, or Cold in the intestines.
   b. Distended abdomen
      (1) Thick skin with blue-gray color: mostly gas. Gas is Yang,

and distention caused by gas is rapid, often starting above and coming down; the patient is able to sleep comfortably.

(2) Thin skin with bright color: mostly water. Water is Yin, and distention caused by water is slow, often starting below and rising, with difficulty breathing and inability to sleep while lying flat.

c. Blood distention. Conspicuous veins or telangiectasia (red streaks of dilated blood vessels) in extremities.

d. Protruded umbilicus. Water retention or Wind in the umbilicus; also infantile umbilical hernia.

e. Distention of both umbilicus and abdomen: accumulation in the abdomen of fluid (ascites), blood, or Qi.

f. Sunken umbilicus. Dehydrated stomach and intestines, generally indicating prolonged, difficult-to-treat illness.

2. Anus and Rectum
   a. Anal itch: pinworm, or Dampness with Heat.
   b. Anal pain: hemorrhoids, or intestinal Heat descending and causing inflammation.
   c. Rectal prolapse: sinking of the Central Qi, childbirth, prolonged diarrhea, or Dampness and Heat localizing below.
   d. Draining hemorrhoids: Heat and Wind in large intestine, or Dryness and Fire in the spleen and kidney, or Yin deficiency allowing strong Fire, or trapped Dampness and Heat.
   e. Rectal prolapse or hemorrhoid: dysentery, sinking of Qi.

3. Defecation
   a. Difficulty in defecation: deficiency of Central Qi, or impedance in the liver. In prolonged illness or in the aged or in women during labor, difficult defecation occurs frequently and is caused by some drying of the blood or body fluids.
   b. Constipation can be due to one of six causes:
      (1) Heat: fever, halitosis, abdominal fullness, dark urine.
      (2) Cold: preference for warmth, pallor of lips, slow pulse.
      (3) Qi impedance: frequent eructation, fullness and swelling of chest and ribs.
      (4) Deficiency: emaciation, dyspnea, perspiration, dizziness.
      (5) Wind: feces and urine both blocked, generalized pruritus, superficial and rapid pulse.
      (6) Drying of blood: weakness, restless heat, aggravation at night.
   c. Diarrhea immediately following cramps, with yellow-brown stool and scanty and dark urine: Heat.
   d. Cold causes three patterns:

   (1) persistent cramps, thin and clear diarrhea, with no desire for
       food or drink;
   (2) urgency with explosive diarrhea, a hot anus, stool like water;
   (3) prolonged diarrhea with pale and cold limbs, undigested food
       in the feces, tiredness and lassitude.
  e. Diarrhea with loss of appetite, chest tightness, greasy tongue
     coating, and limp pulse: Dampness.
  f. Diarrhea with abdominal pain and foul-smelling feces: food
     indiscretion.
  g. Pain and diarrhea, alternating repeatedly, with stools that contain
     specks of blood and pus: dysentery.
  h. Unexpected vomiting, persistent watery diarrhea, numbness in
     the limbs, and perspiration on the head: cholera.
4. Character of Feces
  a. Watery stools, light color: Cold in the intestines.
  b. Watery stools, dark or black: Heat in the intestines.
  c. Very thick: excess Heat, inadequate fluids.
  d. Dry stools: excess Heat, exhausted fluids.
  e. Stool first dry, then watery: internal Qi insufficient.
  f. Loose, with light blood in feces: spleen deficiency.
  g. Diarrhea only at dawn: kidney is weak.
  h. Blood in feces: may be due to Heat damaging the Yin meridians,
     as in intestinal Wind and visceral poisoning, or to the spleen not
     being able to govern blood.
  i. Pus in feces: dysentery; if white, the disease is at the pneuma
     level; if red, at the blood level.
  j. Undigested food in feces: deficiency-induced Cold in spleen and
     kidney, or insufficiency of central Yang.
5. Color of Feces
  a. Light yellow: Heat induced by deficiency.
  b. Dark yellow: Heat evil in the intestines.
  d. Clear white: deficiency of large intestine.
  e. White feces and red urine: jaundice.
  f. Diarrhea with white pus: disease at the pneuma level.
  g. Green: liver evil overcoming the spleen.
  h. Red: Heat in blood, causing internal overflowing, dysentery.
  i. Color of fish brain: diarrhea caused by Dampness and Heat; dys-
     entery.
  j. Clay-colored feces: jaundice, deficiency-induced Cold in the
     large intestine.
  k. Black feces: old blood in feces.

6. Quantity of Feces
    a. Large and several times a day: mostly insufficiency of spleen Qi.
    b. Decreased and constipated: mostly due to Dryness in the intestines; decreased body fluids.

P. Body and Limbs

1. Pain and Aches
    a. Generalized body aching associated with symptoms of exterior illness: usually caused by external factors, such as Wind or Cold; resolves promptly with perspiration.
    b. Joint pain or migratory pain in the limbs, without fever or chills: rheumatism induced by Wind and Cold, often related to weather conditions.
    c. Painful cramps of all four limbs: liver insufficiency and blood unable to nourish the sinews, or invasion by Cold.
    d. Excessive rest, with body aches and discomfort that improve with exercise: disharmony of Qi and blood.
    e. Numbness of hands and feet or some other part of body: Qi deficiency.
    f. Numbness of thumb or index finger extending to elbow: a premonition of Wind invasion.
    g. Fatigue with a heavy feeling in the body and difficulty moving about: most commonly Dampness blocking circulation.
    h. Painful inflammation of the leg: erysipelas; descent of Dampness and Heat.
2. Movement and Mobility
    a. Rhythmic contractions: seizures, tetany.
    b. Difficulty moving, with joint pains: rheumatism resulting from Wind, Cold, and Dampness.
    c. Contracture: solidifying due to Cold, or injury from blood deficiency in the tendons.
    d. One-sided paralysis: Wind invasion.
    e. Flexed and difficult to stretch: disease in Yin.
    f. Stretched and difficult to flex: disease in Yang.
    g. Fixed flexion: disease in the tendons and ligaments.
    h. Fixed stretching: disease in bone.
    i. Tremor: deficiency in Qi and blood.
3. Appearance
    a. Swollen: mostly water, or external evil.

b. Well developed: Proper Qi is full.

c. Poorly developed: Proper Qi is insufficient.

d. Resembling a dry twig: deficiency.

e. Hands stay open (unable to close): Yang Qi dissipated.

f. Closed fist (unable to open): Yin evil hidden internally.

g. Stork knee (knee swollen and large, thin above and below): Wind, Cold, and Dampness evils invading during deficiency in all three foot-Yin meridians. This is an incurable case of externally caused disease.

h. Pestle- or drumstick-shaped finger: chronic disease of the heart and lung.

i. Enlarged joints: rheumatism due to Wind and Dampness.

j. Externally rotated feet: infantile palsy, disease located in the sinews.

k. Internally rotated feet: infantile palsy, disease located in the bones.

l. Unusual shapes: trauma or congenital deformity.

4. Fingernails
   a. Appearance
      (1) Pitted or concave: deficient blood; weak gallbladder.
      (2) Convex: ungual tinea.
      (3) Firm nails: gallbladder strong.
      (4) Soft nails: gallbladder weak.
   b. Color.
      (1) Pale: blood deficiency.
      (2) Red: blood full; Heat disease.
      (3) Green: pain; slow Wind in spleen.

Q. Sleep and Mental Status

1. Sleep
   a. Chronic drowsiness: Heat affecting sensorium.
   b. Excessive sleep: waning of Yang and waxing of Yin, sometimes Phlegm and Dampness.
   c. Increased dreaming: Yin deficiency in liver and kidney; however, also seen in imbalance of Yin-Yang or excess Qi in the Zang viscera, particularly excessive liver Fire.
   d. Brief sleep and easy waking: anxiety, weakness of the heart and gallbladder Qi, or rise of the heart Fire.
   e. Insomnia: dissociation of heart and kidney, insufficiency of heart

and blood, excessive worry, exhaustion of heart and spleen, deficiency of liver and kidney Yin, and organ deficiency states.

    f. Restless sleep: dietary indiscretion causing indigestion, or internal obstruction by Dampness and Phlegm.

    g. Night terrors: deficiency of gallbladder Qi.

2. Mental Status

    a. Forgetfulness has much the same significance as insomnia.

    b. Anxiety: insufficiency of heart and blood, or Yin deficiency permitting strong Fire.

    c. Restlessness can result from many conditions—for example, if the body is unable to perspire when there should be perspiration, when there is constipation, when perspiration has caused damage to the body fluids, where there is Yin deficiency or disease in the Lesser Yang meridian, when Yin waxes and attacks yang.

    d. Abnormal mentation can be seen in delirium, frenzy, seizure, or Dryness in the viscera. In the last case, there may be frequent sadness to the point of shedding tears and restlessness, but the sensorium is usually relatively clear.

R. Urine

1. Urination

    a. Urgency and frequency of urination: Qi deficiency.

    b. Excessive urine: diabetes.

    c. Dripping urine with pain on urination: gonorrhea.

    d. Inability to urinate despite abdominal distention and urgency: urinary retention, with Heat blocking the lower sphincter or dysfunction of all three sphincters.

    e. Urinary incontinence: Qi deficiency, Wind invasion, or Heat disease.

    f. Bed-wetting: weakness of the bladder Qi with Cold in deficiency.

2. Appearance

    a. Clear: Cold disease; waning of kidney Yang or Qi deficiency.

    b. Cloudy: Heat disease, caused by Dampness and Heat descending.

    c. Dark: Heat.

    d. Bloody: Heat accumulation in the bladder (injuring the lower sphincter), or kidney damage from excessive sexual activity.

    e. Urine with white mucus: inflammation of the urethra.

    f. Urine with gravel: stone causing urethral irritation.

3. Odor
   Urine with strong odor: mostly Heat.
4. Color
   a. Light yellow: normal or mild Heat diseases.
   b. Reddish yellow: Heat evil in the liver meridian.
   c. Yellow and cloudy: Dampness and Heat.
   d. Red: Heat in blood.
   e. Dark like soy: if accompanied by swelling, due to fluid retention.
5. Quantity
   a. Excessive amount: commonly due to diabetes. It is normal to see increased urine in those who drink much tea or other liquids, and in winter.
   b. Scanty amount: commonly seen in edema (fluid swelling) states. The urine volume also decreases when the body fluids are damaged by excessive perspiration, vomiting, or diarrhea. In the summer, with increased perspiration, urine is normally decreased.

S. Male Genitalia

1. Itch: Dampness and Heat accumulating below.
2. Swelling: Dampness and Heat, or ulceration.
3. Spastic pain: Cold in the liver meridian.
4. Impotence: excessive sexual indulgence, exhaustion of kidney Yang, or depression and anxiety damaging the heart or the liver.
5. Premature ejaculation: deficiency of kidney Qi, Yin not preserved internally.
6. Night emission with dreaming (wet dream): liver Fire burning internally, or disconnection between heart and kidney.
7. Night emission without dreaming: the seminal gate is insecure.
8. Priapism: depletion of kidney Yin.
9. Scrotal atrophy: liver failure.
10. Pain above the pubes and in the groin, shooting into the testicles: can be caused by Cold, Heat, Dampness with Heat, anger, depression, impedance of Qi, and so forth.

T. Menses

1. Abnormal Menses
   a. Early menses, especially if bright red, generally reflect Heat; late menses, especially if dark purple, generally reflect Cold.

b. Irregular menses may be due to spleen deficiency, depressed Qi, or blood stasis.

c. Excessive menses is usually caused by Heat in the blood or Qi deficiency that is difficult to control. Scanty menses is usually a symptom of blood deficiency, stasis, or obstruction by Phlegm.

d. If the menstrual flow contains clots, there is impedance of Qi and blood.

e. If the patient develops Heat injury during menstruation or the menses come while the patient is ill with Heat, and the sensorium becomes clouded, then the Heat evil has entered the blood level.

f. Bright red flow: Heat.

g. Light color: Qi deficiency with obstruction by Phlegm.

h. Dull purple: impedance of Qi and blood, or Heat blockage.

2. Absence of Menses

Under normal conditions and before menopause, absence of menses should raise the question of pregnancy. Aside from pregnancy, absence of menses may be of several types:

a. Drying of blood: pale and wan face, fatigue, shortness of breath, loss of appetite, and loss of taste.

b. Blood stasis: dry and scaly skin, gray complexion, dryness of mouth but without thirst, pelvic cramps.

c. Congealment by the Cold evil: chills and wind intolerance, greenish-pale complexion, flank aches, abdominal pains.

d. Depletion of body fluids: flushed cheeks, restlessness, high fever at night, bitter taste and parched throat, dry feces and dark urine.

e. Obstruction by Phlegm: obesity, idleness, excessive sputum, greasy tongue coating, recurrent vomiting.

f. Trapped Qi: chest heaviness, loss of appetite, depression.

3. Metrorrhagia

Metrorrhagia, or bleeding from the uterus not associated with menses, may be sudden and gushing or persistent and oozing. There are several types:

a. Deficiency-induced Cold: pale flow, prolonged pelvic pain, cold intolerance, fatigue.

b. Deficiency-induced Heat: bright red and copious flow, often flushed face, warm palms, restlessness, insomnia.

c. Dampness and Heat: purple flow that is viscous and malodorous, gray face and greasy tongue coating, loss of appetite with epigastric bloating, pelvic pressure.

d. Blood stasis: purple and clotted flow that is scanty in amount, pelvic pressure and pain, purple tongue and impeded pulse.

e. Trapped Qi: purple flow with clots, depression, chest tightness and rib pain; pulse is mostly impeded and stringy.

U. Vaginal Discharge

1. White discharge: spleen deficiency and impedance of liver Qi.
2. Yellow discharge: Dampness and Heat.
3. Green discharge: liver meridian invaded by Dampness and Heat, concentrating below.
4. Red and white discharge: Dampness and Heat remaining below with subsequent decay.
5. Scanty but rancid discharge: Cold and Dampness.
6. Thick and fetid discharge: Dampness and Heat.

V. Back

1. Tortoise back (kyphosis). Often due to Wind residing in the backbone, entering the marrow; or insufficiency of the Original Yang or emptiness in the overseer meridian; or caused by improper posture.
2. Flat back. Terminal stage of total body swelling, severe failure of kidney.
3. Arched back. Often due to damage by Wind evil; or high fever burning the brain, disease in overseer meridian—frequently seen in seizures, tetany, Wind in umbilicus, brain diseases.
4. Vertebral deformities. Rickets, abnormal growth; if recent, mostly due to Wind, Cold, and Dampness residing in the joints of the vertebral column; if chronic, usually kidney failure.

W. Pulse

Palpation of the pulse (also called determining the configuration of the pulse) is one of the most important techniques in diagnosis. See chapter 4, section A4 (page 44), for details of technique and descriptions of the basic configurations. The primary implications of the various configurations are as follows:

Superficial: exterior disease. If forceful, strong evil in exterior; if weak, deficiency in exterior.

Deep: internal disease. Forceful means strong evil internally; weak means internal deficiency.

Slow: Cold disease. Forceful means accumulation of Cold evil; weak means Cold invading during deficiency.

Rapid: Heat disease. Forceful indicates virulent Heat evil; weak means Heat injury during deficiency.

Smooth: Phlegm or Heat disease.

Impeded: blood depletion, Cold in blood.

Deficient: deficiency disease, Heat damage.

Strong: strong external evil, virulent Heat evil.

Short: Original Qi deficient.

Tidal: Heat disease; Yang waxing and Yin waning.

Faint: Yang destroyed; both Qi and blood deficient.

Tight: Cold disease; pain.

Even: normal or Dampness.

Hollow: major blood loss.

Stringy: liver Qi; Phlegm accumulation.

Drum: exterior Cold and interior deficiency.

Firm: solidifying of accumulations.

Limp: Yang deficiency, Dampness disease.

Elusive: Yin deficiency.

Small: decreased blood, waning Qi.

Irregular: kidney Qi destroyed.

Hidden: the disease evil is in deep hiding.

Tapping: fright, pain.

Hurried: Fire rising high.

Hesitant: Cold accumulation.

Arrhythmic: the Qi of viscera destroyed.

Very rapid: Yang evil rising to extreme, True Yin about to perish.

Note that the presence of any of the seven strange configurations is an ominous sign. (See chapter 4, section A4e, page 47.)

__10__
Therapeutics

This compendium categorizes the common drugs in accordance with their applicability to various diseases. The formulas of the cited compound drugs are listed in chapter 12, whereas chapter 11 summarizes the most important properties of each of the common drugs. Each illness can be treated by one of many different prescriptions, and with experience the physician can devise his or her own formulas based on an understanding of the nature and efficacy of each herbal drug.

A. *Drugs Contraindicated in Pregnancy*

Many drugs are contraindicated during pregnancy. Some of them, in fact, are abortifacients. All together eighty-seven are known, but of these only the following are still commonly in use. Some may be used judiciously by those with much experience.

1. Plant Herbs

Achyranthes bidentata	*Gleditsia sinensis*
Aconitum carmichaeli	*Hordeum vulgare* sprout
Arisaema consanguineum	*Imperata cylindrica*
Carthamus tinctorius	*Paeonia suffruticosa*
Cinnamomum cassia	*Pharbitis nil*
Coix lachryma-jobi	*Pinellia ternata*
Croton tiglium	*Prunus persica* kernel
Dianthus superbus	*Rubia cordifolia*
Euphorbia pekinensis	*Sophora japonica*

Sparganum stoloniferum
Ulmus macrocarpa

Veratrum nigrum
Zingiber officinale

2. Animal Drugs
    bovine gallstone
    Erinaecus koreanus, hide
    Eumeces quinaque lineatus
    Gryllotalpa africanus
    Hirudo nipponica

Moschus moschiferus
Mylabris phalerata
Scolopendra subspinipes
Snake molt
Tabanus bovinui

3. Mineral Drugs
    arsenolite
    hematite
    mirabilite
    realgar

B. Therapeutic Classification of Drugs

1. Drugs that relieve the exterior
   Their action is to disperse the disease evil from the exterior.
   a. Acrid-warming drugs

   Angelica dahurica
   Angelica pubescens
   Angelica sylvestris
   Asarum heterotropoides
   Cinnamomum cassia branch
   Elsholtzia splendens

   Ephedra sinica
   Gentiana macrophylla
   Perilla frutescens
   Saposhnikovia divaricata
   Schizonepeta tenuifolia

   b. Acrid-cooling drugs

   Bupleurum chinense
   chrysanthemum
   Cimicifuga foetida
   Glycine max, seed and sprout

   Mentha haplocalyx
   Morus alba, leaf
   Pueraria lobata
   Spirodela polyrrhiza

   c. Drugs that drive out Wind and Dampness

   Acanthopanax spinosum
   Angelica dahurica
   Clematis chinensis

   Piper kadsura
   Trachelospermum jasminoides

2. Cathartics
   a. Cold cathartics

   Mirabilite, anhydrous
       crystals

   Rheum palmatum

   b. Warm cathartics
   Croton tiglium

  c. Lubricating cathartics

Cannabis sativa   *Tricosanthes kirilowii*, seed
Prunus japonica, kernel

  d. Water cathartics

Daphne genkwa   *Lepidium apetalum*
Euphorbia kansui   *Pharbitis nil*
Euphorbia pekinensis   *Phytolacca acinosa*

3. Drugs that control Dampness

  a. Fragrant mobilization of Dampness

Agastache rugosa   *Citrus medica, v. sarcodactylis*
Amomum tsao-ko   *Eupatorium fortunei*
Atractylodes spp.   *Magnolia officinalis*

  b. Bland penetrants

Coix lacryma-jobi   *Tetrapanax papyriferus*
Poria cocos

  c. Urine promotion (diuretics)

Akebia quinata   *Plantago asiatica*
Alisma plantago-aquatica *Polygonum aviculare*
Dianthus superbus   *Polyporus umbellatus*
Dioscorea hypoglauca   *Stephania tetrandra*

4. Cooling drugs

  a. Bitter-cold cooling drugs

Anemarrhena asphodeloides *Lonicera japonica*
Artemisia apiacea   *Paeonia suffruticosa*
Coptis chinensis   *Phellodendron amurense*
Forsythia suspensa   *Prunella vulgaris*
Gardenia jasminoides   *Scutellaria baicalensis*
Gentiana scabra

  b. Sweet-cold cooling drugs

Gypsum   *Phyllostachys nigra*, leaf and
Imperata cylindrica, root   stalk lining
Lycium chinense, root skin *Rehmannia glutinosa* (fresh)
Phragmites communis   *Tricosanthes kirilowii*, root

  c. Drugs that cool and undo poisons

Belamcanda chinensis   Rhinoceros horn
Clerodendron cyrtophyllum *Scrophularia ningpoensis*
Isatis indigotica   *Sophora subprostrata*
Lasiosphaera fenzlii   *Viola patrinii*

5. Warming drugs, including those that rescue Yang

  a. Central warming to disperse Cold

Aconitum carmichaeli
Evodia rutaecarpa
Foeniculum vulgare
  b. Supporting Yang and strengthening Fire
Aconitum carmichaeli
Alpinia oxyphylla
Cinnamomum cassia, bark

Syzygium aromaticum
Zingiber officinale

Morinda officinale
Myristica fragrans

6. Emetics
  Alunite (bile treated)
  Tricosanthes kirilowii, seed
  Veratrum nigrum

7. Drugs that promote digestion and strengthen the stomach
  Amomum villosum
  Crataegus pinnatifida
  Gallus gallus domesticus, gizzard lining

  Hordeum vulgare, sprout
  Myristica fragrans
  Raphanus sativus
  Shenqu

8. Drugs that control cough, with the action of smoothing the lung, dissolving Phlegm and relieving difficult breathing
  a. Cooling lung and stopping cough
Arctium lappa
Aristolochia debilis
Eriobotrya japonica, leaf
Fritillaria spp
Lilium brownii
Morus alba, root skin

Peucedanum praeruptorum
Platycodon grandiflorum
Prunus armeniaca, kernel
Stemona japonica
Sterculia scaphigera

  b. Warming lung and stopping cough
Aster tartaricus
Cynanchum stauntoni

Inula brittannica, flower
Tussilago farfara

  c. Dissolving Phlegm and quieting respiration
Arisaema consanguineum
Bambusa textilis
Brassica alba
Laminaria japonica
Perilla frutescens, fruit

Pinellia ternata
Phyllostachys nigra, liquid from roasting stalk
Pumice
Sargassum fusiforme

9. Drugs that regulate Qi
  a. Moving Qi
Citrus medica
Citrus tangerina, fruit peel
Curcuma longa, tuberous root
Cyperus rotundus

Lindera strychnifolia
Melia toosendan
Saussurea lappa

b. Dissipating Qi

Aquilaria aggalocha
Citrus tangerina, unripe fruit peel

Magnolia officinalis
Poncirus trifoliata, tiny fruit

10. Drugs that regulate blood, resolve stagnation, and stop bleeding
   a. To enliven (mobilize) blood

Angelica sinensis
Boswellia carterii
Carthamus tinctorius
Commiphora myrrha

Corydalis yanhusuo
Ligustinum wallichii
Pleropus pselaphon
Spatholobus suberectus

   b. To dissolve stagnation

Artemisia anomala
Curcuma longa, stalk
Hirudo nipponica
Leonurus heterophyllus

Patrinii villosa
Prunus persica
Tabanus bivittatus

   c. To stop bleeding (hemostasis)

Agrimonia pilosa
Biota orientalis
Cephalanoplos segetum
Cirsium japonicum
Euonymous tengyuehensis
human hair ashes
Nelumbo nucifera, root node

Panax pseudoginseng
Rubia cordifolia
Sanguisorba officinalis
Sophora japonica
Trachycarpus wagnerianus
Typha angustata, pollen

11. Restoratives
   a. Qi restoration

Astragalus spp.
Atractylodes macrocephala
Codonopsis pilosula

Dioscorea opposita
Glyccyrrhiza uralensis
Panax ginseng

   b. Blood restoration

Angelica sinensis
Equus asinus, gelatin
Euphoria longan

Paeonia lactiflora, white
Polygonum multiflorum
Rehmannia glutinosa, cooked

   c. Warming restoration

Cervus nippon, antler gelatin
Cervus nippon, young antler
Cibotium barometz
Cistanche salsa
Cuscuta chinensis

Dipsacus japonicus
Eucommia ulmoides
Gekko gecko
Psoralea corylifolia
Schisandra chinensis

   d. Cooling restoration

Adenophora verticillata
Amyda sinensis

Asparagus chochinchinensis
Chinemys reevesii

Dendrobium nobile	*Lycium chinense*, ripe fruit
Ligustrum lucidum	*Ophiopogon japonicus*

12. Drugs to unblock conduits/ostia, stimulate brain, banish filth

Acorus gramineus	*Liquidambar orientalis*
Bos taurus, gallstone	*Moscus moschifera*
Bufo bufo gargarizane	*Styrax benzoin*
Dryobalanops aromatica	

13. Tranquilizers

a. To settle down

Hematite

b. To disperse Wind and submerge Yang

Buthus martensi	*Saiga tartaricus*
Gastrodia elata	*Scolopendra subspinipes*
Haliotis diversicolor	*Uncaria rhynchophylla*
Ostrea rivularis	

c. To sedate

Biota orientalis, kernel	*Polygala tenuifolia*
cinnabar	*Poria cocos*, grown on pine root
fossil teeth	*Ziziphus jujuba*, seed

14. Drugs that solidify and pull back

a. To stop diaphoresis

Ephedra sinica, root	*Triticum aestivum*
Schisandra chinensis	

b. To stop spontaneous or nocturnal seminal emission

Euryale ferox	*Nelumbo nucifera*, seed, stamen,
fossil bones	and pistils
	Rosa laevigata

c. To control diarrhea

halloysite	*Terminalia chebula*
Punica granatum	

15. Drugs that eliminate parasites

Areca catechu, seed	*Quisqualis indica*
Carpesium abrotanoides	realgar
Melia azedarach	*Torreya grandis*
Polyporus mylittae	*Ulmus macrocarpa*

C. Particularly Efficacious Combinations

The following combinations have been found through the ages to be especially efficacious.

1. Mutual Assistance

Aconitum carmichaeli + *Cinnamomum cassia* (to warm kidney, rescue Yang)

Adenophora verticillata + *Ophiopogon japonicus* (to lubricate lung and generate fluid)

Agastache rugosa + *Eupatorium fortunei* (to cool Heat and dissolve Phlegm)

Angelica sinensis + *Ligustinum wallachii* (to restore and mobilize blood and relieve effusions)

Angelica sylvestris + *Angelica pubescens* (to expel Wind and release Dampness)

Biota orientalis, kernel + *Ziziphus jujuba*, seed (to sedate and calm heart)

Boswellia carterii + *Commiphora myrrha* (to regulate Qi, dissolve effusions, and stop pain)

Burned *Hordeum vulgare* + burned *Shenqu* + burned *Crataegus pinnafitida* (to aid digestion and overcome impedance)

Cannabis sativa + *Tricosanthes kirilowii* (to lubricate intestines and promote defecation)

Cimicifuga foetida + *Bupleurum chinense* (to raise Central Qi)

Citrus tangerina, ripe + unripe peel (to regulate liver and stomach Qi)

Citrus tangerina, seed + *Litchi chinensis*, seed (to relieve hernia and stop pain temporarily)

Codonopsis pilosula + *Astragalus* spp. (to restore Qi)

fossil bones + *Ostrea rivularis* (to stop incontinence, to stop diaphoresis)

Laminaria japonica + *Sargassum fusiforme* (to soften the firm and dissolve sputum)

Lonicera japonica + *Forsythia suspensa* (to cool Heat and relieve poison)

Morus alba, leaf + chrysanthemum (to dispel Wind and cool Heat)

Phellodendron amurense + *Anemarrhena asphodeloides* (to dispel Dampness, cool Heat, cool deficiency Fire)

Prunus persica + *Carthamus tinctorius* (to mobilize blood and disperse sputum)

Rosa laevigata + *Euryale ferox* (to stop nocturnal emission)

Scutellaria baicalensis + *Coptis chinensis* (to purge Fire and relieve poison)

Sparganium stoloniferum + *Artemisia* spp. (to mobilize blood and disperse effusions)

Taraxacum mongolicum + *Viola patrinii* (to cool Heat, relieve poison)

Typha angustata + *Pleropus pselaphon* (to disperse effusions and stop pain)

2. Mutual Potentiation

Alpinia katsumadai + *Chaenomeles lagenaria* (to mediate stomach and promote appetite)

Anemarrhena asphodeloides + *Fritillaria* spp. (to cool lung and disperse Phlegm)

Atractylodes spp. + *Magnolia officinalis* (to dry Dampness and eliminate distention)

Coptis chinensis + *Saussurea lappa* (to cool Heat and stop diarrhea)

Cyperus rotundus + *Alpinia officinarum* (to warm stomach and stop pain)

Gardenia jasminoides + fossil teeth (to cool heart and sedate)

Gardenia jasminoides + *Paeonia suffruticosa* (to cool liver and blood)

Inula brittanica + hematite (to lower Qi and stop vomiting)

Panax ginseng + *Aconitum carmichaeli* (to enrich Qi and rescue Yang)

Phellodendron amurense + *Atractylodes* spp. (to dispel Dampness and Heat from the lower position)

Phragmites communis + *Imperata cylindrica*, root (to cool Heat in lung and stomach)

Pinellia ternata + *Citrus tangerina* (to dissolve Phlegm and regulate Qi)

Poncirus trifoliata + *Phyllostachys nigra* (to cool stomach and stop vomiting)

Prunus armeniaca + *Fritillaria* spp. (to stop cough and dissolve sputum)

Rheum palmatum + mirabilite (to purge Heat and promote defecation)

3. Combinations for Different Effects

Amyda sinensis + *Artemisia apiacea* (to nourish Yin and cool Heat)

Astragalus spp. + *Angelica sinensis* (to restore Qi and generate blood)

Astragalus spp. + *Saposhnikovia divaricata* (to firm exterior and stop diaphoresis)

Astragalus spp. + *Stephania tetrandra* (to enrich Qi and disperse swelling)

Atractylodes macrocephala + *Artemisia apiacea* (to enrich Qi and eliminate distention)

Atractylodes macrocephala + *Poncirus trifoliata* (to strengthen spleen and disperse swelling)

Cinnamomum cassia + *Paeonia lactiflora* (to regulate guard and encampment)

Coptis chinensis + *Cinnamomum cassia* (to promote communication between heart and kidney)

Coptis chinensis + *Evodia rutaecarpa* (to purge liver and control acid)

Diospyros kaki + *Syzygium aromaticum* (to warm stomach and stop hiccough)

Lycium chinense + chrysanthemum (to nourish liver and improve vision)

Melia toosendan + *Corydalis yanhusuo* (to regulate Qi, mobilize blood, and stop pain)

Tricosanthes kirilowii + *Allium chinense* (to loosen chest and mobilize Yang)

D. Therapeutic Classification of Prescriptions

1. Dispersion of the Exterior
   a. Acrid-warming dispersion of the exterior: formulas 175, 176, 203, 249, and 293.
   b. Acrid-cooling dispersion of the exterior: formulas 181, 235, 246, 305, and 306.
2. Cooling
   a. Cooling with catharsis of Fire: formulas 91, 92, and 303.
   b. Cooling blood level Heat: formulas 219 and 229.
   c. Cooling and relieving poisoning: formulas 227, 252, and 278.
   d. Cooling visceral Heat: formulas 289, 314, 320, and 326.
   e. Cooling and dissipating Dampness and Heat: formulas 15, 94, 115, 199, 200, 201, and 291.
   f. Cooling Heat and moistening Dryness: formulas 78, 100, 113, 137, 196, 228, and 312.
3. Catharsis
   a. Purging strength Heat: formulas 19, 29, 172, 250, 307, 309, and 325.
   b. Attacking amassed Cold: formula 255.
   c. Driving out accumulated water: formulas 12, 102, and 212.
   d. Moistening intestines and facilitating defecation: formulas 245 and 308.

4. Mediation
   a. Mediating exterior and interior: formulas 23 and 31.
   b. Harmonizing intestines and stomach: formulas 62, 85, and 89.
   c. Harmonizing liver and spleen: formulas 37, 73, 190, and 258.
5. Warming
   a. Central warming and dispersion of exterior: formulas 22, 30, 108, 120, 233, 242, 274, and 287.
   b. Yang rescue: formulas 49, 70, 71, 210, 211, and 318.
   c. Warming meridian and dispersing Cold: formulas 260, 286, 319, and 341.
6. Restoration
   a. Qi restoration: formulas 45, 66, 90, 165, 208, 234, 265, and 324.
   b. Blood restoration: formulas 10, 11, 67, 128, 185, and 288.
   c. Yin restoration: formulas 1, 4, 46, 112, 129, and 243.
   d. Yang restoration: formulas 6, 64, 133, and 321.
7. Dissipation
   a. Dissipation of food and relief of blockage: formulas 138, 146, 147, and 167.
   b. Dissipation of abdominal mass and passing of stones: formulas 110, 158, and 339.
   c. Dissipation of abscess and drainage of pus: formulas 26, 39, 109, 145, 188, 271, 298, and 302.
   d. Killing of parasites: formulas 2, 48, 191, 337, and 338.
8. Regulation of Qi
   a. Mobilization of congealed Qi with pain suppression: formulas 52, 61, 65, 72, 81, 82, 134, 148, 150, and 284.
   b. Lowering Qi and stopping counterflow: formulas 3, 216, 317, and 334.
9. Regulation of Blood
   a. Enlivening (mobilizing) blood and dissolving stagnation: formulas 54, 88, 103, 139, 144, 154, 238, 251, 256, 266, and 301.
   b. Hemostasis (stopping bleeding): formulas 13, 33, 141, 273, 299, and 300.
10. Elimination of Phlegm
   a. Dissolving Phlegm, stopping cough, calming difficult breathing: formulas 7, 16, 36, 57, 63, 74, 111, 159, 173, 221, 222, 244, 254, 294, 316, and 323.
   b. Dissolution of Phlegm and softening of the firm: formula 189.
11. Elimination of Dampness
   Formulas 9, 40, 42, 43, 69, 76, 127, 157, 166, 194, 232, 297, and 333.

12. Solidification or Pulling Back
    a. To secure the exterior and stop perspiration: formulas 79 and 114.
    b. To control lung and stop difficulty of breathing: formulas 5 and 209.
    c. To impede intestines and stop diarrhea: formulas 28, 68, and 313.
    d. To control semen and decrease urine: formulas 124 and 182.
    e. To control uterine bleeding and stop vaginal discharge: formulas 123 and 281.
13. Sedation
    Formulas 87, 98, 179, 267, 279, and 310.
14. Extinction of Wind
    Formulas 53, 231, 236, and 329.

E. *Treatment of Qi, Blood, the Four Levels, and the Six Regions*

1. Diseases of Qi
   a. Qi deficiency
      Method: restoration of Qi.
      Prescription: formula 66. For Qi deficiency of specific organs, see section F.
   b. Qi impedance
      Method: mobilization or breaking of Qi.
      Prescription: formula 150.
   c. Abnormal rise of Qi
      See below, F3 (Spleen) and F4 (Lung).
2. Diseases of Blood
   a. Blood deficiency
      Method: restoration of blood, alone or in combination with enrichment of Qi.
      Prescription: formulas 67 and 288.
   b. Blood stasis or stagnation
      Method: mobilization of blood and dissipation of stagnation.
      Prescription: formulas 103 and 185.
   c. Heat in blood
      Method: cooling of blood and Heat; elimination of poison.
      Prescription: formulas 33 and 219.
3. Diseases at the Guard Level
   a. Wind and Heat in the exterior

Method: acrid-cooling diaphoresis.
Prescription: mild cases, formula 181; more severe, formula 306.

b. Dampness and Heat in the exterior
Method: fragrant dissipation of Dampness.
Prescription: formula 333.

c. Heat in the exterior
Method: diaphoresis with cooling.
Prescription: formula 282.

d. Cold and Dryness in the exterior
Method: warming diaphoresis, dissolution of Phlegm, and lubrication of Dryness.
Prescription: formula 111.

e. Heat and Dryness in the exterior
Method: acrid-cooling diaphoresis, smoothing of lung, and lubrication of Dryness.
Prescription: formula 180.

4. Diseases at the Pneuma Level

a. Heat at the pneuma level
Method: cooling and generation of fluids.
Prescription: formula 91. If perspiration has been excessive, so that the body fluids are injured and Qi exhausted, producing tidal yet forceless pulse, add *Panax ginseng*.

b. Heat accumulation in stomach and intestines
Method: cooling catharsis.
Prescription: formula 19.

c. Heat evil obstructing lung
Method: cooling of lung and calming of difficult breathing.
Prescription: formula 246.

d. Dampness and Heat at the pneuma level
Method: cooling and dissipation.
Prescription: if Dampness is worse than Heat, use formula 15. If Heat is worse than Dampness, use formula 240.

5. Diseases at the Encampment Level

a. Heat at the encampment level
Method: cooling encampment Heat.
Prescription: formula 219.

b. Heat in the pericardium
Method: cooling heart and clearing opening.
Prescription: formula 225 to wash down formula 97 or formula 101. For cooling the heart, 97 is better; for clearing opening, 101 is better. If there are muscular spasms, one may add

Uncaria rhynchophylla, Pheretima aspergillum, Scolopendra subspinipes, Buthus martensi, or *Saiga tatarica.*

   c. Simultaneous disease at the pneuma and encampment levels
   Method: cooling pneuma and encampment.
   Prescription: combine formula 91 and formula 219.
6. Diseases at the Blood Level
   a. Heat at the blood level
   Method: lowering Heat and cooling blood.
   Prescription: formula 229. Use formula 47 if there are rashes, blood in feces, or nosebleed.
   b. Pneuma and blood levels both burning
   Method: cooling both pneuma and blood.
   Prescription: formula 78 or 227, with selected additions or subtractions.
7. Diseases of Greater Yang
   a. Greater Yang meridian illnesses
      (1) Exterior deficiency (Wind injury)
      Method: diaphoresis and dispersion of muscles; mediation of guard and encampment.
      Prescription: formula 175. If there is spastic arching of the neck (opisthotonus), add *Pueraria lobata* root. If constitution is weak, add *Codonopsis pilosus.*
      (2) Exterior strength Cold injury
      Method: diaphoresis.
      Prescription: formula 249. In Wind and Cold in the exterior with spastic arching of the back of the neck, use formula 290. If there is fluid accumulation in the lung, use formula 36; for additional thirst, restlessness, and other symptoms of internal Heat, add gypsum. If exterior Cold is combined with internal Heat, with cold intolerance, fever, no perspiration, body aches, restlessness, dry mouth, and rapid pulse, use formula 25 instead.
   b. Greater Yang Fu organ illnesses
      (1) Water accumulation
      Method: smoothing Qi, facilitating urination, acrid-warming diaphoresis.
      Prescription: formula 42.
      (2) Blood accumulation
      Method: dissolution of stagnation and mobilization of blood.
      Prescription: formula 183 in mild cases; formula 126 in more severe cases.

c. Complications of Greater Yang diseases
   (1) Deficiency resulting from erroneous treatment
       (a) Erroneous diaphoresis: use formula 116 to suppress Yin and support Yang.
       (b) Heart Yang insufficiency following diaphoresis: use formula 177 to strengthen Yang and preserve the internal. If there is abnormal movement of kidney water also, then use formula 160.
   (2) Deficiency restlessness, resulting from residual Heat despite diaphoresis and emesis or catharsis: use formula 152 to cool and sedate.
   (3) Chest blockage. This usually results when there is Phlegm in the interior erroneously treated with catharsis so that Yang Heat submerges and combines with Phlegm, producing symptoms of Dryness and Heat in the stomach and intestines as well as symptoms of Phlegm.
       (a) Severe: formula 24.
       (b) Mild: formula 35.
   (4) Internal stagnation. This results when the Heat evil submerges internally as a result of erroneous treatment (such as emesis or catharsis) or because the stomach Qi has been chronically weak.
       (a) Heat stagnation: formula 27.
       (b) Cold and Heat stagnation: formula 62.
       (c) Water and Heat stagnation in stomach deficiency: formula 89.
       (d) Stomach deficiency: formula 85.
       (e) Yang deficiency with stagnation: formula 119.
       (f) Stagnation of Phlegm and Qi: formula 216.
8. Diseases of Bright Yang
   a. Bright Yang meridian diseases
      Method: cooling with generation of fluids.
      Prescription: formula 91. If the strong Heat damages fluids and Qi, add *Panax ginseng* or *Codonopsis pilosula*.
   b. Bright Yang Fu diseases
      Method: catharsis, or purgation to preserve Yin.
      Prescription: if Dryness and strength are principal, with constipation, heat intolerance, and thirst, use formula 309. If fullness and distention are principal, use formula 29. If all the symptoms are prominent, use formula 19.
   c. Combined Bright Yang diseases

Method: catharsis to eliminate Heat and jaundice, cooling and mobilization of Dampness.

Prescription: formula 200. In Dampness and Heat without abdominal distention or constipation, use formula 151. If there are symptoms of interior and of exterior, use formula 247.

9. Diseases of Lesser Yang
   a. Lesser Yang diseases
   Method: mediation of interior and exterior.
   Prescription: formula 31.
   b. Combined diseases of Lesser Yang
      (1) With exterior symptoms: formula 149.
      (2) With interior symptoms: formula 23.

10. Diseases of Greater Yin
    Method: central warming and supporting spleen.
    Prescription: formula 233. If Cold is particularly strong, add *Aconitum carmichaeli*.

11. Diseases of Lesser Yin
    a. Deficiency Cold in Lesser Yin
       (1) Waxing Yin, waning Yang, cold limbs with diarrhea.
           Method: in general, warming Yang and stopping diarrhea; in severe cases, warming and rescuing Yang.
           Prescription: in general, formula 70; in severe cases, 237.
       (2) Waxing Yin, waning Yang, with overflow of Cold water
           Method: warming Yang, expulsion of Cold, movement of water.
           Prescription: formula 194.
       (3) Yang collapse through external loss
           Method: rapid Yang rescue.
           Prescription: formula 70, with additions (*Panax ginseng*, *Astragalus* spp., fossil bones, *Ostrea rivularis*, and similar drugs).
       (4) Waxing Yin, waning Yang, impure Qi rising against stream
           Method: central warming with clearing of impurities.
           Prescription: formula 108.
       (5) Deficiency Cold with bloody diarrhea
           Method: central warming and intestinal slowing.
           Prescription: formula 184.
    b. Deficiency Heat in Lesser Yin
       (1) Yin deficient, Yang rising abnormally
           Method: restoration of Yin and curbing of Fire.
           Prescription: formula 279.

(2) Yin deficiency with water stoppage
Method: Yin restoration and water mobilization.
Prescription: formula 232.
(3) Yin deficiency with burning Fire
Method: cooling and elimination of poison.
Prescription: formula 84; if severe, use formula 174.
c. Combined Lesser Yin diseases
(1) Lesser Yin and Greater Yang
Method: meridian warming diaphoresis, double dispersion of interior and exterior.
Prescription: formula 248.
(2) Lesser Yin and Bright Yang
Method: purgation to preserve Yin.
Prescription: formula 19.
12. Diseases of Dark Yin
a. Upper Heat, lower Cold (mixed chills and fever)
Method: restoration with warming of Yang.
Prescription: formula 191.
b. Cyclic fluctuation of fever and cold limbs
(1) Cold stage: the basic formula is 70. If there is blood deficiency as well, use formula 286. If interior Cold has been prolonged, add *Zingiber officinale* and *Evodia rutaecarpa*.
(2) Fever stage: the basic formula is 91. For abdominal distention and pain with constipation, one can also use formulas 19 and 29.
c. Vomiting and diarrhea in Dark Yin
(1) Vomiting due to deficiency Cold: formula 108.
(2) Vomiting due to cyclic fluctuations: formula 206.
(3) Diarrhea: formula 94.

F. Treatment of Common Diseases, by Organ

1. Diseases of the Liver
a. Liver deficiency: formula 283. To generate liver blood, use formula 67. To restore liver Yin, use formula 112. If there is dryness of the mouth and throat, add *Ophiopogon japonicus* and *Dendrobium nobile*. If there are numbness and contractions, add *Spatholobus suberectus* and *Uncaria rhychophylla*.
b. Disease of the liver meridian: use formula 55 to loosen the liver and regulate Qi. Use formula 284 to warm and nourish the liver.

   c. Liver Yang rising against stream
     (1) Fire strength in liver meridian: formula 112 or 289, depending on the conditions.
     (2) Pent-up Fire in liver meridian: formula 320.
     (3) Internal movement of liver Wind
       (a) Formula 21 to nourish liver Yin and blood.
       (b) Formula 329 to restore liver Yin.
       (c) Formula 227 or 236 when the Wind is due to extreme Heat. Alternately, formula 335 followed by 168.
       (d) Formula 121 when the Wind is due to blood deficiency.
   d. Disequilibrium of liver Qi: one of the following: formulas 55, 75, 150, 190, 215.
   e. Combined liver diseases
     (1) Liver Fire invading lung: formula 125 or 190.
     (2) Liver Qi invading heart: formula 134 together with 73.
     (3) Liver Qi invading stomach: formula 7 together with 73.
     (4) Disharmony of liver and spleen: formula 190. If the liver is strong and the spleen weak, use formula 258.
     (5) Disquiet of liver and gallbladder: formula 195 or 310.
     (6) Yin deficiency in both liver and kidney: formula 1. Also formula 112, but add *Astragalus* spp. and *Angelica sinensis* for blood deficiency, *Angelica sinensis* and *Leonurus heterophyllus* for decreased menses. Use formula 128 when this is due to damage by Heat.
     (7) Deficient kidney Yin with rising liver Yang: formula 329.
     (8) Dampness and Heat in liver and gallbladder: formula 200. Add *Astragalus rugosa* and *Lycopus lucidus* for nausea and vomiting, *Melia toosendan* and *Corydalis yanhusuo* for flank pain, *Magnolia officinalis* and *Poncirus trifoliata* for abdominal distention.
2. Diseases of the Heart
   a. Heat in heart: formula 98.
   b. Heart deficiency
     (1) Formula 51 to nourish heart and calm spirit.
     (2) Formula 311 to nourish heart Qi and settle spirit.
     (3) Formula 117 to conserve heart Qi.
     (4) Formula 267 to restore heart blood and Yin.
     (5) Formula 66 to restore heart Yang.
     (6) Formula 70 or 210 for heart Yang collapse.
     (7) Formula 128 for hesitant and arrhythmic pulse.
   c. Strength in heart: formula 314 to cool heart Fire.

d. Disease in the heart meridian: formula 81 together with 139.

e. Combined heart diseases

  (1) Heart and spleen both deficient

    (a) Formula 45b for Qi deficiency.

    (b) Formula 324 for heart and spleen injury.

    (c) Formula 265 for spleen deficiency and heart weakness.

  (2) Heart and gallbladder both deficient: formula 254 or 315.

  (3) Heart and kidney disconnected: formula 280; or formula 46 together with 95, adding ripe *Lycium chinense* fruit and chrysanthemum for dizziness, *Rosa laevigata* and *Euryale ferox* for night emission of semen, and *Dipsacus japonicus* and *Loranthus yadoriki* for back pain and limb weakness.

3. Diseases of the Spleen

a. Cold in spleen: formula 120.

b. Heat and Dampness in spleen: formula 200. Use formula 199 for jaundice; eliminate *Cinnamomum cassia* if Heat is excessive; add *Coptis chinensis* and burned *Crataegus pinnitifida* for anorexia and fat intolerance; add *Citrus tangerina* peel and the inner stalk lining of *Phyllostachys nigra* for nausea or vomiting; add *Coix lachryma-jobi* and formula 43 for decreased urine flow and water retention; add *Rheum palmatum* for very dry feces.

c. Spleen deficiency: formula 20 for indigestion and food retention. Formula 208 or 59 for chronic diarrhea or watery feces. Formula 120 for deficiency complicated by Cold. Formula 265 for sinking of spleen Qi. Formulas 42 and 76 for Dampness in spleen deficiency.

d. Combined spleen diseases

  (1) Yang deficiency in spleen and stomach: formula 265 for excessive heart Fire in spleen and stomach deficiency. Formula 50 to raise Yang and nourish stomach. Formula 207 for distention. Formula 45 for chronic deficiency. Alternately, use formula 30, but add *Astragalus* spp. for Qi deficiency; add *Aconitum carmichaeli* for cold limbs with cold intolerance; add *Alpinia officinarum, Corydalis yanhusuo,* and *Cyperus rotundus* for severe abdominal pain; add *Syzygium aromaticum* and *Diospyros kaki* for hiccoughs; add *Citrus tangerina* and ginger-treated *Pinellia ternata* for vomiting; add the lining of *Gallus gallus* gizzard and stir-fried sprouts of *Oryza sativa* and *Hordeum vulgare* for anorexia; add *Myristica fragrans* and halloysite for prolonged diarrhea.

(2) Yang deficiency in spleen and kidney: formula 120 together with formula 68 if abdominal distention and diarrhea are the principal features. Formula 194 together with formula 42 if swelling is the principal feature; add *Areca catechu* fruit peel for abdominal fluid accumulation.

(3) Spleen and lung both deficient: formula 66.

4. Diseases of the Lung

   a. Cold in lung: formula 107. Also, formula 36; add *Perilla frutescens* fruit and *Raphanus sativus* for severe shortness of breath; add *Aster tartaricus* and *Stemona japonica* for severe cough. Use formulas 8 and 244 together for Cold transforming into Heat.

   b. Heat in lung: use formula 221 or 326. For Heat transformed from Wind, use formula 217. For Cold trapping Heat inside, use formula 246. Use formula 302 for lung abscesses.

   c. Dryness in lung: formula 113 or 222. For chronic cough, use formula 312; add *Stemona japonica*, *Cryptotympana atrata*, and *Uncaria rhynchophylla* for persistent dry cough.

   d. Lung Yin deficiency: formula 83, 141, or 262. Also formula 99; add fossil bones and *Ostrea rivularis* for night sweats; add *Stemona japonica* and *Uncaria rhynchophylla* for severe cough; add *Bletilla striata*, *Ophicalcite*, and *Imperata cylindrica* root for blood-streaked sputum.

   e. Lung Qi deficiency: formula 268; add *Ephedra sinica* root and floating *Triticum aestivum* for spontaneous perspiration; add *Aster tartaricus*, *Tussilago farfara*, and *Pinellia ternata* for severe productive cough. Use formula 336 for coughing up of blood.

   f. Stasis of Phlegm and Dampness in lung: formula 34, 142, or 334.

   g. Deficiency in both lung and kidney: formula 90 if Qi and fluids are damaged by Heat. To restore lung and kidney, use formula 243.

5. Diseases of the Kidney

   a. Kidney Yin deficiency: formula 277. Also formula 46; add *Lycium chinense* ripe fruit and chrysanthemum for marked dizziness and blurred vision; add *Anemarrhena asphodeloides* and *Phellodendron amurense* for severe deficiency Heat.

   b. Insufficiency of kidney Yang: formula 272 for incontinence and other conditions due to senility. To restore kidney Yang use formula 133; add *Cibotium barometz* and *Dipsacus japonicus* for waist and back pain; add *Curculigo orchioides*, *Epimedium gran-*

diflorum, Morinda officinale, and actinolite for impotence; add *Euryale ferox* and *Rosa laevigata* for premature ejaculation.

c. Kidney deficiency with water retention: formula 321; add *Areca catechu* fruit peel and *Benincasa hispida* melon rind for abdominal distention; add *Polygala tenuifolia* and *Biota orientalis* kernel for palpitations.

d. Kidney deficiency with diarrhea: formula 68; add toasted *Zingiber officinale* for abdominal coldness; add *Lindera strychnifolia* and *Saussurea lappa* for abdominal cramps; add *Astragalus* and *Cimicifuga foetida* for rectal prolapse.

e. Kidney unable to receive Qi: formula 4.

f. Insecure kidney Qi: formula 135 for spontaneous emission of semen. Formula 197 for spontaneous emission and cloudy penile discharge. Formula 322 to restore kidney and control urine.

6. Diseases of the Gallbladder

a. Cold in gallbladder deficiency: formula 304.

b. Heat in gallbladder: formula 198 or 320.

7. Diseases of the Stomach

a. Cold in stomach: formula 3, 108, or 205.

b. Heat in stomach: formula 226. Use formula 187 if there is Dryness.

c. Stomach Yang deficiency: formula 138.

d. Stomach Yin deficiency: formula 244; add *Phragmites communis, Dendrobium nobile, Tricosanthes kirilowii* root, and *Polygonatum odoratum* for dry mouth and tongue; add *Phyllostachys nigra* (inner stalk lining) for dry heaves; add hematite and *Inula brittanica* for hiccoughs; add *Cannabis sativa* kernel and *Prunus japonica* kernel for constipation; add *Adenophora verticillata* and fried gizzard lining of *Gallus gallus domesticus* for loss of appetite.

e. Strength in stomach: formula 138.

8. Diseases of the Small Intestine

a. Cold in the small intestine: formula 108 for severe pain around the umbilicus and cold sweats. Formula 140 for pain with pus and blood in diarrhea.

b. Heat in the small intestine: formula 56. Use formula 314 for strong Fire in small intestine with blood in the urine and restless insomnia.

c. Small-intestine pain: formula 14 for abdominal pain. Formula 202 for inguinal and scrotal pain.

9. Diseases of the Large Intestine
   a. Heat and Dryness in large intestine: formula 38.
   b. Heat and Dampness in large intestine: formula 94; add *Lonicera japonica* and *Forsythia suspensa* for poisoning from extreme Heat; add *Saussurea lappa* and *Paeonia lactiflora* for abdominal pain; add *Areca catechu* seed, burned *Crataegus pinnatifida*, and fried *Raphanus sativus* for indigestion; add formula 101 or 261 for somnolence.
   c. Large-intestine deficiency: formula 193.
   d. Strength in large intestine: formula 26, 153, or 213.
10. Diseases of the Bladder
   a. Cold in bladder deficiency: formula 239.
   b. Heat in bladder: formula 126 or 183.
   c. Dampness and Heat in bladder: formula 9; add *Rehmannia glutinosa*, *Imperata cylindrica* root, *Cirsium japonicum*, and *Cephalanoplos segetum* for blood in the urine; add *Lygodium japonicum*, *Glechoma longituba*, and the inner gizzard lining of *Gallus gallus domesticus* for stones; add *Melia toosendan* and *Lindera strychnifolia* for pain above the pubis; add *Lonicera japonica* and *Forsythia suspensa* for fever.

G. Treatment of Common Diseases, by Cause

1. Diseases of Wind
   a. Wind injury: formulas 111, 143, or 175.
   b. Wind invasion
      (1) Formula 32 for one-sided paralysis.
      (2) Formula 106 for red and painful eyes, cough, abdominal fullness.
      (3) Formula 17 for sudden loss of consciousness with sputum. Use formula 259 for milder cases.
   c. Internal Wind
      (1) Due to blood deficiency: formula 60 or 121.
      (2) Due to extreme Heat: formula 236.
      (3) Due to Yin deficiency: formula 21.
   d. Wind and Cold: formula 293 for mild injury. Formula 170 for more severe cases.
   e. Wind and Heat: formula 306 for early or mild cases. Formula 276 if there are red eyes, decreased hearing, and dry mouth. Also formula 181.

f. Wind and Dampness: formula 333 for the interior. Formula 257 for the exterior.

g. Wind and water: formula 270. If the exterior is cold, delete gypsum, double the amount of *Ephedra sinica*, and add *Schizonepeta tenuifolia* and *Saposhnikovia divaricata*.

h. Wind and Phlegm: formula 315.

2. Diseases of Cold

a. Cold injury: formula 249, caution if the constitution is weak, or the Cold injury occurs in the summer. Formula 333 if the Cold is superimposed on Heat.

b. Cold rheumatism: formula 192.

c. Cold invasion

(1) Formula 233. If Cold is especially strong, add *Alpinia officinarum*, *Piper longum*, *Zanthoxylum bungeanum* fruit, and *Cinnamomum cassia* bark.

(2) Formula 93 if Yang Qi is obstructed.

(3) Formula 70 if Cold has entered the three Yin regions.

(4) Formula 237 if Yang has collapsed.

d. Internal Cold

(1) Formula 64 or 233.

(2) Formula 70 if Cold is in the three Yin regions.

(3) Formula 93b for true Cold, false Heat.

(4) Formula 118 for severe cases.

3. Diseases of Heat

a. Heat injury: formula 168 or 296. Also formula 80, if Qi and fluids are damaged, add *Codonopsis pilosula* and *Polygonatum odoratum* to restore and nourish them. Use formula 333 if Heat is followed by Cold.

b. Heat invasion

(1) Formula 97, 104, or 261 for sudden loss of consciousness.

(2) Formula 91 for high fever with somnolence.

(3) Formula 220 for Qi damage.

(4) Formula 90 for Qi and fluid damage.

(5) Formula 18 if true Yin is injured.

4. Diseases of Dampness

a. External Dampness: formula 163.

b. Internal Dampness in the middle position: formula 76, 77, or 332.

c. Internal Dampness in the lower position: formula 9 or 42.

d. Cold and Dampness: formula 162, 178, or 340.

e. Dampness and Heat

(1) In general, use formula 218 or 223.

(2) For more Dampness than Heat, use formula 15 or 132.

(3) For more Heat than Dampness, use formula 161 or 303.

(4) Upper and middle positions: formula 86.

(5) Middle position: formula 240.

(6) At the pneuma level: formula 86 or 275.

(7) In the spleen: formula 44.

(8) With indigestion: formula 171 or 172.

5. Diseases of Dryness
   a. External Dryness
      (1) Cool Dryness: formula 169.
      (2) Warm Dryness: formula 222.
   b. Internal Dryness
      (1) Dryness in lung: formula 113.
      (2) Dryness and Heat: formula 180.
      (3) Lung Dryness, intestine Heat: formula 122.
      (4) Dryness due to blood deficiency: formula 285.
      (5) Dryness due to exhaustion of fluids by Heat: formula 307.

6. Diseases of Fire
   a. Strength Fire: formula 278. Use formula 19 if there is abdominal distention with guarding and constipation.
   b. Heart Fire: formula 314. Use formula 265 if there is deficiency of the spleen and stomach as well.
   c. Pericardium Fire: formula 58 or 101.
   d. Lung Fire: formula 217 or 326.
   e. Liver Fire: formula 320 or 327.
   f. Spleen Fire: formula 328.
   g. Stomach Fire: formula 226.
   h. Fire due to Yin deficiency: formula 137 or 196. Use formula 129 for kidney Yin deficiency.
   i. Fire due to Qi deficiency: formula 265.

7. Epidemic Diseases
   a. In general
      (1) Formula 224 if more exterior than interior.
      (2) Formula 227 if more interior than exterior.
      (3) Formula 330 if both exterior and interior.
      (4) Formula 295 if Damp impurities are heavy.
   b. Pestilence expressed in the jaws: formula 252.
   c. Virulent epidemic
      (1) Formula 333 in the early stages.

(2) Formula 101 or 261 during high fever and delirium.

(3) Formula 131 if there are impurities and Heat.

  d. Epidemic dysentery

    (1) Cold dysentery: formula 120.

    (2) Heat dysentery: formula 342.

    (3) Bloody and purulent diarrhea with painful straining: formula 94, 155, or 214.

8. Diseases of the Passions
Excess passion causing scrofula or Phlegm nodules (tubercles) in the neck: formula 65 or 186.

9. Diseases of Phlegm

  a. Phlegm accumulation: formula 159.

  b. Phlegm in the heart: formula 331.

  c. Wind and Phlegm: formula 63, 111, or 315. Use formula 136 for sudden loss of consciousness with one-sided paralysis.

  d. Heat and Phlegm: formula 221.

  e. Cold and Phlegm: formula 36 or 156.

  f. Dampness and Phlegm: formula 7.

  g. Dryness and Phlegm: formula 212 or 331.

  h. Phlegm and Fire: formula 331.

10. Diseases caused by Food and Drink

  a. Dietary indiscretion: formula 138.

  b. Food indigestion and retention: formula 20.

  c. Food retention and blockage: formula 146.

11. Diseases of Water Accumulation

  a. Water accumulation under the axillae: formula 12.

  b. Water accumulation in the entire body (anasarca): formula 25 or 36.

  c. Swelling with difficulty breathing on lying down: formula 294.

12. Diseases Caused by Parasites.

  a. Vomiting of *Ascaris*: formula 191.

  b. Acute abdominal pain: formula 230.

  c. Parasites in spleen and stomach weakness: formula 130.

  d. Parasites causing impedance of Qi and blood, with abdominal distention, abdominal mass, guarding: formula 292.

  e. Cold and parasites, with abdominal pain, cold limbs, pallor: formula 253.

  f. Stomach Heat with craving for strange foods: formula 241.

  g. Parasites with Qi impedance: formula 204.

11

Common Drugs Used in Chinese Medicine

Of more than 5,767 currently described drugs in Chinese medicine, fewer than 10 percent are commonly used. Most of these common drugs are briefly described here. The drugs are listed alphabetically by their Latin names, or English names where more appropriate. Each entry is organized as follows:

Latin/English Name/(common name if available)
Chinese name

    P: part used
  T&N: taste and nature (whether or not poisonous)
    M: meridian or organ affinity if known
  Act: actions
  A&F: amount and form of use
  C&C: cautions and contraindications
  Msc: miscellaneous comments
  For: used in the formulas listed by number

Acanthopanax spp., esp *A. spinosum*
Wujiapi 五加皮

    P: root epidermis
  T&N: acrid; warm
    M: liver, kidney
  Act: to dissipate Wind and Dampness, to strengthen the sinews and bones, to mobilize blood and disperse hematoma

  A&F: 4–9 grams as decoction, elixir, pill, powder
  C&C: Yin deficiency with strong Fire; not to be used with *Scrophularia ningpoensis* or with snake molt

Achyranthes bidentata
Niuqi 牛膝

P: root
T&N: sweet, bitter, and acid;
neither warm nor cool
M: liver, kidney
Act: (raw) to dissolve clots and
release stagnation
(dry-stirfried) to restore
liver and kidney, strengthen
sinews
A&F: 9–15 grams as decoction, pill,
gel, elixir
C&C: sinking of central Qi, spleen
deficiency with diarrhea,
nocturnal emission, polyme-
norrhea (excessive menses),
pregnancy
For: 75, 78, 103, 319, 321, 329

Aconitum carmichaeli (monkshood)
Wutou 乌头
P: tuberous root
T&N: acrid; hot; poisonous
M: spleen, kidney
Act: to dispel Cold and Dampness, to disperse Wind, to
warm meridians, to stop pain
A&F: 2–6 grams as decoction, pill,
powder
C&C: Yin deficiency and Yang waxing, Heat diseases, pregnancy
For: 17, 32, 64, 70, 93, 107, 116,
118, 119, 120, 133, 136, 162,
178, 191, 192, 194, 201, 210,
211, 231, 237, 248, 255, 263,
272, 273, 297, 340

Aconitum carmichaeli (monkshood)
Fuzi 附子
P: secondary root
T&N: acrid and sweet; hot; poison-
ous
M: heart, spleen, kidney

Act: to rescue Yang and restore
Fire, to disperse Cold and
expel Dampness
A&F: 3–9 grams as decoction, pill,
powder
C&C: Yin deficiency with Yang
waxing, genuine Heat/false
Cold, pregnancy
For: 17, 136

Acorus gramineus (Japanese sweet
flag)
Shichangpu 石菖蒲
P: root stalk
T&N: acrid; slightly warm
M: heart, liver, spleen
Act: to open ostia and conduits, to
eliminate sputum, to regulate
Qi, to mobilize blood, to dis-
perse Wind, to excrete
Dampness
A&F: 3–6 grams (fresh: 9–24
grams) as decoction, pill,
powder
C&C: waning Yin with waxing Yang,
restlessness with diaphoresis,
cough, vomiting of blood,
spontaneous semen emission
For: 45b, 86, 155, 182, 240, 315

Actinolite
Yangqishi 阳起石
T&N: salty; warm
M: kidney
Act: to warm and restore kidney
A&F: 3–5 grams as pill or powder
C&C: Yin deficiency with strong
Fire

Adenophora tetraphylla, and other
species (lady bells)
Shashen 沙参

P: root
T&N: sweet, slightly bitter; cool
M: lung, liver
Act: to support Yin and cool lung, to expel Phlegm and stop cough
A&F: 9–15 grams (fresh: 30–90 grams) as decoction, pill, powder
C&C: Wind and Cold diseases
For: 1, 83, 180, 198, 222

Agastache rugosa (giant hyssop)
Huoxiang 藿香
P: whole herb
T&N: acrid; slightly warm
M: lung, spleen, stomach
Act: to facilitate Qi, to mediate centrally, to ward off the impure, to dispel Dampness
A&F: 45–90 grams as decoction, pill, powder
C&C: Yin deficiency with strong Fire, stomach weakness or stomach Heat, strong Fire in middle position, Heat diseases
For: 44, 75, 77, 86, 132, 161, 238, 328, 332, 333

Agkistrodon acutus (viper)
Baihuashe 白花蛇
P: sundried eviscerated carcass (without head or tail)
T&N: sweet and salty; warm; strongly poisonous
M: liver, spleen
Act: to dissipate Wind and Dampness, to penetrate sinews and bones, to stop convulsion and tetany
A&F: 2–9 grams as decoction, elixir, gel, pill, powder

C&C: Yin deficiency with internal Heat

Agrimonia pilosa (agrimony)
Xianhecao 仙鹤草
P: whole herb
T&N: bitter and acrid; neither warm nor cold
M: lung, liver, spleen
Act: hemostasis, spleen nourishment
A&F: 9–15 grams (fresh: 15–30 grams) as decoction, pressed juice, powder

Akebia quinata
Mutong 木通
P: stalk
T&N: bitter; cool
M: heart, small intestine, bladder
Act: catharsis of Fire, movement of water, to facilitate circulation
A&F: 3–6 grams as decoction, pill, powder
C&C: fluid depletion, Qi deficiency, spontaneous emission, polyuria, pregnancy
For: 9, 33, 56, 86, 286, 314, 320

Alisma plantago-aquatica (water plantain)
Zexie 泽泻
P: bulbous stalk
T&N: sweet; cold
M: kidney, bladder
Act: to induce urine flow, to excrete Dampness, to expel Heat
A&F: 6–12 grams as decoction, pill, powder

C&C: kidney deficiency, spontaneous emission
For: 4, 42, 46, 50, 55, 69, 133,
146, 164, 220, 223, 232, 263,
264, 320, 332

Allium chinense
Xiebai 薤白
P: stalk
T&N: acrid and bitter; warm
M: liver, lung, heart
Act: to regulate Qi, to loosen
chest, to mobilize Yang, to
disperse accumulation
A&F: 4–9 grams as decoction
(fresh: 30–60 grams); pill,
powder
C&C: Qi deficiency, Yin deficiency
with Heat
For: 81, 148

Allium fistolosum
Congbai 葱白
P: stalk
T&N: acrid; warm
M: lung, stomach
Act: to disperse exterior, to facili-
tate Yang, to relieve poison
A&F: 9–15 grams as decoction or
elixir
C&C: exterior deficiency with dia-
phoresis
For: 93, 169, 238, 293

Allium sativum (Chinese chive)
Dasuan 大蒜
P: stalk
T&N: acrid; warm; somewhat
poisonous
M: spleen, stomach, lung
Act: to mobilize blocked Qi, to
warm spleen and stomach,

to eliminate poison, to kill
parasites
A&F: 4–9 grams as decoction, or
eat raw or roasted
C&C: Yin deficiency with strong
Fire; diseases of the eye,
mouth, throat, teeth, tongue;
seasonal diseases
For: 338

Aloe vera, A. ferox (aloe)
Luhui 芦荟
P: liquid from the leaf, dried
T&N: bitter; cold
M: liver, heart, spleen
Act: to cool fever, to promote
defecation, to kill parasites
A&F: 1–5 grams as pill or powder;
externally, paste from powder
C&C: pregnancy
For: 289

Alpinia katsumadai
Caodoukou 草豆蔻
P: seed cluster
T&N: acrid; warm
M: spleen, stomach
Act: to warm centrally, to expel
Cold, to move Qi, to dry
Dampness
A&F: 2–5 grams as decoction, pill,
powder
C&C: Yin deficiency, blood deple-
tion, fluid depletion, absence
of Cold and Dampness
For: 28, 55, 75

Alpinia officinarum (galanga)
Gaoliangjiang 高良姜
P: root stalk
T&N: acrid; warm
M: spleen, stomach

Act: to warm stomach, to dispel Wind, to dissipate Cold, to move Qi, to stop pain

A&F: 2–5 grams as decoction, pill, powder

C&C: Yin deficiency with Heat

For: 14, 52, 156, 205, 281

Alpinia oxyphylla

Yizhiren 益智仁

P: fruit

T&N: acrid; warm

M: spleen, kidney

Act: to warm spleen and kidney, to conserve Qi, to impede seminal flow

A&F: 3–9 grams as decoction, pill, powder

C&C: Yin deficiency with strong Fire, spontaneous emission and uterine bleeding due to Heat

For: 55, 322

Alunite

Baifan 白矾

Kufan 枯矾

P: crystals

T&N: acid and astringent; cold; poisonous

M: lung, spleen, stomach, large intestine

Act: to dissolve sputum, to dry Dampness, to stop diarrhea, to stop bleeding, to eliminate poison, to kill parasites (refined crystals are more potent in pulling in and generating flesh)

A&F: 0.6–3.0 grams as pill, powder

C&C: Yin deficiency with weak stomach, absence of Damp-

ness and Heat; not to be used with *Ostrea* or *Ephedra*

For: 107, 259

Amber

Hupo 琥珀

T&N: sweet; neither warm nor cool

M: heart, liver, small intestine

Act: to control convulsion and sedate, to dissolve effusion and stop bleeding, to induce urine flow and stop dribbling

A&F: 1–2 grams as pill, powder

C&C: Yin deficiency with internal Heat

For: 101

Amomum cardamomum (cardamom)

Baidoukou 白豆蔻

P: fruit

T&N: acrid; warm

M: lung, spleen

Act: to mobilize Qi, to warm stomach, to aid digestion, to loosen centrally

A&F: 1–6 grams

C&C: Yin deficiency with decreased blood but not Cold or Dampness

For: 15, 132, 218, 275, 332

Amomum tsao-ko

Caoguo 草果

P: fruit

T&N: acrid; warm

M: spleen, stomach

Act: to dry Dampness and expel Cold, to eliminate sputum and stop contagion, to aid digestion and dissolve accumulation

A&F: 2–5 grams as decoction, pill, powder

C&C: Qi deficiency or blood depletion

For: 295, 297, 339

Amomum villosum, A. xanthioides

Sharen 砂仁

P: ripe fruit or seed

T&N: acrid; warm

M: spleen, stomach

Act: to move Qi and regulate centrally, to mediate stomach, to activate spleen

A&F: 3–6 grams as decoction

C&C: Yin deficiency with Heat

For: 14, 75, 165, 166, 167, 208, 253

Ampelopsis japonica

Bailian 白蘞

P: root

T&N: sweet, bitter and acrid; cool

M: heart, liver, spleen

Act: to cool fever, to eliminate poison, to generate flesh, to stop pain

A&F: 3–9 grams as decoction; externally as powder or paste

C&C: deficiency Cold of spleen and stomach, absence of Fire strength

Ref: 56, 211

Amyda sinensis (turtle)

Biejia 鳖甲

P: dorsal exoskeleton

T&N: salty; neither warm nor cool

M: liver, spleen

Act: to generate Yin and cool Heat, to calm liver and Wind, to soften firm and disperse accumulation

A&F: 9–24 grams as decoction, gel, pill, powder

C&C: Yang deficiency in spleen and stomach, anorexia with diarrhea, pregnancy

For: 18, 21, 137, 196, 228, 339

Anemarrhena asphodeloides

Zhimu 知母

P: root stalk

T&N: bitter; cold

M: lung, stomach, kidney

Act: to enrich Yin and lower Fire, to moisten Dryness and lubricate intestines

A&F: 6–15 grams as decoction, pill, powder

C&C: deficiency Cold in spleen and stomach with diarrhea

For: 6, 47, 78, 91, 129, 137, 196, 217, 224, 227, 228, 262, 295, 310

Angelica dahurica

Baizhi 白芷

P: root

T&N: acrid; warm

M: lung, spleen, stomach

Act: to disperse Wind and Dampness, suppress swelling and stop pain

A&F: 2–6 grams as decoction, pill, powder

C&C: Yin deficiency, Heat in blood; not to be used with *Inula*

For: 75, 188, 257, 333

Angelica pubescens

Duhuo 独活

P: root and root stalk

T&N: acrid and bitter; warm

M: kidney, bladder

Act: to expel Wind, to excrete Dampness, to dissipate Cold, to stop pain

A&F: 3–6 grams as decoction,
elixir, pill, powder
C&C: Yin deficiency and blood
drying
For: 50, 203, 260, 283, 319,
340

Angelica sinensis
Danggui 当归
P: root
T&N: sweet and acrid; warm
M: heart, liver, spleen
Act: to restore and mediate blood,
to regulate menses and stop
pain, to moisten dryness and
lubricate intestines
A&F: 4–9 grams as decoction,
elixir, gel, pill, powder
C&C: blockage by Dampness with
central fullness, watery diarrhea; not to be used with
Acorus, Sargassum, Zingiber
For: 1, 6, 33, 51, 54, 55, 56, 67,
88, 98, 99, 103, 105, 106,
109, 115, 140, 153, 154, 182,
188, 190, 191, 193, 195, 196,
205, 220, 226, 251, 256, 260,
265, 266, 267, 272, 276, 277,
283, 284, 285, 286, 287, 288,
289, 298, 300, 301, 308, 311,
313, 319, 320, 324, 327, 330,
334, 340, 341

Angelica sylvestris
Qianghuo 羌活
P: root stalk
T&N: acrid and bitter; warm
M: kidney, bladder
Act: to dispel Wind, to eliminate
Dampness, to stop pain, to
disperse Cold from exterior
A&F: 3–9 grams as decoction,
elixir, pill, powder

C&C: Yin deficiency, blood depletion
For: 50, 75, 105, 163, 164, 203,
224, 257, 260, 308, 327, 340,
341

Aquilaria aggallocha, A. sinensis
Chenxiang 沉香
P: resinous wood
T&N: acrid and bitter; warm
M: kidney, spleen, stomach
Act: to lower Qi and warm cen-
trally, to warm kidney and
enable it to accept Qi
A&F: 1–3 grams as decoction,
pressed juice, pill, powder
C&C: Yin depletion with strong
Fire, deficient Qi sunk low
For: 14, 75, 195, 261, 284, 331,
335

Arctium lappa (great burdock)
Niubangzi 牛蒡子
P: fruit
T&N: acrid and bitter; cool
M: lung, stomach
Act: to disperse Wind and Heat,
to facilitate lung and pene-
trate rashes, to suppress
swelling and eliminate
poisons
A&F: 4–9 grams as decoction or
powder
C&C: Qi deficiency with diarrhea
For: 143, 252, 305

Areca catechu (betel palm)
Binglang 槟榔
P: seed
T&N: bitter and acrid; warm
M: spleen, stomach, large intes-
tine

Act: to kill parasites, to break
accumulation, to lower Qi, to
move water
A&F: 4–9 grams as decoction, pill,
powder (if used alone to kill
parasites, may use up to 90
grams)
C&C: Qi deficiency with sinking
For: 2, 48, 52, 56, 96, 102, 115,
130, 153, 202, 204, 230,
241, 253, 292, 295, 337,
338, 339

Areca catechu (betel palm)
Dafupi 大腹皮
P: fruit peel
T&N: acrid; slightly warm
M: spleen, stomach, large and
small intestines
Act: to lower Qi and relieve cen-
trally, to move water
A&F: 6–9 grams as decoction or
pill
C&C: Qi deficiency or weak consti-
tution
For: 40, 77, 275, 297, 333

Arisaema consanguineum (jack-in-
the-pulpit)
Tiannanxing 天南星
P: tuberous stalk
T&N: bitter and acrid; warm; poi-
sonous
M: lung, liver, spleen
Act: to dry Dampness and dissolve
sputum, suppress swelling
and disperse Wind
A&F: 2–5 grams as decoction, pill,
powder
C&C: Yin deficiency, pregnancy;
not to be used with *Aconi-
tum, Zingiber*
For: 17, 34, 136, 257

Arisaema consanguineum (jack-in-
the-pulpit)
Dannanxing 胆南星
P: tuberous root treated with
bovine bile
T&N: bitter; cool
M: liver, gallbladder
Act: to cool Fire and dissolve
Phlegm, to sedate and stop
convulsion
A&F: 3–6 grams as decoction or
pill
For: 75, 107, 221, 315

Aristolochia debilis, A. contosta
Madouling 马兜铃
P: ripe fruit
T&N: bitter; cold
M: lung
Act: to cool lung and lower Qi, to
dissolve sputum and stop
cough
A&F: 3–9 grams as decoction
C&C: cough due to deficiency Cold,
spleen deficiency with diar-
rhea

Arsenolite, arsenopyrite
Pishi 砒石
P: treated mineral
T&N: acrid and acid; hot; poisonous
M: intestines, stomach
Act: to expel Phlegm and stop
contagion, to kill parasites, to
dissipate necrotic tissue
A&F: 3–8 milligrams as pill, pow-
der; externally as ground
powder, paste, ointment
C&C: weak constitution, pregnancy

Artemisia anomala (wormwood)
Liujinu 刘寄奴

P: whole herb
T&N: bitter; warm
 M: heat, spleen
 Act: to mobilize blood and facilitate circulation, to resorb
   abscesses and suppress swelling
A&F: 4–9 grams as decoction or
   powder
C&C: Qi and blood deficiency,
   spleen deficiency with diarrhea

Artemesia apiacea, A. annua
(sagebrush)
Qinghao 青蒿
 P: whole herb
T&N: bitter and mildly acrid;
   cold
 M: liver, gallbladder
 Act: to cool fever, expel Heat
A&F: 4–9 grams as decoction, pill,
   powder
C&C: postpartum blood deficiency,
   internal Cold, indigestion
   with diarrhea
 For: 137, 218, 228, 296, 329

Artemisia argyi
Aiye 艾叶
 P: dry leaf
T&N: bitter and acrid; warm
 M: spleen, liver, kidney
 Act: to regulate Qi and blood, to
   expel Cold and Dampness, to
   warm meridians, to stop
   bleeding; to calm fetus
A&F: 3–9 grams as decoction, pill,
   powder, pressed juice
C&C: Yin deficiency and Heat in
   blood
 For: 21, 156, 169

Artemisia capillaris
Yinchenhao 茵陈蒿
 P: tender stalk with leaf
T&N: bitter and acrid; cool
 M: liver, spleen, bladder
 Act: to cool Heat and excrete
   Dampness
A&F: 9–15 grams as decoction
C&C: jaundice not due to Damp-
   ness and Heat
 For: 86, 158, 162, 199, 200, 201,
   204

Asarum heterotropoides, A. sieboldi
(wild ginger)
Xixin 细辛
 P: whole herb, including root
T&N: acrid; warm
 M: lung, kidney
 Act: to expel Wind, to disperse
   Cold, to move water, to open
   ostia
A&F: 1–3 grams as decoction
C&C: Qi deficiency with diaphore-
   sis, blood deficiency with
   headaches, Yin deficiency
   with cough
 For: 2, 36, 75, 107, 156, 173, 191,
   248, 286, 319, 340

Asparagus chochinchinensis
Tianmendong 天门冬
 P: tuberous root
T&N: sweet and bitter; cold
 M: lung, kidney
 Act: to nourish Yin, to moisten
   Dryness, to cool lung, to
   lower Fire
A&F: 6–12 grams as decoction, gel,
   pill, powder
C&C: deficiency Cold with diar-
   rhea, external Wind and Cold
 For: 51, 267, 329

Aster tartaricus (tartarian aster)
Ziwan 紫菀
   P: root and root stalk
T&N: bitter; warm
   M: lung
   Act: to warm lung, to lower Qi, to
      dissipate Phlegm, to stop
      cough
A&F: 1–9 grams as decoction, pill,
      powder
C&C: strength Heat diseases
   For: 57, 107, 173, 262, 268, 336

Astragalus complanatus
Shayuanzi 沙苑子
   P: seed
T&N: sweet; warm
   M: liver, kidney
   Act: to restore and nourish liver
      and kidney, to brighten eyes
      and make Jing firm
A&F: 6–9 grams as decoction, pill,
      powder
C&C: strong liver Fire, waxing Yang
      rising readily
   For: 124, 135

Astragalus spp.
Huangqi 黄耆
   P: dried root
T&N: sweet; slightly warm
   M: lung, spleen
   Act: (raw) to strengthen exterior,
      to move water and reduce
      edema
      (moist-stir-fried) to restore
      centrally and enrich Qi
A&F: 9–15 grams (max. 60 grams)
      as decoction, pill, powder,
      gel
C&C: strength diseases, Yin defi-
      ciency with waxing Yang

For: 11, 32, 79, 114, 117, 123,
      192, 220, 224, 265, 266, 268,
      274, 288, 311, 324, 339, 340,
      341

Atractylodes macrocephala
Baizhu 白朮
   P: root stalk
T&N: bitter and sweet; warm
   M: spleen, stomach
   Act: to restore spleen and enrich
      stomach, to dry Dampness,
      to mediate centrally
A&F: 4–9 grams as decoction, gel,
      pill, powder
C&C: Yin deficiency, Qi blockage
   Msc: *Atractylodes* grown in Che-
      kiang is better at restoring
      centrally and enriching Qi,
      but less potent at drying
      Dampness
   For: 20, 42, 50, 55, 59, 63, 66, 69,
      75, 79, 96, 106, 118, 123,
      140, 146, 147, 156, 159, 162,
      164, 178, 190, 193, 194, 201,
      207, 208, 220, 223, 233, 258,
      265, 269, 272, 273, 283, 297,
      303, 304, 313, 316, 324, 330,
      333, 335, 339

Atractylodes, other spp.
Cangzhu 苍朮
   P: root stalk
T&N: bitter and acrid; warm
   M: spleen, stomach
   Act: to strengthen spleen, to dry
      Dampness, to release block-
      age
A&F: 4–9 grams as decoction, gel,
      pill, powder
C&C: Yin deficiency with internal
      Heat

For: 74, 76, 77, 162, 163, 164, 218, 220, 223, 257, 272, 333, 340

Bambusa textilis

Tianzhuhuang 天竹黄
  P: resin
  T&N: sweet; cold
  M: heart, liver, gallbladder
  Act: to cool Heat, expectorate sputum, cool heart, calm convulsion
  A&F: 3–9 grams as decoction, pill, powder
  For: 75

Belamcanda chinensis (blackberry lily)

Shegan 射干
  P: root stalk
  T&N: bitter; cold; poisonous
  M: lung, liver
  Act: to suppress Fire, to eliminate poison, to disperse blood, to dissolve sputum
  A&F: 2–5 grams as decoction, powder, pressed juice
  C&C: pregnancy
  For: 86, 173

Benincasa hispida (winter melon)

Dongguazi 冬瓜子
  P: seed
  T&N: sweet; cool
  M: foot Dark Yin
  Act: to lubricate lung, to dissolve sputum, to drain abscess, to move water
  A&F: 3–12 grams as decoction or ground powder
  C&C: excessive use chills centrally
  For: 26, 109, 145

Benincasa hispida (winter melon)

Dongguapi 冬瓜皮
  P: melon rind
  T&N: sweet; cool
  M: spleen, lung
  Act: to move water and suppress swelling
  A&F: 9–30 grams as decoction or powder
  C&C: edema due to malnutrition
  For: 302

Biota orientalis

Cebaiye 侧柏叶
  P: young twigs and leaves
  T&N: bitter and astringent; cold
  M: heart, liver, large intestine
  Act: to cool blood, to stop bleeding, to expel Wind and Dampness, to disperse swelling and poison
  A&F: 6–12 grams as decoction, pill, powder
  For: 13, 299

Biota orientalis

Baiziren 柏子仁
  P: seed kernel
  T&N: sweet; neither warm nor cool
  M: heart, liver, spleen
  Act: to support heart and sedate Shen, to lubricate intestines and promote defection
  A&F: 3–9 grams as decoction, pill, powder
  C&C: watery feces, Phlegm
  For: 38, 51, 195, 267, 311

Bletilla striata

Baiji 白及
  P: bulbous stalk
  T&N: bitter and sweet; cool

M: lung

Act: to restore lung, to stop blood, to suppress swelling, to generate flesh, to heal sores

A&F: 3–9 grams as decoction, pill, powder

C&C: hemoptysis (coughing up blood), lung abscess, strength Heat in lung and stomach

For: 75

Bombyx mori (silkworm)

Baijiangcan 白僵蚕

P: dry body of the silkworm dying from infestation by the fungus *Beauveria bassiana*

T&N: acrid and salty; neither warm nor cool

M: liver, lung, stomach

Act: to expel Wind and control convulsion, to dissolve Phlegm and release accumulation

A&F: 4–9 grams as decoction, pill, powder

C&C: not to be used with *Paratenodera, Platycodon, Poria, Dioscorea*

For: 75, 186, 231, 252

Bombyx mori (silkworm)

Cansha 蚕砂

P: droppings of the (normal) larva

T&N: sweet and acrid; warm

Act: to expel Wind and Dampness, to dissolve Dampness and impurities

A&F: 6–12 grams as decoction

For: 342

Borax

Pengsha 硼砂

P: crystals

T&N: sweet and salty; cool

M: lung, stomach

Act: to cool Heat and dissipate Phlegm, to relieve poison and prevent necrosis

A&F: 1–3 grams as pill or powder; externally as ground powder

C&C: Yin deficiency and fluid depletion

For: 104

Bos taurus domesticus (domesticated cow)

Niuru 牛乳

P: milk

T&N: sweet; neither warm nor cool

M: heart, lung, stomach

Act: to restore deficiency, to enrich lung and stomach, to generate fluid and lubricate intestines

A&F: boiled milk, drink while warm

C&C: deficiency Cold of spleen and stomach, internal Phlegm and Dampness

For: 187

Bos taurus domesticus (domesticated cow)

Niuhuang 牛黄

P: gallstone

T&N: bitter and sweet; cool

M: heart, liver

Act: to cool heart, to dissolve sputum, to promote gallbladder function, to control convulsion

A&F: 0.15–0.45 gram as pill, powder

C&C: pregnancy; not to be used with fossil bones, *Rehmannia, Achyranthes*

For: 58, 97, 101, 104, 131

Boswellia carterii
Ruxiang 乳香
  P: tree resin
  T&N: acrid and bitter; warm
    M: heart, liver, spleen
    Act: to regulate Qi and mobilize
      blood
  A&F: 3–9 grams as decoction, pill,
      powder; externally as paste
      from ground powder
  C&C: pregnancy
  For: 14, 75, 144, 154, 188, 260,
      340

Brassica alba (white mustard)
Baijiezi 白芥子
  P: seed
  T&N: acrid; warm
    M: lung, stomach
    Act: to facilitate Qi and expecto-
      rate sputum, to warm cen-
      trally and disperse Cold, to
      promote circulation and stop
      pain
  A&F: 3–9 grams as decoction, pill,
      powder
  C&C: lung deficiency with cough,
      Yin deficiency with Fire
  For: 16, 212, 271

Bufo bufo gargarizans (toad)
Chansu 蟾酥
  P: dried skin venom
  T&N: sweet and acrid; warm; poi-
      sonous
    M: foot Bright Yang, foot Lesser
      Yin
    Act: to relieve poison, to reduce
      swelling, to strengthen heart
  A&F: 15–30 milligrams as pill or
      powder; externally as paste or
      ointment

  C&C: pregnancy; not to be applied
      to eyes

*Bupleurum chinense, B. scorzoneri-
folium* (thoroughwax)
Chaihu 柴胡
  P: root
  T&N: bitter; cool
    M: liver, gallbladder
    Act: to mediate exterior and inte-
      rior, to clear liver, to raise
      Yang
  A&F: 2–5 grams as decoction, pill,
      powder
  C&C: depletion of true Yin, rising
      of liver Yang
  For: 23, 31, 50, 55, 72, 75, 103,
      125, 127, 149, 150, 163, 190,
      196, 203, 214, 251, 252, 265,
      320

Buthus martensi (scorpion)
Quanxie 全蝎
  P: whole body, dried
  T&N: salty and acrid; neither warm
      nor cool; poisonous
    M: foot Dark Yin
    Act: to dispel Wind, to stop con-
      vulsion, to improve circula-
      tion, to eliminate poison
  A&F: 2–5 gram (tail only: 1–1.5
      grams) as decoction, pill,
      powder
  C&C: blood deficiency giving rise to
      Wind
  For: 231, 315

Caesalpinia sappan (sappan wood)
Sumu 苏木
  P: branch center
  T&N: sweet and salty; neither warm
      nor cool

M: heart, liver

Act: to move blood, to dissolve clot, to suppress swelling, to stop pain

A&F: 3–9 grams as decoction, ground powder, gel

C&C: blood deficiency without clots, pregnancy

For: 153

Cannabis sativa (hemp, marijuana)

Huomaren 火麻仁

P: seed kernel

T&N: sweet; neither warm nor cool

M: spleen, stomach, large intestine

Act: to moisten, to lubricate intestines, to cure urinary dribbling, to improve blood circulation

A&F: 9–15 grams as decoction, pill, powder

C&C: not to be used with *Ostrea rivularis, Cynanchum, Poria cocos*

For: 18, 21, 60, 128, 222, 245, 308

Carpesium abrotanoides

Heshi 鹤虱

P: fruit

T&N: bitter and acrid; neither warm nor cool; mildly poisonous

M: liver

Act: to kill parasites

A&F: 9–15 grams as decoction, pill, powder

For: 48

Carthamus tinctorius (safflower)

Honghua 红花

P: flower

T&N: acrid; warm

M: heart, liver

Act: to mobilize blood and improve circulation, to dissolve clots

A&F: 3–6 grams as decoction, powder, elixir, pressed juice

C&C: pregnancy

For: 103, 139, 185, 238, 251, 257, 266, 301

Cephalanoplos segetum

Xiaoji 小蓟

P: root or whole herb

T&N: sweet; cool

M: liver, spleen

Act: to cool blood, to dissolve hematoma and effusion, to stop bleeding

A&F: 4–9 grams (fresh: 100–200 grams) as decoction, pressed juice, ground powder

C&C: deficiency Cold of spleen and stomach

For: 13, 33

Cervus nippon, C. elaphus (deer)

Lurong 鹿茸

P: antler velvet

T&N: sweet and salty; warm

M: liver, kidney

Act: to strengthen Original Yang, to restore Qi and blood, to enrich Jing and marrow, to strengthen sinews

A&F: 1–3 grams as ground powder, pill, elixir

C&C: Yin deficiency with rising Yang

For: 272

Cervus nippon, C. elaphus (deer)

Lujiaojiao 鹿角胶

P: gelatin extracted from antler
T&N: sweet and salty; warm
  M: liver, kidney
  Act: to restore blood, to enrich kidney Yang
A&F: 4–9 grams as decoction, pill, powder
C&C: Yin deficiency with rising Yang
  For: 271

Chaenomeles lagenaria (Chinese quince)
Mugua 木瓜
  P: fruit
T&N: acid; warm
  M: liver, spleen
  Act: to calm liver and mediate stomach, to dissipate Dampness and soothe sinews
A&F: 4–9 grams as decoction, pill, powder
C&C: deficiency of Jing and blood, indigestion with spleen and stomach not deficient
  For: 44, 75, 283, 297, 342

Chinemys reevesii (tortoise)
Guiban 龟版
  P: ventral exoskeleton
T&N: salty and sweet; neither warm nor cool
  M: liver, kidney
  Act: to enrich Yin, to submerge Yang, to restore kidney, to strengthen bone
A&F: 9–24 grams dissolved in boiling water or wine
C&C: pregnancy, Cold and Dampness in the stomach
  For: 18, 21, 75, 182, 329

Chinemys reevesii (tortoise)
Guibanjiao 龟版胶
  P: glue extracted by boiling the exoskeleton
T&N: sweet and salty; neither warm nor cool
  M: liver, kidney
  Act: to enrich Yin, to restore blood, to stop bleeding
A&F: 3–9 grams dissolved in boiling water or wine
C&C: Cold and Dampness in the stomach

Chlorite-schist, mica-schist
Mengshi 礞石
T&N: salty; neither warm nor cool
  M: liver, lung, stomach
  Act: to eliminate Phlegm, to aid digestion, to lower Qi, to calm liver
A&F: 9–15 grams as decoction, pill, powder
C&C: spleen and stomach deficiency, pregnancy
  For: 331

Chrysanthemum indicum, C. boreale, C. lavandulaefolium
Yejuhua 野菊花
  P: flower
T&N: bitter and acrid; cool
  M: lung, liver
  Act: to disperse Wind and cool Heat, to reduce swelling and eliminate poison
A&F: 6–12 grams as decoction (fresh: 30–60 grams)
  For: 39, 112, 181, 236, 276

Chrysanthemum morifolium
Juhua 菊花

P: flower

T&N: sweet and bitter; cool

M: lung, liver

Act: to dissipate Wind, to cool Heat, to improve vision, to eliminate poison

A&F: 4–9 grams as decoction, tea, pill, powder

C&C: Qi deficiency, stomach Cold

For: 304

Cibotium barometz

Gouji 狗脊

P: root stalk

T&N: bitter and sweet; warm

M: liver, kidney

Act: to restore liver and kidney, to expel Wind and Dampness, to strengthen waist, legs, and smooth joints

A&F: 4–9 grams as decoction, gel, pill

C&C: Yin deficiency with Heat, difficulty with urine

Cimicifuga foetida (bugbane, snakeroot)

Shengma 升麻

P: root stalk

T&N: acrid and sweet, slightly bitter; cool

M: lung, spleen, stomach

Act: to raise Yang, to disperse the exterior, to eliminate poison

A&F: 1–9 grams as decoction, pill, powder

C&C: upper strength lower deficiency, Yin deficiency with strong Fire, rash at its height

For: 55, 163, 220, 224, 226, 252, 261, 265

Cinnabar

Zhusha 朱砂

T&N: sweet; cool; poisonous

M: heart

Act: to sedate, to control convulsion, to improve vision, to relieve poison

A&F: 0.3–1.0 gram as ground powder

For: 58, 75, 98, 101, 117, 131, 261, 335

Cinnamomum cassia (Chinese cinnamon)

Rougui 肉桂

P: bark

T&N: acrid and sweet; hot

M: kidney, spleen, bladder

Act: to restore Original Yang, warm spleen and stomach, dispel accumulated Cold, restore blood movement through the meridians

A&F: 1–5 grams as decoction, pill, powder

C&C: Yin deficiency with Fire, pregnancy

For: 11, 54, 64, 75, 95, 115, 133, 193, 253, 263, 271, 272, 284, 311, 313, 334

Cinnamomum cassia (Chinese cinnamon)

Guizhi 桂枝

P: tender branch

T&N: acrid and sweet; warm

M: bladder, heart, lung

Act: diaphoresis to relieve exterior, warm and facilitate meridians

A&F: 1–6 grams as decoction, pill, powder

C&C: Heat diseases, waning Yin
with waxing Yang, pregnancy
For: 25, 30, 32, 36, 42, 105, 128,
148, 149, 159, 160, 175, 177,
178, 179, 183, 191, 202, 205,
249, 256, 257, 260, 286, 290,
304, 319, 336, 340

Cirsium japonicum
Daji 大薊
P: whole herb or root, dried
T&N: sweet; cool
M: liver, spleen
Act: to cool blood, to stop bleed-
ing, to dissolve effusion and
hematoma, to suppress
swelling
A&F: 4–9 grams as decoction or
ground powder
C&C: deficiency Cold of spleen and
stomach
For: 13

Cistanche salsa, C. deserticola,
C. ambigua
Roucongrong 肉苁蓉
P: stalk
T&N: sweet, acid and salty; warm
M: kidney, large intestine
Act: to restore kidney, to enrich
Jing, to moisten Dryness, to
lubricate intestine
A&F: 6–9 grams as decoction, pill
C&C: stomach weakness with
watery feces, liver Fire strong
For: 272

Citrus medica, C. wilsonii (citron)
Xiangyuan 香橼
P: ripe fruit
T&N: acrid, bitter, acid; warm
M: liver, lung, spleen

Act: to regulate Qi, to loosen
blockage, to dissolve Phlegm
A&F: 3–6 grams as decoction, pill,
powder
C&C: Yin deficiency, blood depletion, pregnancy, Qi deficiency
For: 14

Citrus medica L. v. *sacrodactylis*
Foshougan 佛手柑
P: fruit
T&N: acrid, bitter, acid; warm
M: liver, stomach
Act: to regulate Qi, to dissolve
Phlegm
A&F: 2–9 grams as decoction or tea
C&C: Yin deficiency with Fire
For: 75

Citrus tangerina, C. erythrosa
(tangerine)
Qingpi 青皮
P: skin of the unripe fruit
T&N: bitter and acrid; slightly
warm
M: liver, gallbladder
Act: to clear out liver and break
out Qi, to disperse accumula-
tion and dissolve sputum
A&F: 3–9 grams as decoction, pill,
powder
C&C: Qi deficiency
For: 52, 55, 75, 102, 125, 202, 220

Citrus tangerina, C. erythrosa
(tangerine)
Chenpi 陈皮
P: ripe fruit peel
T&N: acrid and bitter; warm
M: spleen, lung
Act: to regulate Qi, to modulate
centrally, to dry Dampness,
to dissolve sputum

A&F: 3–9 grams as decoction, pill,
  powder
C&C: Qi or Yin deficiency, hema-
  temesis
  For: 7, 20, 38, 40, 44, 45, 50, 57,
   59, 74, 75, 76, 77, 96, 102,
   109, 138, 156, 164, 169, 170,
   188, 207, 208, 220, 221, 234,
   252, 258, 265, 298, 317, 333,
   339

Citrus tangerina, C. erythrosa
(tangerine)
Juhong 橘红
  P: the orange scraping from the
   peel
T&N: acrid and bitter; warm
  Act: to dissolve Phlegm, to facilitate Qi, to loosen centrally, to
   dissipate accumulation
A&F: 2–5 grams as decoction, pill,
  powder
C&C: Yin deficiency with dry
  cough, Qi deficiency with
  chronic cough
  For: 143, 161, 186, 315, 334

Citrus tangerina, C. erythrosa
(tangerine)
Juhe 橘核
  P: seed
T&N: bitter; neither warm nor cool
  M: liver, kidney
  Act: to regulate Qi, to stop pain
A&F: 3–9 grams as decoction, pill,
  powder
C&C: deficiency diseases
  For: 202

Clematis chinensis
Weilingxian 威灵仙
  P: root

T&N: acrid and salty; warm; mildly
  poisonous
  M: bladder
  Act: to expel Wind and Dampness,
   to open meridians, to dissipate sputum and saliva, to
   dissipate accumulation
A&F: 6–9 grams as decoction,
  elixir, pill, powder
C&C: Qi deficiency and blood
  weakness, Dampness without
  Wind and Cold
  For: 75, 257, 340

Clerodendron cyrtophyllum
Daqingye 大青叶
  P: leaf
T&N: bitter; cold
  M: liver, heart, stomach
  Act: to cool, to eliminate poison,
   to stop bleeding
A&F: 9–15 grams as decoction or
  pressed juice
C&C: deficiency Cold of spleen and
  stomach

Clerodendron cyrtophyllum
Daqinggen 大青根
  P: root
T&N: bitter; cold
  Act: to cool fever and relieve
   poison, to expel Wind and
   eliminate Dampness
A&F: 9–15 grams (fresh: 30–60
  grams) as decoction
  For: 155

Cnidium monnieri
Shechuangzi 蛇床子
  P: fruit
T&N: acrid and bitter; warm
  M: kidney, spleen

Act: to warm kidney and aid Yang, to expel Wind, to dry Dampness, to kill parasites
A&F: 3–9 grams as decoction or pill
C&C: Dampness and Heat in lower position, deficiency of kidney Yin, liver Fire easily perturbed, spontaneous seminal emission
For: 239

Codonopsis pilosula
Dangshen 党参
P: root
T&N: sweet; neither warm nor cool
M: Greater Yin meridians
Act: to restore centrally, to enrich Qi, to generate fluids
A&F: 9–15 grams (up to 60 grams) as decoction, gel, pill, powder
C&C: strength diseases
For: 3, 5, 22, 31, 49, 62, 66, 89, 100, 108, 128, 183, 191, 208, 216, 233, 244, 255, 256, 265, 267, 313, 317, 319, 324

Coix lacryma-jobi (Job's tears)
Yiyiren 薏苡仁
P: seed kernel
T&N: sweet; cool
M: spleen, lung, kidney
Act: to enrich spleen, to restore lung, to cool Heat, to excrete Dampness
A&F: 9–30 grams as decoction or powder
C&C: spleen deficiency with constipation, pregnancy
For: 15, 132, 145, 208, 218, 264, 302, 332, 342

Commiphora myrrha
Meiyao 没药
P: resin of the tree
T&N: bitter; neither warm nor cool
M: liver
Act: to disperse blood and dissolve effusion, to suppress swelling and stop pain
A&F: 3–9 grams as decoction, pill, powder; external: paste from powder
C&C: pregnancy
For: 54, 75, 144, 154, 188, 340

Coptis chinensis and other spp.
Huanglian 黄连
P: root stalk
T&N: bitter; cold
M: heart, liver, stomach, large intestine
Act: to purge Fire, to dry Dampness, to relieve poison, to kill parasites
A&F: 1–3 grams as decoction, pill, powder
C&C: Yin deficiency with fever and restlessness, stomach deficiency with vomiting, spleen deficiency with diarrhea
For: 27, 35, 50, 58, 62, 73, 75, 85, 89, 94, 95, 97, 98, 115, 119, 122, 130, 140, 146, 168, 171, 187, 191, 206, 219, 223, 224, 226, 227, 240, 242, 252, 253, 276, 277, 278, 279, 280, 289, 291, 325, 342

Cornus officinalis (bunchberry)
Shanzhuyu 山茱萸
P: fruit
T&N: acid; mildly warm
M: liver, kidney

Act: to restore liver and kidney, to conserve spirit and Qi, to prevent collapse
A&F: 4–9 grams as decoction, pill, powder
C&C: excessive kidney Fire, strong Yang, chronic Dampness and Heat, dribbling of urine; do not use with *Platycodon grandiflorum*, *Saposhnikovia divaricata*, or *Stephania tetrandra*
For: 27, 46, 64, 123, 133, 239, 263, 283

Corydalis yanhusuo

Yanhusuo 延胡索

P: tuberous stalk
T&N: acrid and bitter; warm
M: liver, stomach
Act: to overcome indigestion, to disperse blood stagnation, to kill parasites
A&F: 6–12 grams as decoction, pill, powder
C&C: spleen and stomach deficiency
For: 14, 54, 75, 134, 202, 301

Crataegus pinnatifida, C. cuneata (Chinese hill haw)

Shancha 山楂

P: fruit
T&N: acid and sweet; slightly warm
M: spleen, stomach, liver
Act: to aid indigestion, to disperse stagnated blood, to eliminate parasites
A&F: 6–12 grams as decoction, pill, powder
C&C: spleen and stomach deficiency
For: 20, 44, 138, 207

Croton tiglium

Badoushuang 巴豆霜

P: seed kernel; after removal of the covering, grind and press in absorbent paper to remove the oil, repeat until all oil is removed
T&N: acrid; hot; strongly poisonous
M: stomach, large intestine
Act: catharsis of Cold accumulation, opening of blockage, elimination of Phlegm, movement of water, parasiticide
A&F: 0.15–0.3 gram as pill, powder
C&C: absence of Cold accumulation, pregnancy, weak constitution
Msc: the oil from the kernel is a violent purgative and emetic
For: 52

Cryptotympana atrata (cicada)

Chantui 蝉蜕

P: molt
T&N: sweet and salty; cool
M: lung, liver
Act: to disperse Wind and Heat, to soothe lung, to stop convulsion
A&F: 3–6 grams as decoction, pill, powder
C&C: pregnancy

Cucurbita moschata (pumpkin)

Nanguazi 南瓜子

P: seed
T&N: sweet; neither warm nor cool
Act: to treat parasites; to control postpartum edema, whooping cough, hemorrhoids
A&F: 30–60 grams as decoction or ground powder
For: 337

Curculigo orchioides

Xianmao 仙茅

P: root stalk
T&N: acrid; warm; poisonous
M: kidney, liver
Act: to warm kidney Yang, to strengthen sinews and bones
A&F: 4–9 grams as decoction, pill, powder
C&C: Yin deficiency, strong Fire
For: 6

Curcuma longa

Jianghuang 姜黄

P: root stalk
T&N: acrid and bitter; warm
M: spleen, liver
Act: to mobilize blood, to move Qi, to open meridians, to stop pain
A&F: 3–9 grams as decoction, pill, powder
C&C: blood deficiency without blockage; can stimulate contractions of the gravid uterus
For: 58, 97, 158, 276, 341

Curcuma zeodaria

Eshu 莪朮

P: root
T&N: acrid and bitter; warm
Act: to move Qi and stop pain, to mobilize blood and disperse accumulation, to aid digestion
A&F: 3–9 grams as decoction
For: 202, 292

Cuscuta chinensis, C. japonica

Tusizi 菟丝子

P: seed
T&N: acrid and sweet; neither warm nor cool

M: liver, kidney
Act: to restore liver and kidney, to enrich Jing and marrow
A&F: 9–15 grams as decoction, pill, powder
C&C: kidney Fire, strong Yang, pregnancy, uterine bleeding, constipation, Yin deficiency with Fire
For: 197

Cyathula officinalis

Chuanniuqi 川牛膝

P: root
T&N: sweet and slightly bitter; neither warm nor cool
M: liver, kidney
Act: to drive out Wind, to mobilize Dampness, to facilitate circulation
A&F: 4–9 grams as decoction, elixir, pill, powder
C&C: excessive uterine bleeding, pregnancy
For: 53, 110

Cynanchum stauntoni,
C. glaucessens

Baiqian 白前

P: root and root stalk
T&N: acrid and sweet; mildly warm
M: lung
Act: to clear lung and lower Qi, to dissolve sputum and stop cough
A&F: 4–9 grams as decoction
C&C: Qi deficiency, Qi not returning to its abode
For: 57

Cyperus rotundus

Xiangfu 香附

P: root stalk
T&N: acrid, slightly bitter, and
    sweet; neither warm nor cool
M: liver, the three sphincters
Act: to regulate Qi and release
    blockage, to stop pain and
    regulate circulation
A&F: 4–9 grams as decoction, pill,
    powder
C&C: Qi deficiency without block-
    age, Yin deficiency with
    blood Heat
For: 14, 75, 150, 169, 170, 202,
    301, 335

Dalbergia odorifera
Jiang(zhen)xiang 降（真）香
    P: heart of root
T&N: acrid; warm
    M: liver, spleen
Act: to regulate Qi, to stop bleed-
    ing, to mobilize effusion, to
    stop pain
A&F: 2–5 grams as decoction, pill,
    powder
C&C: Heat in blood, multiple
    draining ulcers, Yin deficiency
    with Fire
For: 14, 139

Daphne genkwa
Yuanhua 芫花
    P: flower bud
T&N: acrid and bitter; warm;
    poisonous
    M: lung, spleen
Act: to induce urine flow, to clear
    sputum
A&F: 1–3 grams as decoction, pill,
    powder
C&C: weak constitution, pregnancy
For: 12, 102

Dendrobium nobile
Shihu 石斛
    P: stalk
T&N: sweet and mildly salty; cold
    M: stomach, lung, kidney
Act: to generate fluid, to nourish
    stomach, to cool fever and
    generate Yin
A&F: 6–12 grams as decoction, gel,
    pill, powder
C&C: deficiency of stomach and
    kidney without Fire
For: 83, 272

Dianthus superbus, D. chinensis
(China rainbow pink)
Qumai 瞿麦
    P: whole herb with flower
T&N: bitter; cold
    M: heart, kidney, small intestine,
    bladder
Act: to cool Heat and excrete
    water, to mobilize blood and
    open meridians
A&F: 4–9 grams as decoction, pill,
    powder
C&C: spleen or kidney deficiency,
    pregnancy
For: 9

Dictamnus dasycarpus (burning
bush)
Baixianpi 白鲜皮
    P: root skin
T&N: bitter and salty; cold
    M: spleen, stomach
Act: to dispel Wind, to dry
    Dampness, to cool Heat, to
    relieve poison
A&F: 6–15 grams as decoction
C&C: deficiency Cold
For: 198

Dioscorea hypoglauca and other spp.

Beixie 萆薢

P: bulbous stalk
T&N: bitter; neither warm nor cool
M: liver, stomach, bladder
Act: to expel Wind, to excrete Dampness
A&F: 9–15 grams as decoction, pill, powder
C&C: kidney deficiency, Yin depletion
For: 264

Dioscorea opposita (Chinese yam)

Shanyao 山药

P: stalk
T&N: sweet; neither warm nor cool
M: lung, spleen, kidney
Act: to nourish spleen, to restore lung, to strengthen kidney, and to enrich Shen
A&F: 9–18 grams as decoction, pill, powder
C&C: strength diseases, avoid using with *Euphorbia kansui*
For: 4, 46, 64, 117, 133, 197, 208, 263, 283, 322

Diospyros kaki (Japanese persimmon)

Shidi 柿蒂

P: calyx
T&N: bitter and astringent; neither warm nor cool
M: lung, stomach
Act: to lower the abnormally risen Qi
A&F: 6–12 grams as decoction or powder
For: 3

Dipsacus japonicus, asper

Xuduan 续断

P: root
T&N: bitter and acrid; mildly warm
M: liver, kidney
Act: to restore liver and kidney, to rejoin sinews and bones, to regulate blood and meridians
A&F: 6–12 grams as decoction, pill, powder
C&C: suppressed anger

Dolichos lablab

Biandou 扁豆

P: white seed (occasionally, fresh flower, as specified); white seed skin is about twice as potent
T&N: sweet; neither warm nor cool
M: spleen, stomach
Act: to enrich spleen and mediate centrally, to disperse Heat and Dampness
A&F: 9–18 grams as decoction, pill, powder
C&C: diseases of Cold and Heat
For: 44, 113, 168, 208, 296; 282

Dryobalanops aromatica (Borneo camphor tree)

Longnaoxiang 龙脑香

P: resin from the tree
T&N: acrid and bitter; cool
M: heart, lung
Act: to open all ostia, to disperse all trapped Fire, to improve vision, to suppress swelling and stop pain
A&F: 0.15–0.3 gram as pill or powder; externally applied as powder or paste
C&C: deficiency of blood or Qi, pregnancy

For: 58, 75, 97, 101, 104, 131, 335

Dryopteris crassirhizoma (wood fern)

Guanzhong 贯众

P: root stalk
T&N: bitter; cool
M: liver, stomach
Act: to kill parasites, to cool fever and relieve poison, to cool blood, to stop bleeding
A&F: 4–9 grams as decoction, pill, powder
C&C: Yin deficiency with internal Heat, deficiency Cold of spleen and stomach, pregnancy
For: 338

Elsholtzia splendens

Xiangru 香薷

P: whole herb, including flower
T&N: acrid; slightly warm
M: liver, stomach
Act: to disperse exterior by diaphoresis, to induce urine flow and dissipate Dampness, to warm stomach and mediate centrally
A&F: 3–9 grams as decoction or ground powder
C&C: deficiency in the exterior
For: 44, 168, 282

Ephedra sinica and other spp.

Mahuang 麻黄

P: stalk
T&N: acrid and bitter; warm
M: lung, bladder
Act: to induce diaphoresis, to calm dyspnea, to excrete water

A&F: 1–6 grams as decoction, pill, powder
C&C: spontaneous perspiration, night sweats, or dyspnea due to chronically weak constitution
For: 25, 32, 36, 114, 173, 192, 246, 247, 248, 249, 269, 270, 271, 290, 330

Ephedra sinica and other spp.

Mahuanggen 麻黄根

P: root and root stalk
T&N: sweet; neither warm nor cool
Act: to stop spontaneous perspiration and night sweats
A&F: 1–6 grams as decoction, pill, powder
C&C: exterior evil diseases
For: 106, 107

Epimedium grandiflorum and other spp. (barren wort)

Yinyanghuo 淫羊藿

P: stalk leaf
T&N: acrid and sweet; warm
M: liver, kidney
Act: to restore kidney and strengthen Yang, to expel Wind and eliminate Dampness
A&F: 3–9 grams as decoction, elixir, gel, pill, powder
C&C: Yin deficiency, liver Fire easily perturbed
For: 6

Equus asinus (ass)

Ejiao 阿胶

P: gelatin from the skin, dried
T&N: sweet; neither warm nor cool
M: lung, liver, kidney

Act: to nourish Yin and restore blood, to calm fetus
A&F: 4–9 grams dissolved in wine or boiled water, or as pill, powder
C&C: spleen and stomach deficiency
For: 5, 18, 21, 60, 121, 122, 128, 222, 232, 256, 262, 273, 279, 280

Eragrostis tenella (love grass)
Xiangfeicao 香榧草
  P: whole herb
T&N: salty; neither warm nor cool
Act: to cool Heat and blood
A&F: 30–60 grams as decoction
For: 14

Eretmochelys imbricata
Daimao(xie) 玳瑁（屑）
  P: exoskeleton
T&N: sweet and salty; cold
  M: hand Lesser Yin, foot Dark Yin
Act: to cool Heat and relieve poison, to control convulsion
A&F: 3–6 grams as decoction, pill, powder
For: 101

Eriobotrya japonica (loquat)
Pipaye 枇杷叶
  P: leaf
T&N: bitter; cool
  M: lung, stomach
Act: to cool lung and mediate stomach, to lower Qi and dissolve sputum
A&F: 4–9 grams (fresh: 15–30 grams) as decoction, pill, powder

C&C: stomach Cold with vomiting, Wind and Cold in lung with cough
For: 125, 132, 218, 222

Eucommia ulmoides
Duzhong 杜仲
  P: bark
T&N: sweet, mildly acrid; warm
  M: liver, kidney
Act: to restore liver and kidney, to strengthen sinews and bone, to calm fetus
A&F: 9–15 grams as decoction, elixir, pill, powder
C&C: Yin deficiency with strong Fire
For: 53, 64, 272, 319

Euonymous tengyuehensis
Baipi 白芨
  P: bark
T&N: bland; neither warm nor cool
Act: to stop bleeding
A&F: externally as ground powder or juice

Eupatorium fortunei (mist flower)
Peilan 佩兰
  P: stalk and leaf
T&N: acrid; neither warm nor cool
  M: spleen, stomach
Act: to cool Heat, to ward off contagion, to dissolve Dampness, to regulate the meridians
A&F: 4–9 grams (fresh: 9–15 grams) as decoction
C&C: Yin or Qi deficiency
For: 132

Euphorbia kansui
Gansui 甘遂

P: root
T&N: bitter and sweet; cold; poisonous
M: spleen, lung, kidney
Act: to excrete accumulated
water, to disperse stagnation
and effusion, to promote
urination and defecation
A&F: 1–3 grams as decoction, pill,
powder
C&C: Qi deficiency, Yin damage,
spleen and stomach weak-
ness, pregnancy
For: 12, 24, 102, 212

Euphorbia pekinensis
Daji 大戟
P: root
T&N: bitter and acrid; cold; poi-
sonous
M: lung, spleen, kidney
Act: to eliminate accumulated
water, to facilitate urination
and defecation
A&F: 1–3 grams as decoction, pill,
powder
C&C: deficiency Cold, Yin water, or
pregnancy
For: 12, 102, 212

Euphoria longan
Longyanrou 龙眼肉
P: flesh of the fruit
T&N: sweet; warm
M: heart, spleen
Act: to nourish heart and spleen, to
restore Qi and blood, to sedate
A&F: 6–15 grams as decoction, gel,
elixir, pill
C&C: internal Phlegm and Fire,
Dampness accumulation with
anorexia
For: 324

Euryale ferox
Qianshi 芡实
P: seed kernel
T&N: sweet and astringent; neither
warm nor cool
M: spleen, kidney
Act: to firm up kidney and impede
seminal flow; to restore
spleen and stop diarrhea
A&F: 9–15 grams as decoction, pill,
powder
For: 28, 124, 135

Evodia rutaecarpa
Wuzhuyu 吴茱萸
P: unripe fruit
T&N: acrid and bitter; warm;
somewhat poisonous
M: liver, stomach
Act: to warm centrally, to stop
pain, to regulate Qi, to dry
Dampness
A&F: 1–6 grams as decoction, pill,
powder
C&C: Yin deficiency with strong Fire
For: 55, 68, 73, 108, 171, 256, 342

Fecal filtrate
Jinzhi 金汁
P: aqueous filtrate of human
excrement
T&N: bitter; cool
Act: to cool Heat and relieve
poison
A&F: 15–30 grams as filtrate or
mixed with other decoctions
C&C: not to use except for strength
Heat or Fire poison diseases
For: 155

Foeniculum vulgare (fennel)
(Xiao)huixiang (小) 茴香

P: fruit
T&N: acrid; warm
  M: kidney, bladder, stomach
  Act: to warm kidney and disperse
    Cold, to mediate stomach
    and regulate Qi
A&F: 3–9 grams as decoction, pill,
    powder
C&C: Yin deficiency with strong Fire
  For: 52, 54, 202, 284

Forsythia suspensa (weeping
golden bell)

Lianqiao 连翘
  P: fruit
T&N: bitter; cool
  M: heart, liver, gallbladder
  Act: to cool fever and eliminate
    poison, to release blockage
    and suppress swelling
A&F: 9–15 grams as decoction, pill,
    powder
C&C: spleen and stomach defi-
    ciency, Qi deficiency with
    fever, draining abscess
  For: 8, 20, 86, 106, 109, 138, 145,
    153, 172, 181, 186, 219, 227,
    252, 276, 282, 296, 305, 330

Forsythia suspensa (weeping
golden bell)

Lianqiaoxin 连翘心
  P: seed
T&N: bitter; cold
  Act: to cool heart, excrete Fire,
    strengthen stomach, stop
    vomiting
A&F: 6–15 grams as decoction
  For: 225

Forsythia suspensa (weeping
golden bell)

Lianqiaogen 连翘根

P: root
T&N: bitter; cold
  Act: for Cold injury, effusion with
    early jaundice
A&F: 60 grams as decoction
  For: 225

Fossil bones

Longgu 龙骨

T&N: sweet and astringent; neither
    warm nor cool
  M: heart, liver, kidney, large
    intestine
  Act: sedation, impedance of
    perspiration and seminal out-
    flow, hemostasis, generation
    of flesh and absorption of
    abscess
A&F: 9–15 grams as decoction, pill,
    powder
C&C: Dampness and Heat, evil
    strength
  For: 123, 124, 135, 140, 179, 182,
    211, 329

Fossil teeth

Longchi 龙齿

T&N: astringent; cool
  M: heart, liver
  Act: sedation, cooling
A&F: 9–15 grams as decoction
C&C: conflicts with gypsum
  For: 195

Fraxinus bungeana and other spp.

Qinpi 秦皮
  P: bark
T&N: bitter; cold
  M: liver, gallbladder
  Act: to cool Heat and dry Damp-
    ness, to calm dyspnea and
    stop cough, to improve vision

A&F: 4–9 grams as decoction or
 pill
C&C: deficiency Cold of spleen and
 stomach; not to be used with
 Evodia
For: 94

Fritillaria cirrhosa, F. delavayi
Chuanbeimu 川贝母
 P: underground stalk
 T&N: bitter and sweet; cool
  M: lung
  Act: to cool or lubricate lung, to
   dissolve sputum and control
   coughing
 A&F: 3–9 grams as decoction, pill,
  powder; externally as powder
  or cream
 C&C: deficiency Cold in spleen and
  stomach; Dampness and
  Phlegm; not to be used with
  Aconitum
 For: 5, 86, 99, 143, 180, 217, 236,
  262, 312

Fritillaria verticillata
Zhebeimu 浙贝母
 P: stalk
 T&N: very bitter; cold
  M: hand Greater Yin and Lesser
   Yang, foot Bright Yang and
   Dark Yin
  Act: to cool fever and dissolve
   sputum, to dissipate accumu-
   lation and eliminate poison
 A&F: 4–9 grams as decoction, pill,
  powder
 For: 5, 86, 99, 188, 189

Gallus gallus domesticus (chicken)
Jizihuang 鸡子黄
 P: egg yolk

T&N: sweet; neither warm nor cool
 M: heart, kidney
 Act: to nourish Yin and moisten
  Dryness, to generate blood
  and calm Wind
C&C: excess causes constipation
For: 21, 121, 290

Gallus gallus domesticus (chicken)
Jineijin 鸡内金
 P: internal lining of the gizzard
 T&N: sweet; neither warm nor cool
  M: spleen, stomach
  Act: to dissipate accumulations,
   to strengthen spleen and
   stomach
 A&F: 3–9 grams as decoction, pill,
  powder

Gardenia jasminoides and other
spp. (gardenia)
Zhizi 栀子
 P: fruit
 T&N: bitter; cold
  Act: to cool fever and sedate, to
   disperse Heat and Dampness, to cool blood and
   relieve poison
 A&F: 6–9 grams as decoction
 For: 8, 9, 13, 33, 37, 53, 58, 83,
  97, 106, 141, 151, 152, 161,
  172, 180, 186, 200, 217, 227,
  240, 276, 278, 289, 320, 327,
  328, 330, 342

Gastrodia elata
Tianma 天麻
 P: root and stalk
 T&N: sweet; neither warm nor
  cool
  M: liver
  Act: to disperse Wind

A&F: 4–9 grams as decoction, pill, powder
For: 53, 63, 315, 316

Gekko gecko
Gejie 蛤蚧
    P: dried eviscerated carcass
T&N: salty; neither warm nor cool
    M: lung, kidney
Act: to restore lung and kidney, to calm dyspnea and stop cough
A&F: 3–6 grams as decoction, pill, powder
C&C: cough due to external Wind and Cold evils
For: 209

Gentiana macrophylla, G. crassicaulis (gentian)
Qinjiao 秦艽
    P: root
T&N: bitter and acrid; neither warm nor cool
    M: liver, stomach, gallbladder
Act: to expel Wind and Dampness, to mediate blood and soothe sinews, to cool Heat and promote urine
A&F: 4–9 grams as decoction, elixir, pill, powder
C&C: chronic pain and emaciation, excessive urine, diarrhea
For: 105, 196, 260, 285, 319

Gentiana scabra, G. triflora (rough gentian)
Longdancao 龙胆草
    P: root
T&N: bitter; cold
    M: liver, gallbladder
Act: to eliminate strength Fire from liver and gallbladder, to

eliminate Dampness and Heat from the lower position
A&F: 3–9 grams as decoction, pill, powder
C&C: spleen and stomach deficient and weak
For: 228, 257, 289, 320, 327

Glechoma longituba
Jinqiancao 金钱草
    P: whole herb, may include root
T&N: bitter and acrid; cool
Act: to cool Heat, to induce urine flow, to control cough, to relieve swelling, to eliminate poison
A&F: 9–15 grams (fresh: 30–60 grams) as decoction, elixir, pressed juice
For: 110, 158

Gleditsia sinensis
Zaojia 皂荚
    P: fruit
T&N: acrid; warm; slightly poisonous
Act: to dispel Wind and Phlegm, to eliminate Dampness and poison, to kill parasites
A&F: 1–1.5 grams as ground powder, pill
C&C: pregnancy
For: 107, 131, 259

Gleditsia sinensis
Zaojiaoci 皂角刺
    P: thorns
T&N: acrid; warm
Act: to control Wind and remove poison, to suppress swelling and drain pus
A&F: 3–9 grams as decoction, pill, powder

C&C: draining abscess, pregnancy
For: 34, 188, 204

Glehnia littoralis
Beishashen 北沙参
  P: root
T&N: sweet, bitter; cool
  M: lung, spleen
  Act: to generate Yin and cool
    lung, to dissipate Phlegm and
    stop cough
A&F: 9–15 grams as decoction, gel,
    pill
C&C: Wind and Cold causing
    cough; deficiency Cold of
    lung, stomach
For: 113

Glycine max
Douchi 豆豉
  P: seed
T&N: sweet; neither warm nor cool
  M: spleen, kidney
  Act: to mobilize blood, to excrete
    water, to repel Wind, to
    relieve poison
A&F: 9–30 grams as decoction, pill,
    powder
C&C: not to be used with *Panax
    ginseng, Magnolia, Gentiana*
For: 152, 155, 169, 180, 240, 293,
    305, 332

Glycine max
Dadoujuan 大豆卷
  P: sprouting seed
T&N: sweet; neither warm nor cool
  M: spleen, stomach
  Act: to disperse and cool exterior,
    to dissipate Dampness and
    Heat
A&F: 9–15 grams as decoction, pill,
    powder

C&C: not to be used with *Zingiber,
    Gentiana*
For: 132, 342

Glycyrrhiza uralensis (Chinese
licorice)
Gancao 甘草
  P: root stalk (sometimes termi-
    nal branches of root)
T&N: sweet; neither warm nor cool
  M: spleen, stomach, lung
  Act: to mediate centrally, to lubri-
    cate lung, to eliminate poison,
    to harmonize various drugs
A&F: 1–9 grams as decoction, pill,
    powder
C&C: abdominal distention due to
    strength disease
For: 7, 8, 9, 18, 25, 30, 31, 32, 33,
    36, 43, 44, 47, 49, 50, 56, 57,
    59, 60, 62, 64, 66, 70, 72, 76,
    80, 84, 85, 87, 88, 89, 91, 98,
    99, 100, 103, 105, 106, 107,
    109, 113, 115, 116, 117, 121,
    125, 128, 145, 149, 150, 151,
    159, 160, 162, 164, 170, 172,
    174, 175, 177, 179, 181, 183,
    186, 188, 190, 192, 193, 198,
    203, 208, 214, 216, 217, 220,
    222, 223, 224, 227, 228, 233,
    236, 237, 244, 246, 247, 249,
    251, 252, 255, 256, 260, 262,
    265, 269, 270, 271, 272, 273,
    277, 285, 286, 290, 291, 295,
    296, 297, 301, 305, 309, 310,
    311, 312, 313, 314, 317, 319,
    320, 324, 326, 328, 329, 330,
    333, 334, 339, 341

Gold (native)
Jinbo 金箔
T&N: acrid and bitter; neither
    warm nor cool

M: heart, liver

Act: to calm heart, to sedate, to relieve poison

A&F: generally used as coating for pills

C&C: Yang deficiency with sunken Qi

For: 101, 131, 261

Grain syrup

Yitang 饴糖

P: fermented syrup from *Oryza, Hordeum*, and other grains

T&N: sweet; warm

M: spleen, stomach, lung

Act: to slow centrally, to restore deficiency, to generate fluid, to moisten Dryness

A&F: 30–60 grams in decoction, gel, pill

C&C: Heat and Dampness trapped internally, central distention with vomiting

For: 22, 30

Gryllotalpa africana (mole cricket)

Lougu 蝼蛄

P: dried whole insect

T&N: salty; cold

M: stomach, bladder

Act: to induce or promote urine flow

A&F: 3–5 grams as decoction or powder

C&C: Qi deficiency, weak constitution, pregnancy

Gypsum

Shigao 石膏

T&N: acrid and sweet; cold

M: lung, stomach

Act: to disperse the exterior and cool fever, to sedate restlessness and quench thirst

A&F: 9–30 grams as decoction, pill, powder; may use up to 240 grams; externally as roasted powder or paste

C&C: deficiency Cold of spleen and stomach, blood deficiency, fever due to Yin deficiency

For: 25, 47, 78, 80, 91, 100, 106, 142, 222, 224, 227, 246, 261, 264, 269, 270, 328, 330

Hair

Xueyuhui 血余炭

P: fired human hair

T&N: bitter; warm

M: heart, liver, kidney

Act: to stop bleeding or disperse effusion

A&F: 1–3 grams each time as ground powder or pill; externally as snuff for nosebleed, as powder or paste on skin wounds

Haliotis diversicolor, gigantea discus (sea-ear)

Shijueming 石决明

P: shell

T&N: salty; neither warm nor cool

M: liver, kidney

Act: to calm liver and submerge Yang, to eliminate Heat, to improve vision

A&F: 9–30 grams as decoction, pill, powder; externally fine suspension as eye drops

C&C: not to be used with *Inula*

For: 53, 121

Halloysite

Chishizhi 赤石脂

T&N: sweet and astringent; warm

M: stomach, large intestine
Act: to impede intestinal flow, to
stop bleeding, to pull in
Dampness, to generate flesh
A&F: 9–12 grams as decoction, pill,
powder
C&C: accumulated Dampness and
Heat, pregnancy
For: 28, 184

Hematite
Daizheshi 代赭石
T&N: bitter and sweet; neither
warm nor cool
M: liver, stomach, pericardium
Act: to calm liver and control
abnormal flow, to cool blood,
to stop bleeding
A&F: 9–30 grams as decoction, pill,
powder
C&C: pregnancy
For: 216, 329

Hirudo nipponica (leech)
Shuizhi 水蛭
P: dried whole worm
T&N: salty and bitter; neither warm
nor cool; poisonous
M: liver, bladder
Act: to mobilize blood and dis-
solve effusion, to facilitate
circulation
A&F: 1–3 grams as pill, powder
C&C: weak constitution with blood
deficiency, pregnancy,
absence of clotting and
effusion
For: 126

Homalomena occulta
Qiannianjian 千年健
P: root and stalk

T&N: acrid; warm
M: liver, lung
Act: to drive out Wind and
Dampness, to strengthen
bones and sinews, to sup-
press swelling; analgesia
A&F: 4–9 grams as decoction,
elixir; externally as cream
C&C: Yin deficiency with internal
Heat; not to be used with
Raphanus
For: 340

Hordeum vulgare (wheat)
Maiya 麦芽
P: sprouting grain
T&N: sweet; slightly warm
M: spleen, stomach
Act: to aid digestion, to mediate
centrally, to lower Qi
A&F: 9–15 grams as decoction, pill,
powder
C&C: spleen deficiency, Phlegm
and Fire causing dyspnea,
pregnancy
For: 44, 130, 207, 329

Imperata cylindrica (Japanese
blood grass)
Baimaohua 白茅花
P: flower
T&N: sweet; warm
Act: hemostasis, analgesic
A&F: 9–15 grams as decoction;
externally as paste or nasal
packing

Imperata cylindrica v. *major*
Baimaogen 白茅根
P: root stalk
T&N: sweet; cold
M: lung, stomach, small intestine

Act: to cool blood, to stop bleeding, to cool Heat, to promote
urine
A&F: 9–15 grams (fresh: 30–60
grams) as decoction
C&C: deficiency Cold of spleen and
stomach, excessive urine
without thirst
For: 13

Inula britannica, I. linariaefolia
(elecampane)
Xuanfuhua 旋复花
  P: flower
T&N: salty; warm
  M: lung, liver, stomach
  Act: to dissolve sputum, to lower
  Qi, to soften the firm, to
  move water
A&F: 4–9 grams as decoction, pill,
  powder
C&C: Yin deficiency and chronic
  cough, Wind and Dampness
For: 215, 216

Isatis indigotica
Qingdai 青黛
  P: the pigment from the leaf
T&N: salty; cold
  M: liver, lung, stomach
  Act: to cool fever and blood, to
  relieve poison
A&F: 1–2 grams as decoction, pill,
  powder
C&C: central Cold
For: 141, 289, 323

Juncus effusus (bog rush)
Dengxincao 灯芯草
  P: whole herb
T&N: sweet; cold
  M: heart, lung, small intestine

Act: to cool heart and lower Fire,
to promote urine and resolve
dribbling
A&F: 1–2 grams if used fresh and
alone; 15–30 grams as decoction, pill, powder
C&C: deficiency Cold, central Cold
with excessive urine, Qi deficiency with excessive urine
For: 9, 131

Laminaria japonica and other spp.
(seaweed)
Kunbu 昆布
  P: whole herb
T&N: salty; cold
  M: spleen, stomach
  Act: to soften the firm, to induce
  urine
A&F: 4–9 grams as decoction, pill,
  powder
C&C: deficiency Cold and Damp-
  ness in spleen and stomach
For: 202

Lasiophaera fenzlii
Mabo 马勃
  P: fruit
T&N: acrid; neither warm nor cool
  M: lung
  Act: to cool lung and lubricate
  throat, to eliminate poison, to
  stop bleeding
A&F: 1–3 grams as decoction, pill,
  powder
C&C: chronic cough with hoarse-
  ness due to Wind and Cold
For: 252

Lead oxide
Mituoseng 密陀僧
T&N: salty and acrid; neither warm
  nor cool; poisonous

M: liver, spleen
Act: to reduce swelling, to kill
parasites, to draw in and prevent necrosis, to control convulsion
A&F: externally as ground powder
or paste; internally 0.3–1.0
gram as ground powder or
pill
C&C: weak constitution

Leonurus heterophyllus
Yimucao 益母草
P: whole herb
T&N: acrid and bitter; cool
M: pericardium, liver
Act: to mobilize blood, to dispel
hematoma and effusion, to
regulate menses, to excrete
water
A&F: 9–18 grams as decoction, gel,
pill, powder
C&C: Yin deficiency, blood deple-
tion
For: 53

Lepidium apetalum, L. virginicum
Tinglizi 葶苈子
P: seed
T&N: acrid and bitter; cold
M: lung, bladder
Act: to lower Qi and move water
A&F: 4–9 grams as decoction, pill,
powder
C&C: lung deficiency, spleen defi-
ciency
For: 294

*Ligusticum sinense, L. jeholense, L.
tenuissimum*
Gaoben 藁本
P: root stalk or root

T&N: acrid; warm
M: bladder
Act: to disperse Wind, Cold,
Dampness
A&F: 3–9 grams as decoction
C&C: blood deficiency with
headache
For: 163, 239

Ligustinum wallichii
Chuanxiong 川芎
P: root and stalk
T&N: acrid; warm
M: liver, gallbladder
Act: to move Qi and release
blockage, to drive out Wind
and dry Dampness to facilitate circulation
A&F: 3–6 grams as decoction, pill,
powder; externally as powder
or cream
C&C: Yin deficiency with strong Fire
For: 32, 54, 67, 75, 88, 103, 106,
139, 150, 153, 203, 214, 238,
256, 257, 260, 266, 276, 283,
301, 310, 311, 319, 327, 330,
339

Ligustrum lucidum (Japanese wax
privet)
Nuzhenzi 女贞子
P: fruit
T&N: bitter and sweet; neither
warm nor cool
M: liver, kidney
Act: to restore liver and kidney,
to strengthen the waist and
knees
A&F: 4–9 grams as decoction, gel,
pill
C&C: deficiency Cold of spleen and
stomach with diarrhea, Yang
deficiency

Lilium brownii, L. pumilum, L. longiflorum

Baihe 百合
P: bulb petals
T&N: sweet and mildly bitter; neither warm nor cool
M: heart, lung
Act: to lubricate lung and stop cough, to cool heart and sedate
A&F: 9–30 grams as decoction, or eat steamed
C&C: cough due to Wind and Cold, central Cold with diarrhea
For: 83, 99

Lindera strychnifolia

Wuyao 乌药
P: root
T&N: acrid; warm
M: spleen, lung, kidney, bladder
Act: to smooth Qi, to overcome blockage, to disperse Cold, to stop pain
A&F: 4–9 grams as decoction, pill, powder, juice obtained by grinding
C&C: Qi deficiency, internal Heat
For: 14, 52, 75, 284, 298, 301, 322

Liquidambar orientalis

Suhexiang 苏合香
P: resin from the tree
T&N: acrid; warm
M: lung, liver
Act: to open ostia, to stimulate, to expel sputum
A&F: 1–3 grams as pill
C&C: Yin deficiency with Fire
For: 335

Litchi chinensis

Lizhihe 荔枝核
P: seed
T&N: sweet and astringent; warm
M: liver, kidney
Act: to warm centrally, to regulate Qi, to stop pain
A&F: 4–9 grams as decoction, pill, powder
For: 202

Lithospermum erythrorhizon and other spp.

Zicao 紫草
P: root
T&N: bitter; cold
M: pericardium, liver
Act: to cool and mobilize blood, to cool Heat, to relieve poison
A&F: 3–9 grams as decoction or powder
C&C: stomach and intestine weakness, diarrhea
For: 155

Lonicera japonica (Japanese honeysuckle)

Jinyinteng 金银藤
P: stalk and leaf
T&N: sweet; cold
M: heart, lung
Act: to cool Heat, to relieve poison, to open meridians
A&F: 9–30 grams as decoction, pill, powder, elixir

Lonicera japonica (Japanese honeysuckle)

Jinyinhua 金银花
P: flower buds
T&N: sweet; cold

M: lung, stomach

Act: to cool fever and relieve poison

A&F: 9–15 grams as decoction, pill, powder

C&C: deficiency Cold of spleen and stomach, Qi deficiency with carbuncles with clear drainage

For: 39, 109, 145, 155, 188, 219, 282, 305

Loranthus yadoriki, L. parasiticus

Sangjisheng 桑寄生

P: branch and stalk

T&N: bitter and sweet; neither warm nor cool

M: liver, kidney

Act: to restore liver and kidney, to strengthen sinews, to expel Wind and Dampness, to facilitate circulation, to enrich blood, to calm fetus

A&F: 9–18 grams as decoction, powder, elixir, pressed juice

For: 53, 75, 319, 340

Lycium chinense (Chinese wolfberry)

Digupi 地骨皮

P: root skin

T&N: sweet; cold

M: lung, liver, kidney

Act: to cool fever and blood

A&F: 9–15 grams as decoction, pill, powder

C&C: deficiency Cold of spleen and stomach

For: 196, 198, 228, 326

Lycium chinense (Chinese wolfberry)

Gouqizi 枸杞子

P: ripe fruit

T&N: sweet; neither warm nor cool

M: liver, kidney

Act: to nourish kidney, to lubricate lung, to restore liver, to improve vision

A&F: 6–12 grams as decoction, gel, elixir, pill, powder

C&C: external Heat disease, spleen deficiency with Dampness

For: 1, 64, 112, 284

Lycopus lucidus

Zelan 泽兰

P: whole herb

T&N: bitter and acrid; mildly warm

M: liver, spleen

Act: to mobilize blood, to induce urine flow

A&F: 4–9 grams as decoction, pill, powder

C&C: blood deficiency

Lygodium japonicum (fern)

Haijinsha 海金沙

P: seed

T&N: sweet; cold

M: small intestine, bladder

Act: to cool Heat and eliminate poison, to move water and facilitate urination

A&F: 4–9 grams as decoction, pill, gel

C&C: watery diarrhea and spontaneous emission, Dampness and Phlegm

For: 14, 110

Mactra quadrangularis (clam)

Gelifen 蛤蜊粉

P: ground fired shell
T&N: salty; cold
  M: lung, kidney
  Act: to cool Heat, excrete Dampness, dissolve Phlegm, soften the firm
  A&F: 3–9 grams as pill or powder; externally as powder
  C&C: deficiency Cold in spleen and stomach
  For: 34

Magnolia officinalis, M. biloba
Houpo 厚朴
  P: bark or root skin
T&N: bitter and acrid; warm
  M: spleen, stomach, large intestine
  Act: to warm centrally, to lower Qi, to dry Dampness, to dissolve sputum
  A&F: 3–9 grams as decoction, pill, powder
  C&C: pregnancy
  For: 14, 15, 19, 29, 44, 55, 61, 74, 75, 76, 77, 140, 148, 168, 205, 218, 240, 245, 250, 253, 282, 295, 297, 332, 333, 334, 339

Manis pentadactyla (anteater)
Chuanshanjia 穿山甲
  P: scales
T&N: salty; cool
  M: liver, stomach
  Act: to relieve swelling and drain abscess, to improve circulation, to promote milk flow
  A&F: 4–9 grams as decoction, powder
  C&C: Qi or blood insufficiency, draining abscess
  For: 188, 202, 251

Melaphis chinensis, M. paitan
Wubeizi 五倍子
  P: cocoon
T&N: acid; neither warm nor cool
  M: lung, stomach, large intestine
  Act: to collect lung, to impede intestinal flow, to stop bleeding, to eliminate poison
  A&F: 1–6 grams as ground powder or pill
  C&C: Wind and Cold diseases, cough due to strength Heat, diarrhea due to intestinal accumulation
  For: 51, 123

Melia azedarach, M. toosendan
(chinaberry tree)
Kuliangenpi 苦楝根皮
  P: root skin
T&N: bitter; cold; slightly poisonous
  Act: to cool Heat, to dry Dampness, to kill parasites
  A&F: 6–9 grams (fresh: 30–60 grams) as decoction, pill, powder
  C&C: weak constitution, deficiency Cold of spleen and stomach
  For: 2, 48

Melia toosendan (Chinaberry tree)
Chuanlianzi 川楝子
  P: fruit
T&N: bitter; cold; mildly poisonous
  M: liver, stomach, small intestine
  Act: to eliminate Dampness and Heat, to cool liver Fire, to kill parasites, to stop pain
  A&F: 4–9 grams as decoction, pill, powder; externally as cream
  C&C: deficiency Cold in spleen and stomach

Msc: use *Foeniculum vulgare* as its
    steward
For: 1, 52, 134, 202, 204, 298, 329

Mentha haplocalyx (mint)

Bohe 薄荷

    P: whole herb or leaf

T&N: acrid; cool

    M: lung, liver

    Act: to disperse Wind, to dissipate
        Heat, to ward off the impure,
        to relieve poison

A&F: 2–6 grams as decoction, pill,
        powder

C&C: Yin deficiency and blood
        depletion, liver Yang rising
        abnormally, exterior defi-
        ciency with diaphoresis

For: 8, 86, 106, 143, 172, 181,
       190, 203, 252, 276, 305, 312,
       330

Mercury

Shuiyin 水银

T&N: acrid; cold; highly poisonous

    M: heart, liver, kidney

    Act: to kill parasites, to attack
        poison

A&F: used externally only

C&C: highly poisonous

Mirabilite

Hanshuishi 寒水石

    P: crystals (sometimes refined
        crystals or anhydrous
        crystals)

T&N: acrid and salty; cold

    M: heart, stomach, kidney

    Act: to cool Heat and reduce Fire,
        to facilitate openings, to
        reduce swelling

A&F: 9–15 grams as decoction, pill,
        powder

C&C: deficiency Cold in spleen and
        stomach

For: 2, 19, 24, 26, 48, 80, 106,
       172, 183, 250, 261, 307, 309

Morinda officinale

Bajitian 巴戟天

    P: root

T&N: acrid and sweet; warm

    M: liver, kidney

    Act: to restore kidney Yang, to
        strengthen sinews and bones,
        to drive out Wind and
        Dampness

A&F: 4–9 grams as decoction, pill,
        powder, elixir, gel

C&C: Yin deficiency with strong Fire;
        not to be used with *Polyporus*

For: 6

Morus alba (white mulberry)

Sangye 桑叶

    P: leaf

T&N: bitter and sweet; cold

    M: lung, liver

    Act: to expel Wind and cool Heat,
        to cool blood and improve
        vision

A&F: 4–9 grams as decoction, pill,
        powder

For: 113, 143, 180, 181, 222, 236

Morus alba (white mulberry)

Sangzhi 桑枝

    P: tender branches

T&N: bitter; neither warm nor cool

    M: liver

    Act: to expel Wind and Damp-
        ness, to facilitate joints, to
        move water Qi

A&F: 30–60 grams as decoction or
        gel

For: 260

Morus alba (white mulberry)

Sangbaipi 桑白皮

P: root skin
T&N: sweet; cold
 M: lung, spleen
 Act: to dissipate lung and calm
  dyspnea, to move water and
  reduce swelling
A&F: 6–12 grams as decoction
C&C: lung deficiency without Fire,
  excessive urine, cough due to
  Wind and Cold
 For: 5, 8, 40, 125, 217, 247, 268,
  326, 336

Moschus moschiferus (muskdeer)

Shexiang 麝香

P: dried secretion from the pre-
  putial glands
T&N: acrid; warm
 M: heart, spleen, liver
 Act: to open ostia, to ward off the
  impure, to open meridians,
  to disperse effusion
A&F: 9–15 milligrams as pill,
  powder
C&C: pregnancy
 For: 58, 97, 101, 104, 117, 131,
  261, 289, 335

Mylabris phalerata, M. cichorii

Banmao 斑蝥

P: dried whole insect
T&N: acrid; cold; highly poisonous
 M: large and small intestines,
  liver, kidney
 Act: to expel poison, to disperse
  effusion (topically applied for
  persistent sores, rashes)
A&F: 30–60 milligrams as stir-fried
  powder, pill, powder
C&C: weak constitution, pregnancy

Myristica fragrans (nutmeg)

Rou(dou)kou 肉（豆）蔻

P: seed
T&N: acrid; warm
 M: spleen, large intestine
 Act: to warm centrally, to lower
  Qi, to aid digestion, to
  strengthen intestines
A&F: 1–6 grams as decoction, pill,
  powder
C&C: Heat diseases causing diar-
  rhea
 For: 68, 86, 130, 140, 193, 313

Nelumbo nucifera (lotus)

Lianzi 莲子

P: fruit, seed
T&N: sweet and astringent; neither
  warm nor cool
 M: heart, spleen, kidney
 Act: to enrich heart and kidney, to
  restore spleen, to impede
  intestines
A&F: 6–12 grams as decoction, pill,
  powder
 For: 28, 135, 199, 208, 277

Nelumbo nucifera (lotus)

Lianxu 莲须

P: stamen and pistils
T&N: sweet and astringent; neither
  warm nor cool
 M: heart, kidney
 Act: to cool heart, to enrich kidney, to impede seminal flow,
  to stop bleeding
A&F: 2–5 grams as decoction, pill,
  powder
C&C: difficulty with urination; not
  to be used with *Rehmannia*,
  leek, garlic
 For: 124, 135, 293

Nelumbo nucifera (lotus)

Lianxin 莲心

P: the green sprout of the ripe
seed
T&N: bitter; cold
M: heart, lung, kidney
Act: to cool heart and dispel Heat,
to stop bleeding, to impede
semen flow
A&F: 1–3 grams as decoction or
powder
For: 225

Nelumbo nucifera (lotus)

Heye 荷叶

P: leaf
T&N: bitter and astringent; neither
warm nor cool
M: heart, liver, spleen
Act: to cool Heat and excrete
Dampness, to raise the clear
Yang, to stop bleeding
A&F: 3–9 grams (fresh: 15–30 grams)
as decoction, pill, powder
C&C: upper strength diseases; not
to be used with *Poria*
For: 13

Nelumbo nucifera (lotus)

Ou(zhi) 藕 (汁)

P: root stalk
T&N: sweet; cold
M: heart, spleen, stomach
Act: to cool fever, to cool blood,
to disperse effusion
A&F: eat raw or cooked, or
squeezed juice
For: 33, 187

Niter

Xiaoshi(huoxiao) 消石 (火硝)

P: distilled crystals

T&N: bitter and salty; warm; poisonous
M: heart, spleen
Act: to break solid and disperse
accumulation, to facilitate
urination and defecation, to
relieve poison and reduce
swelling
A&F: 1–3 grams as pill, powder
C&C: weak constitution, pregnancy
For: 104

Ophicalcite

Huaruishi 花蕊石

T&N: acid and astringent; neither
warm nor cool
M: Dark Yin
Act: to dissolve clots and effusion,
to stop bleeding
A&F: 3–9 grams as powder
C&C: pregnancy

Ophiopogon japonicus (creeping
lily-turf)

Maimendong 麦门冬

P: bulbous root
T&N: sweet, slightly bitter; cold
M: lung, stomach, heart
Act: to generate Yin and lubricate
lung, to cool heart and
sedate, to support stomach
and generate fluid
A&F: 6–12 grams as decoction, pill,
powder
C&C: deficiency Cold in spleen
and stomach with diarrhea,
stomach with Phlegm and
Dampness, acute Wind and
Cold diseases
For: 1, 18, 21, 51, 60, 78, 83, 90,
99, 100, 113, 128, 198, 219,
220, 222, 225, 243, 244, 256,
267, 307, 312, 336

Oryza sativa (rice)

Guya 谷芽

   P: sprouting grain
T&N: sweet; warm
   M: spleen, stomach
   Act: to strengthen spleen and
      improve appetite, to mediate
      centrally and aid digestion
A&F: 9–15 grams as decoction
For: 44, 77, 326

Oryza sativa (rice)

Jingmi 粳米

   P: rice seed
T&N: sweet; neither warm nor cool
   M: spleen, stomach
   Act: to restore centrally and
      enrich Qi, to strengthen
      spleen and mediate stomach,
      to stop diarrhea
A&F: as decoction
For: 47, 91, 100, 184, 244, 336

Ostrea rivularis (oyster)

Muli 牡蛎

   P: shell
T&N: salty and astringent; cool
   M: liver, kidney
   Act: to pull back Yin, to submerge
      Yang, to stop perspiration, to
      impede semen flow, to dissolve
      sputum, to soften the firm
A&F: 9–30 grams as decoction, pill,
   powder
C&C: deficiency and Cold diseases;
   not to be used with *Ephedra*,
   Magnolia
For: 18, 21, 114, 121, 123, 124,
   135, 179, 186, 189, 211, 329

Paeonia lactiflora (Chinese peony)

Baishaoyao 白芍药

   P: root of the *white* peony
T&N: bitter and acid; cool
   M: liver, spleen
   Act: to generate blood and soften
      liver, to soothe centrally and
      stop pain, to conserve Yin
      and decrease perspiration
A&F: 6–12 grams as decoction, pill,
   powder
C&C: deficiency Cold with abdominal pain and diarrhea
For: 18, 21, 23, 30, 32, 36, 50, 60,
   67, 72, 99, 106, 109, 115,
   116, 118, 121, 122, 123, 149,
   150, 175, 190, 192, 193, 194,
   213, 224, 236, 245, 256, 258,
   272, 279, 280, 281, 285, 286,
   290, 295, 312, 313, 319, 329,
   330, 339

Paeonia lactiflora, P. veitchii
(Chinese peony)

Chishaoyao 赤芍药

   P: root of the *red* peony
T&N: acid and bitter; cool
   M: liver, spleen
   Act: to mobilize stagnant blood, to
      stop pain, to cool blood, to
      suppress swelling
A&F: 4–9 grams as decoction, pill,
   powder
C&C: blood deficiency
For: 44, 54, 56, 103, 109, 139,
   144, 145, 153, 186, 188, 227,
   229, 238, 250, 264, 266, 298,
   301, 341

Paeonia suffruticosa (tree peony)

Mudanpi 牡丹皮

   P: skin of the root
T&N: acrid and bitter; cool
   M: heart, liver, kidney
   Act: to cool fever and blood, to

mediate blood, to dissolve
effusion

A&F: 4–9 grams as decoction, pill,
powder

C&C: blood deficiency with Cold,
pregnancy, excessive uterine
bleeding

For: 4, 13, 26, 37, 46, 133, 137,
153, 226, 227, 229, 256, 263,
264, 298, 301, 312

Panax ginseng (ginseng)

Renshen 人参

P: root

T&N: sweet, slightly bitter; warm

M: spleen, lung

Act: to restore Original Qi, to preserve fluids, to calm the spirit

A&F: 1–9 grams as decoction; in
severe cases, 30–100 grams

C&C: strength diseases, Heat
diseases

For: 8, 32, 49, 50, 51, 59, 66, 71,
75, 90, 92, 100, 117, 118, 193,
195, 206, 207, 209, 210, 211,
214, 220, 224, 262, 267, 268,
272, 277, 304, 311, 318, 336

Panax pseudoginseng

(Renshen)sanqi （人参）三七

P: root

T&N: sweet, slightly bitter; warm

M: liver, stomach, large intestine

Act: hemostasis, dispersion of
effusion, suppression of swelling, analgesia

A&F: 4–9 grams as decoction, 5–10
grams as powder

C&C: pregnancy

Panax quinquefolium

Xiyangshen 西洋参

P: root

T&N: sweet, mildly bitter; cool

M: heart, lung, kidney

Act: to enrich lung Yin, to cool
deficiency Fire, to generate
fluid and quench thirst

A&F: 2–6 grams as decoction

C&C: weakened central Yang, Cold
and Dampness in stomach

Papaver somniferum (opium poppy)

Yinsuke 罂粟壳

P: dried fruit skin

T&N: acid; neither warm nor cool

M: lung, kidney, large intestine

Act: to stop cough, to impede
intestinal flow, to stop pain

A&F: 2–6 grams as decoction, pill,
powder

For: 5, 193, 313

Paratenodera sinensis and other
spp. (praying mantis)

Sangpiaoxiao 桑螵蛸

P: chrysalis

T&N: salty and sweet; neither warm
nor cool

M: liver, kidney

Act: to restore kidney, to conserve
Jing

A&F: 4–9 grams as decoction

C&C: Yin deficiency with strong
Fire, Heat in bladder

For: 182

Patrinii villosa, P. scabiosaefolia

(Shan)baijiang （山）败酱

P: whole herb, including root

T&N: bitter; neither warm nor cool

M: liver, stomach, large intestine

Act: to cool Heat and relieve poison, to drain pus and disperse
effusion

A&F: 9–15 grams (fresh: 60–120
grams) as decoction; externally as powder
C&C: stomach and spleen deficiency, diarrhea with
anorexia, deficiency Cold
For: 145

Perilla frutescens (beefsteak plant)
Zisuzi 紫苏子
P: fruit
T&N: acrid; warm
M: lung, large intestine
Act: to lower Qi, to dissolve spu-
tum, to lubricate lung, to
loosen intestines
A&F: 4–9 grams as decoction,
pressed juice, pill, powder
C&C: Qi, Yin, or spleen deficiency
For: 16, 334

Perilla frutescens (beefsteak plant)
Zisuye 紫苏叶
P: leaf
T&N: acrid; warm
M: lung, spleen
Act: to disperse exterior, to dissi-
pate Cold, to regulate Qi, to
mediate encampment level
A&F: 6–9 grams as decoction
C&C: Heat diseases, Qi weakness
with deficiency in exterior
For: 44, 61, 70, 333

Perilla frutescens (beefsteak plant)
Zisugeng 紫苏梗
P: stalk
T&N: acrid and sweet; slightly
warm
M: spleen, stomach, lung
Act: to regulate Qi, to relieve
blockage, to stop pain, to
calm fetus

A&F: 4–9 grams as decoction
For: 111, 169

*Peucedanum praeruptorum, P.
decursivum*
Qianhu 前胡
P: root
T&N: bitter and acrid; cool
M: lung, spleen
Act: to disperse Wind and Heat,
to lower Qi, to dissipate
Phlegm
A&F: 4–9 grams as decoction, pill,
powder
C&C: Qi deficiency and blood
insufficiency
For: 111, 143, 203, 214, 217, 304,
334

Pharbitis nil
Qianniuzi 牵牛子
P: seed
T&N: bitter, acrid; cold; mildly poi-
sonous
M: lung, kidney, large and small
intestines
Act: catharsis of water, lowering
of Qi, parasiticide
A&F: 0.3–1.0 gram as pill, powder;
4–9 grams as decoction
C&C: pregnancy, weak stomach,
deficient Qi
For: 48, 102, 204, 230, 292

Phaseolus calcaratus, P. angularis
Chixiaodou 赤小豆
P: seed
T&N: sweet and acid; neither warm
nor cool
M: heart, small intestine
Act: to induce urine flow and
eliminate Dampness, to

mediate blood and drain pus,
to suppress swelling and
eliminate poison
A&F: 9–30 grams as decoction or
powder
For: 247

Phaseolus radiatus

Ludou 绿豆

P: seed
T&N: sweet; cool
M: heart, stomach
Act: to cool Heat and eliminate
poison, to induce urine flow
A&F: 15–30 grams as decoction,
ground powder, or juice
obtained by grinding
C&C: deficiency Cold of spleen and
stomach; dangerous if used
with the shell of *Torreya
grandis*

*Phellodendron amurense, P.
chinense* (Amur cork tree)

Huangbai 黄柏

P: bark
T&N: bitter; cold
M: kidney, bladder
Act: to cool Heat, to dry Dampness, to purge Fire, to relieve
poison
A&F: 4–9 grams as decoction, pill,
powder
C&C: spleen deficiency with diarrhea, stomach weakness with
anorexia
For: 6, 94, 127, 129, 151, 191,
220, 223, 241, 257, 264, 276,
278, 281, 289

Pheretima aspergillum (earthworm)

Qiuyin 蚯蚓

P: whole worm
T&N: salty; cold
M: liver, spleen, lung
Act: to cool Heat, to calm liver, to
control dyspnea, to facilitate
circulation
A&F: 4–9 grams as decoction, pill,
powder
For: 266

Phragmites communis (reed grass)

Lugen 芦根

P: root stalk
T&N: sweet; cold
M: lung, stomach
Act: to cool fever, to generate
fluid, to sedate, to stop
vomiting
A&F: 15–30 grams (fresh: 60–120
grams) as decoction or
pressed juice
C&C: deficiency Cold of spleen and
stomach
For: 161, 181, 240, 302, 306

Phyllostachys nigra

Zhuye 竹叶

P: leaf; also new leaves, still
curled
T&N: sweet; cold
M: heart, lung, gallbladder,
stomach
Act: to cool and sedate, to generate fluid and induce urine
flow; new leaves, still curled,
are stronger in cooling ability, esp. heart Heat
A&F: 6–12 grams as decoction
For: 15, 33, 100, 219, 225, 305,
314, 327; 227 (new leaves)

Phyllostachys nigra

Zhuli 竹沥

22

6 COMPENDIA

P: liquid obtained by roasting
stalk
T&N: sweet and bitter; cold
M: heart, stomach
Act: to cool and loosen sputum, to
sedate
A&F: 30–60 grams as drink
C&C: cough due to Cold, spleen
deficiency with watery feces
For: 164

Phyllostachys nigra
Zhuru 竹茹
P: inner lining of the stalk
T&N: sweet; cool
M: stomach, gallbladder
Act: to cool fever and blood, to
dissolve sputum, to stop
vomiting
A&F: 4–9 grams as decoction
C&C: vomiting due to stomach
Cold
For: 236, 254, 315, 317

Phytolacca acinosa (pokeweed)
Shanglu 商陆
P: root
T&N: bitter; cold; poisonous
M: spleen, bladder
Act: to promote defecation and
urination, to excrete water, to
release blockage
A&F: 4–9 grams as decoction or
powder
C&C: spleen deficiency with
edema, pregnancy

*Picrorhiza kurrooa, P. scrophu-
lariaeflora*
Huhuanglian 胡黄连
P: root stalk
T&N: bitter; cold

M: liver, stomach, large intestine
Act: to cool fever and blood, to
dry Dampness
A&F: 1–5 grams as decoction, pill,
powder
C&C: spleen and stomach defi-
ciency
For: 228, 241

Pinellia ternata
Banxia 半夏
P: tuberous stalk
T&N: acrid; warm; poisonous
M: spleen, stomach
Act: to dry Dampness and dissolve
Phlegm, to lower abnormal
upflow and stop vomiting
A&F: 4–9 grams as decoction, pill,
powder
C&C: blood diseases, Yin defi-
ciency, injury to body fluids;
not to be used with realgar,
*Fraxinus, Aconitum, Chi-
nemys*
For: 15, 35, 45, 50, 55, 61, 62, 82,
85, 100, 107, 125, 136, 138,
149, 173, 186, 216, 240, 244,
256, 272, 315, 332, 342

Pinellia ternata
Banxiaqu 半夏曲
P: tuberous stalk, treated with
flour, ginger juice, etc.
T&N: bitter and acrid; neither
warm nor cool
Act: to dissolve sputum, to stop
cough, to aid digestion, to
stop diarrhea
A&F: 6–9 grams as decoction
C&C: internal Heat
For: 7, 23, 31, 36, 74, 88, 221,
311, 333, 334

Pinus koraiensis

(Hai)songzi （海）松子

  P: seed kernel

  T&N: sweet; warm

    M: liver, lung, large intestine

    Act: to generate fluid, to calm
Wind, to moisten lung, to
lubricate intestines

  A&F: 4–9 grams as decoction, gel,
pill

  C&C: watery diarrhea, Dampness,
and Phlegm

  For: 38

Piper kadsura

Haifengteng 海风藤

  P: vine stalk

  T&N: acrid and bitter; slightly
warm

    M: heart, kidney

    Act: to expel Wind and Damp-
ness, to open meridians, to
regulate Qi

  A&F: 6–15 grams as decoction or
elixir

  For: 260, 340

Piper longum (long pepper)

Biba 荜茇

  P: unripe fruit

  T&N: acrid; hot

    Act: to warm centrally and dis-
perse Cold

  A&F: 1–5 grams as decoction, pill,
powder

  For: 156

Piper nigrum (black pepper)

Hujiao 胡椒

  P: fruit

  T&N: acrid; hot

    M: stomach, large intestine

    Act: to warm centrally, to lower
Qi, to dissolve Phlegm, to
relieve poison

  A&F: 1–3 grams as decoction, pill,
powder

  C&C: Yin deficiency with Fire

  For: 156

Piper wallichii, P. puberulum

Fengteng 风藤

  P: stalk with leaf

  T&N: acrid; warm

    M: liver, spleen, small intestine

    Act: to dispel Wind and Damp-
ness, to open meridians, to
strengthen waist and legs, to
stop pain

  A&F: 3–9 grams as decoction, elixir

  C&C: Yin deficiency with strong Fire

  For: 340

Plantago asiatica

Cheqianzi 车前子

  P: seed

  T&N: sweet; cold

    M: kidney, bladder

    Act: to promote water excretion,
to cool fever, to improve
vision, to eliminate sputum

  A&F: 4–9 grams as decoction, pill,
powder

  C&C: internal injury and exhaustion, sinking of Yang Qi, kidney deficiency

  For: 9, 127, 320, 321

Plantago asiatica

Cheqiancao 车前草

  P: whole herb

    As above, but can cool lung
and stop cough as well.

  For: 56

Platycodon grandiflorum (balloon flower)

Jiegeng 桔梗

P: root
T&N: bitter and acrid; neither warm nor cool
M: lung, stomach
Act: to open lung Qi, to expel sputum and drain pus
A&F: 3–6 grams as decoction, pill, powder
C&C: Yin deficiency with chronic cough, Qi counterflow, coughing up blood
For: 5, 8, 44, 51, 57, 59, 99, 103, 106, 111, 117, 143, 174, 181, 203, 208, 213, 214, 217, 227, 252, 262, 267, 276, 305, 330, 333

Pleropus pselaphon (bat)

Wulingzhi 五灵脂

P: dried feces
T&N: bitter and sweet; warm
M: liver, spleen
Act: (raw) to mobilize blood and stop pain (dry-stir-fried) hemostasis
A&F: 4–9 grams as decoction, pill, powder
C&C: blood deficiency, excessive bleeding during labor; not to be used with *Panax ginseng*
For: 14, 54, 301

Polygala tenuifolia (milkwort)

Yuanzhi 远志

P: root
T&N: bitter and acrid; warm
M: heart, kidney
Act: to sedate, to improve mentation, to expel sputum, to release blockage

A&F: 3–9 grams as decoction, elixir, pill, powder
C&C: Fire in heart and kidney, waning Yin and waxing Yang
For: 45b,51, 117, 182, 267, 277, 304, 311, 324

Polygonatum odoratum (fragrant Solomon's seal)

Yuzhu 玉竹

P: root stalk
T&N: sweet; neither warm nor cool
M: lung, stomach
Act: to generate Yin, to moisten Dryness, to sedate, to quench thirst
A&F: 6–9 grams as decoction, gel, pill, powder
C&C: Phlegm, Dampness or Qi impedance in stomach
For: 83, 113

Polygonatum, other spp. (Solomon's seal)

Huangjing 黄精

P: root stalk
T&N: sweet; neither warm nor cool
M: spleen, lung, kidney
Act: to restore centrally and enrich Qi, to moisten heart and lung, to strengthen sinews and bones
A&F: 9–15 grams (fresh: 30–60 grams) as decoction, gel, pill, powder
C&C: central Cold, blocked-up Phlegm and Dampness
For: 49

Polygonum aviculare (knotweed)

Bianxu 萹蓄

P: whole herb

T&N: bitter; cold
  M: bladder
  Act: to induce urine flow, to cool
    Heat, to kill parasites
  A&F: 6–9 grams as decoction or
    pressed juice
  C&C: excessive use causes loss of
    Jing and Qi
  For: 9

Polygonum multiflorum
Heshouwu 何首乌
  P: tuberous root
  T&N: bitter, sweet, and astringent;
    slightly warm
  M: liver, kidney
  Act: to restore liver, to enrich
    kidney, to generate blood, to
    dispel Wind
  A&F: 9–15 grams as decoction, gel,
    elixir, pill, powder
  C&C: watery diarrhea, Dampness
    and Phlegm disease
  For: 53, 75

Polyporus mylittae
Leiwan 雷丸
  P: fungal body
  T&N: bitter; cold; slightly poison-
    ous
  M: stomach, large intestine
  Act: to dissolve accumulation, to
    kill parasites
  A&F: 6–9 grams as decoction, pill,
    powder
  C&C: deficiency Cold of spleen and
    stomach
  For: 48, 204, 241, 292

Polyporus umbellatus
Zhuling 猪苓
  P: dried fungal body

T&N: sweet; neither warm nor
    cool
  M: spleen, kidney, bladder
  Act: to induce urine flow and
    excrete Dampness
  A&F: 6–12 grams as decoction, pill,
    powder
  C&C: absence of water accumula-
    tion
  For: 42, 69, 232, 275, 332

Poncirus trifoliata (trifoliate
orange)
Zhike 枳壳
  P: almost ripe fruit
  T&N: bitter and acrid; cool
  M: lung, spleen, large intestine
  Act: to break Qi, to move sputum,
    to dissipate accumulation
  A&F: 3–9 grams as decoction, pill,
    powder (max. 60 grams)
  C&C: spleen and stomach defi-
    ciency, pregnancy
  For: 2, 8, 44, 75, 103, 146, 147,
    148, 150, 153, 158, 214, 250,
    299, 300, 301, 304

Poncirus trifoliata (trifoliate
orange)
Zhishi 枳实
  P: tiny fruit
  T&N: bitter; cold
  M: spleen, stomach
  Act: to break Qi, to disperse effu-
    sion, to eliminate Phlegm, to
    dissipate accumulation
  A&F: 3–6 grams as decoction, pill,
    powder
  C&C: spleen and stomach defi-
    ciency, pregnancy
  For: 19, 23, 29, 72, 111, 161, 203,
    207, 213, 221, 245, 253, 254,
    315

Poria cocos

Fuling 茯苓

P: fungal body
T&N: sweet; neither warm nor cool
M: heart, spleen, lung
Act: to mobilize Dampness and induce urine flow; to enrich spleen and mediate stomach; to calm and sedate
A&F: 9–15 grams as decoction, pill, powder
C&C: deficiency Cold, deficient and sunken Qi
For: 4, 7, 20, 28, 42, 46, 50, 51, 55, 59, 61, 66, 69, 75, 77, 109, 117, 118, 133, 138, 146, 159, 160, 162, 164, 190, 194, 197, 203, 208, 214, 221, 223, 232, 262, 263, 267, 272, 275, 284, 296, 297, 310, 311, 315, 319, 332, 333

Poria cocos

Chifuling 赤茯苓

P: pink part near outer skin
T&N: sweet; neither warm nor cool
M: heart, spleen, bladder
Act: to induce urine flow, to mobilize Dampness and Heat
A&F: 6–12 grams as decoction, pill, powder
C&C: deficiency Cold with spontaneous semen emission, Qi deficiency with sinking
For: 105

Poria cocos

Fulingpi 茯苓皮

P: skin of the fungus
T&N: sweet; neither warm nor cool

Act: to induce urine flow, to reduce swelling
A&F: 9–15 grams as decoction, pill, powder
For: 40, 96

Poria cocos

Fushen 茯神

P: fungal body, but grown around pine root
T&N: sweet; neither warm nor cool
M: heart, spleen
Act: to sedate and calm heart, to induce urine flow
A&F: 9–15 grams as decoction, pill, powder
For: 53, 117, 121, 182, 195, 198, 236, 277, 304, 324

Prunella vulgaris (self-heal)

Xiakucao 夏枯草

P: fruit
T&N: bitter and acrid; cold
M: liver, gallbladder
Act: to cool liver, to disperse accumulation
A&F: 6–15 grams as decoction, gel, pill, powder
C&C: deficiency of spleen and stomach, Qi deficiency

Prunus armeniaca (apricot)

Xingren 杏仁

P: ripe seed
T&N: bitter; warm; poisonous
M: lung, large intestine
Act: to dispel sputum and stop cough, to calm dyspnea, to lubricate intestines
A&F: 4–9 grams as decoction, pill, powder

C&C: cough due to Yin deficiency, watery diarrhea
For: 8, 15, 25, 32, 38, 83, 105, 107, 111, 125, 142, 180, 181, 218, 221, 222, 245, 246, 247, 249

Prunus japonica
Yuliren 郁李仁
P: seed
T&N: acrid, bitter, sweet; neither warm nor cool
M: spleen, large and small intestines
Act: to moisten Dryness, to lubricate intestines, to lower Qi, to induce urine flow
A&F: 3–9 grams as decoction, pill, powder
C&C: Yin deficiency and fluid deficiency, pregnancy
For: 38

Prunus mume
Wumei 乌梅
P: unripe fruit (sun-dried)
T&N: acid; warm
M: liver, spleen, lung, large intestine
Act: to generate fluid, to calm stomach, to kill parasites
A&F: 2–5 grams as decoction, pill, powder
C&C: strength evil diseases
For: 5, 191, 196, 241, 253, 339

Prunus mume
Wumei 乌梅
P: calyx
T&N: acid and astringent; neither warm nor cool
Act: to loosen liver and relieve blockage, to improve appetite and raise fluids

A&F: 3–6 grams as decoction
For: 2

Prunus persica, P. davidiana (peach)
Taoren 桃仁
P: nut kernel
T&N: bitter and sweet; neither warm nor cool
M: heart, liver, large intestine
Act: to disperse blood and resolve effusion and hematoma, to moisten Dryness and lubricate intestines
A&F: 4–9 grams as decoction, pill, powder
C&C: pregnancy
For: 26, 38, 88, 102, 110, 126, 144, 153, 183, 184, 202, 238, 250, 251, 257, 266, 301, 302, 308, 332

Pseudosciaena crocea, P. polyactis
Yunaoshi 鱼脑石
P: otoliths
T&N: salty; neither warm nor cool
Act: to dissolve stones, to treat dribbling, to suppress inflammation
A&F: 3–9 grams as powder
For: 110

Psoralea corylifolia
Buguzhi 补骨脂
P: fruit
T&N: acrid; warm
M: kidney
Act: to restore kidney and aid Yang
A&F: 4–9 grams as decoction, pill, powder
C&C: Yin deficiency with strong Fire
For: 68, 202

Pteria magaritifera, P. martensii
(oyster)

Zhenzhumu 珍珠母

P: shell
T&N: salty; cool
M: heart, liver
Act: to calm liver, to submerge
Yang, to stop convulsion, to
stop bleeding
A&F: 9–30 grams as decoction, pill,
powder
C&C: stomach Cold
For: 195

Pteria magaritifera, P. martensii
(oyster)

Zhenzhu 珍珠

P: pearl
T&N: sweet and salty; cold
M: heart, liver
Act: to tranquilize, to enrich Yin
and calm Wind, to cool Heat,
to improve vision, to generate flesh and eliminate poison
A&F: 0.6–0.9 gram as pill or powder; externally as ground
powder or eye drop
For: 58, 97, 104

Pueraria lobata (kudzu vine)

Gegen 葛根

P: bulbous root
T&N: sweet and acrid; neither
warm nor cool
M: spleen, stomach
Act: to raise Yang and disperse
exterior, to resolve rashes
and stop diarrhea, to sedate
and quench thirst
A&F: 4–9 grams as decoction or
pressed juice
For: 105, 176, 220, 224, 276, 290,
291

Pulsatilla chinensis (nodding
anemone)

Baitouweng 白头翁

P: root
T&N: bitter; cold
M: large intestine, liver, stomach
Act: to cool Heat and blood, to
eliminate poison
A&F: 9–15 grams (fresh: 50–100
grams) as decoction, pill,
powder
C&C: deficiency Cold with diarrhea
For: 94

Pumice

Haifushi 海浮石

T&N: salty; cold
M: lung, kidney
Act: to cool lung Fire, to dissolve
old sputum, to soften the
firm, to cure dribbling
A&F: 9–15 grams as decoction, pill,
powder
C&C: cough due to deficiency Cold
For: 141

Punica granatum (pomegranate)

Shiliupi 石榴皮

P: fruit rind
T&N: acid and astringent; warm;
mildly poisonous
M: large intestine, kidney
Act: to impede intestinal movement, to stop bleeding, to
drive out parasites
A&F: 2–5 grams as decoction or
powder

Pyrrosia lingua and other spp.

Shiwei 石苇

P: leaf
T&N: bitter and sweet; cool

M: lung, bladder
Act: to induce urine flow and clear
dribbling, to cool lung and
Heat
A&F: 4–9 grams as decoction or
powder
C&C: Yin deficiency, absence of
Heat and Dampness
For: 110

Quartz
Baishiying 白石英
T&N: sweet; warm
M: lung, kidney, heart
Act: to warm lung and kidney, to
calm heart and Shen, to facil-
itate urine
A&F: 9–15 grams as decoction, pill,
powder
For: 336

Quisqualis indica (Rangoon creeper)
Shijunzi 使君子
P: ripe fruit
T&N: sweet; warm
M: spleen, stomach
Act: to kill parasites, to disperse
accumulation, to strengthen
spleen
A&F: 9–15 grams as decoction, pill,
powder
C&C: not to be taken with hot tea
or food
For: 2, 48, 130

Raphanus sativus (radish)
Laifuzi 莱菔子
P: ripe seed
T&N: acrid and sweet; neither
warm nor cool
M: lung, stomach
Act: to lower Qi and control dys-

pnea, to aid digestion and
dissolve sputum
A&F: 4–9 grams as decoction, pill,
powder
C&C: Qi deficiency
For: 16, 20, 34, 138, 250

Realgar
Xionghuang 雄黄
T&N: acrid and bitter; warm; poi-
sonous
M: heart, liver, stomach
Act: to dry Dampness, to dispel
Wind, to kill parasites, to
relieve poison
A&F: 0.3–1.2 gram as pill, powder
C&C: Yin depletion, blood defi-
ciency, pregnancy
For: 58, 97, 101, 104, 230

Rehmannia glutinosa
Gandihuang 干地黄
P: root and stalk
T&N: sweet and bitter; cool
M: heart, liver, kidney
Act: nourishment of Yin and
generation of blood
A&F: 9–15 grams as decoction
(max. 200 grams); also as gel,
pill, powder
C&C: spleen deficiency with diarrhea, stomach deficiency with
anorexia, excessive sputum in
the chest
For: 1, 18, 21, 33, 51, 60, 98, 99,
103, 121, 122, 128, 137, 155,
158, 187, 219, 224, 226, 227,
229, 236, 267, 277, 285, 307,
312, 314, 320

Rehmannia glutinosa
Shudihuang 熟地黄

P: cooked root stalk
T&N: sweet; slightly warm
  M: liver, kidney
  Otherwise, as above.
  For: 4, 46, 64, 67, 75, 78, 99, 195,
    263, 268, 271, 272, 273, 283,
    304, 319

Rheum palmatum, R. officinale
(rhubarb)
Dahuang 大黄

P: root and stalk
T&N: bitter; cold
  M: stomach, large intestine, liver
  Act: catharsis of Heat poison, dis-
    sipation of effusion and accu-
    mulation
A&F: 3–12 grams as decoction, pill,
    powder
C&C: exterior not yet clear, blood
    deficiency and Qi weakness,
    deficiency Cold in spleen and
    stomach, puerperium
  For: 8, 9, 13, 14, 19, 23, 24, 26,
    27, 29, 48, 102, 106, 115,
    118, 126, 142, 146, 153, 172,
    183, 186, 200, 230, 245, 250,
    251, 255, 276, 289, 307, 308,
    309, 325, 327, 331

Rhinoceros horn
Xijiao 犀角

T&N: acid and salty; cold
  M: heart, liver
  Act: to cool Heat and blood, to
    control convulsion, to relieve
    poison
A&F: 1–2 grams as ground powder;
    1.5–6.0 grams as decoction,
    pill, powder
C&C: pregnancy; not to be used
    with *Polyporus*

For: 47, 58, 97, 101, 155, 195,
    218, 225, 227, 229, 261, 335

Rhododendron sinense
Yangzhizhu 羊踯躅

P: flower
T&N: acrid; warm; poisonous
  M: spleen
  Act: to dispel Wind, to eliminate
    Dampness, to reduce swel-
    ling
A&F: 1–3 grams as decoction or
    elixir
C&C: not to be used with flour,
    Gardenia
  For: 131

Rosa laevigata (Cherokee rose)
Jinyingzi 金樱子

P: fruit
T&N: acid and astringent; neither
    warm nor cool
  M: kidney, bladder, large intes-
    tine
  Act: to firm Jing and impede
    intestinal flow, to decrease
    urine
A&F: 4–9 grams as decoction, pill,
    powder, gel
C&C: strength Fire, Heat evil

Rubia cordifolia (India madder)
Qiancaogen 茜草根

P: root and root stalk
T&N: bitter; cold
  M: heart, liver
  Act: to mobilize blood and stop
    bleeding, to facilitate circula-
    tion, to stop cough and expel
    Phlegm
A&F: 6–9 grams as decoction, pill,
    powder

C&C: deficiency Cold in spleen and
stomach
For: 13, 123

Saiga tatarica (goat)
Lingyangjiao 羚羊角
P: horn
T&N: salty; cold
M: liver, heart
Act: to calm liver and Wind, to
cool Heat and control con-
vulsion, to eliminate poison
A&F: 1–1.5 grams as ground juice;
1.5–3.0 grams as decoction,
pill, powder
For: 56, 75, 198, 235, 236, 261

Salvia miltiorrhiza (sage)
Danshen 丹参
P: root
T&N: bitter; slightly warm
M: heart, liver
Act: to mobilize blood and dis-
perse effusion, to sedate, to
drain pus, to stop pain
A&F: 4–9 grams as decoction, pill,
powder; external: ointment
or solution
C&C: bleeding tendency; not to be
used with vinegar, *Veratrum
nigrum*
For: 51, 109, 139, 154, 219,
267

Sanguisorba officinalis (garden
burnet)
Diyu 地榆
P: root and root stalk
T&N: bitter and acid; cold
M: liver, large intestine
Act: to cool blood, to stop bleed-

ing, to cool fever and elimi-
nate poison
A&F: 6–9 grams as decoction, pill,
powder
C&C: deficiency Cold
For: 300

Santalum album (sandalwood)
Tanxiang 檀香
P: wood from branches
T&N: acrid; warm
M: spleen, stomach, lung
Act: to regulate Qi, to mediate
stomach
A&F: 3–6 grams as decoction, pill,
powder
C&C: Yin deficiency with strong
Fire
For: 14, 44, 75

Saposhnikovia divaricata
Fangfeng 防风
P: root
T&N: acrid and sweet; warm
M: bladder, lung, spleen
Act: to disperse exterior, to dispel
Wind, to overcome Damp-
ness
A&F: 4–9 grams as decoction, pill,
powder
C&C: blood deficiency, headache
not due to Wind
For: 32, 50, 75, 79, 105, 106, 163,
188, 203, 214, 239, 258, 285,
300, 304, 319, 327, 328, 330,
340, 341

Sargassum fusiforme, S. pallidum
(rockweed)
Haizao 海藻
P: whole herb

T&N: bitter and salty; cold
  M: lung, spleen, kidney
  Act: to soften the firm, to dissolve Phlegm, to induce urine flow, to purge Heat
  A&F: 4–9 grams as decoction, elixir, pill, powder
  C&C: deficiency Cold in spleen and stomach, especially if also Dampness

Sargentodoxa cureata
Hong(xue)teng 红（血）藤
  P: vine
T&N: bitter; cool
  Act: to cool Heat and relieve poison, to treat mammary abscess
  A&F: 9–30 grams as decoction
  For: 338

Saussurea lappa (costus)
Muxiang 木香
  P: root
T&N: acrid and bitter; warm
  M: lung, liver, spleen
  Act: to mobilize Qi and stop pain, to warm centrally and mediate stomach
  A&F: 1–5 grams as decoction, pill, powder, pressed juice
  C&C: Yin deficiency and fluid insufficiency
  For: 2, 14, 17, 28, 44, 52, 55, 75, 102, 115, 117, 130, 140, 158, 165, 166, 167, 171, 193, 202, 204, 253, 260, 261, 289, 292, 297, 313, 324, 335

Schisandra chinensis
Wuweizi 五味子
  P: fruit
T&N: acid; warm

M: lung, kidney
  Act: to collect lung, to nourish kidney, to generate fluids, to decrease perspiration, to impede semen flow
  A&F: 1–6 grams as decoction, pill, powder
  C&C: evil in exterior, Heat strength internally, at the onset of cough, at the onset of rashes; not to be used with *Polygonatum officinale*
  For: 4, 5, 21, 36, 68, 90, 127, 173, 197, 220, 243, 262, 267, 268, 272, 283, 311, 336

Schizonepeta tenuifolia
Jingjie 荆芥
  P: whole herb
T&N: acrid; warm
  M: lung, liver
  Act: to dissipate exterior, to expel Wind, to regulate blood; the ashes are used to stop bleeding
  A&F: 4–9 grams as decoction, pill, powder
  C&C: exterior deficient with spontaneous perspiration, Yin deficiency with headache
  For: 57, 106, 131, 203, 214, 299, 305, 330

Scolopendra subspinipes, S. mutilans (centipede)
Wugong 蜈蚣
  P: dried whole worm
T&N: acrid; warm; poisonous
  Act: to dispel Wind, to control convulsion, to attack poison, to disperse accumulation
  A&F: 1.5–5.0 grams as decoction, pill, powder
  C&C: pregnancy

Scrophularia ningpoensis (figwort)
Xuanshen 玄参
  P: root
T&N: bitter and salty; cool
  M: lung, kidney
  Act: to nourish Yin, to lower Fire,
    to sedate, to eliminate poison
A&F: 9–15 grams as decoction, pill,
  powder
C&C: Dampness in spleen and
  stomach, spleen deficiency
  with diarrhea
  For: 47, 51, 99, 155, 186, 189,
    219, 225, 227, 252, 261, 267,
    276, 307, 312, 329

Scutellaria baicalensis (baical skullcap)
Huangqin 黄芩
  P: root
T&N: bitter; cold
  M: heart, lung, gallbladder, large
  intestine
  Act: to purge Fire, to dissipate
  Dampness and Heat, to stop
  bleeding, to calm fetus
A&F: 3–9 grams as decoction, pill,
  powder
C&C: deficiency diseases; not to be
  used with leek, *Paeonia*
  For: 8, 23, 31, 50, 53, 56, 58, 62,
    85, 86, 89, 105, 106, 109,
    115, 119, 122, 125, 127, 144,
    146, 149, 155, 161, 172, 186,
    206, 217, 221, 227, 252, 273,
    275, 276, 278, 279, 280, 285,
    289, 291, 295, 300, 320, 325,
    330, 331, 342

Senecio nudicaulis (groundsel)
Zibeitiankui 紫背天葵
  P: whole herb

T&N: acrid; neither warm nor cool
  Act: to disperse effusion, to mobilize blood, to regulate
  menses
A&F: 9–15 grams as decoction or
  elixir
  For: 39

Sepiella maindroni (cuttlefish)
Sepia esculenta
Haipiaoxiao 海螵蛸
  P: endoskeleton
T&N: salty; slightly warm
  M: liver, kidney
  Act: to eliminate Dampness, to
  control acid, to stop bleeding
A&F: 4–9 grams as decoction, pill,
  powder; externally as powder
  or paste
C&C: Heat in blood; do not use
  with *Ampelopsis japonica*,
  Bletilla striata, *Aconitum*
  carmichaeli
  For: 123

Shenqu
Shenqu 神曲
  P: fermented product from mixture of flour or wheat husk
  with *Prunus armeniaca*, *Arte-*
  misia apiacea, etc.
T&N: sweet and acrid; warm
  M: spleen and stomach
  Act: to strengthen spleen and
  mediate stomach, to aid
  digestion, to regulate centrally
A&F: 6–12 grams as decoction, pill,
  powder
C&C: spleen Yin deficiency,
  stomach Fire; may induce
  miscarriage

For: 20, 44, 107, 130, 138, 146, 207, 220, 257

Silver (native)

Yinbo 银箔

T&N: strong cold
  M: heart, liver
  Act: to sedate, to control convulsion
  A&F: pill or powder; generally used as coating for pills
  For: 19

Snake molt

Shetui 蛇蜕

T&N: sweet and salty; neither warm nor cool; poisonous
  M: liver, (spleen)
  Act: to repel Wind, to control convulsion, to remove blindness, to reduce swelling, to kill parasites
  A&F: 1–3 grams as decoction or ground powder
  C&C: pregnancy

Sophora japonica (pagoda tree)

Huaihua 槐花
  P: flower, bud
T&N: bitter; cool
  M: liver, large intestine
  Act: to cool Heat and blood, to stop bleeding
  A&F: 6–15 grams as decoction, pill, powder
  C&C: deficiency Cold of spleen and stomach
  For: 299

Sophora japonica (pagoda tree)

Huaijiao 槐角
  P: fruit
T&N: bitter; cold

  M: liver, large intestine
  Act: to cool Heat, to lubricate liver, to cool blood, to stop bleeding
  A&F: 6–15 grams as decoction, pill, powder
  C&C: deficiency Cold of spleen and stomach, pregnancy
  For: 300

Sophora subprostrata

Shandougen 山豆根
  P: root
T&N: bitter; cold
  M: heart, lung, large intestine
  Act: to cool Fire, eliminate poison, suppress swelling; analgesia
  A&F: 9–15 grams as decoction or pressed juice
  C&C: deficiency Cold of spleen and stomach, with diarrhea

Sparganium stoloniferum,
S. simplex

Sanleng 三棱
  P: bulbous stalk
T&N: bitter and acrid; neither warm nor cool
  M: liver, spleen
  Act: to mobilize blood, to move Qi, to dissipate accumulation, to stop pain
  A&F: 4–9 grams as decoction, pill, powder
  C&C: Qi deficiency, weak constitution, blood depletion and amenorrhea, pregnancy
  For: 110, 292

Spatholobus suberectus

Jixueteng 鸡血藤
  P: stalk
T&N: bitter and sweet; warm

M: heart, spleen

Act: to mobilize blood, to soothe sinews

A&F: 9–15 grams (max. 30 grams) as decoction or elixir

For: 109, 286, 298

Spirodela polyrrhiza (duckweed)

Fuping 浮萍

P: whole herb

T&N: acrid; cold

M: lung

Act: to induce diaphoresis, to expel Wind, to move water, to cool Heat, to eliminate poison

A&F: 3–6 grams (fresh: 15–30 grams) as decoction, pressed juice, pill, powder

C&C: exterior Qi deficiency with spontaneous perspiration, blood deficiency, Qi deficiency

Stachys baicalensis (betony)

Shuisu 水苏

P: whole herb

T&N: acrid; mildly warm

M: intestines, stomach, lung

Act: to disperse Wind, to regulate Qi, to stop bleeding, to relieve inflammation

A&F: 9–15 grams (fresh: 15–30 grams) as decoction, pressed juice, pill, powder

C&C: dispersion of genuine Qi

For: 132

Stalactite

Zhongrushi 钟乳石

T&N: sweet; warm

Act: to aid Yang, to warm lung, to dissolve Phlegm

A&F: 9–15 grams as decoction, pill, powder

C&C: Yin deficiency with Heat

For: 336

Stellaria dichotoma

Yinchaihu 银柴胡

P: root

T&N: sweet and bitter; cool

M: liver, stomach

Act: to cool Heat and blood

A&F: 3–9 grams as decoction, pill, powder

C&C: exterior Wind and Cold, blood deficiency without fever

For: 228

Stellera chamaejasme

Langdu 狼毒

P: root

T&N: bitter and acrid; neither warm nor cool; poisonous

M: hand Greater Yin and Lesser Yin

Act: to expel water and Phlegm, to release accumulation, to kill parasites

A&F: 1–3 grams as decoction, pill, powder

C&C: weak constitution, pregnancy

Stemona japonica, S. sessilifolia, S. tuberosa

Baibu 百部

P: tuberous root

T&N: sweet and bitter; slightly warm

M: lung

Act: to warm and lubricate lung Qi, to stop cough, to kill parasites

A&F: 3-9 grams as decoction,
   elixir, pill, powder
C&C: cough due to Heat, fluid
   depletion
For: 57

Stephania tetrandra

Fangji 防己

P: root
T&N: bitter; cold
   M: bladder, spleen, kidney
   Act: induction of urine flow,
      catharsis of Dampness and
      Heat in the lower position
A&F: 4-9 grams as decoction, pill,
   powder
C&C: Yin deficiency but without
   Dampness or Heat
For: 32, 257

Sterculia scaphigera

Pangdahai 胖大海

P: seed
T&N: sweet; cool
   Act: to cool fever, to lubricate
      lung and throat, to relieve
      poison
A&F: 4-9 grams as decoction or tea

Stove soil

Fulonggan 伏龙肝

P: the soil from the floor in an
   earthen stove
T&N: acrid; warm
   M: spleen, stomach
   Act: to warm centrally and dry
      Dampness, to stop vomiting,
      to stop bleeding
A&F: 30-60 grams (wrapped in
   cloth) as decoction, or use
   the decoction to prepare
   other drugs

C&C: Yin deficiency, blood loss,
   vomiting due to Heat
For: 28, 273

Styrax benzoin, S. tonkinensis

Anxixiang 安息香

P: tree resin
T&N: acid and bitter; warm
   M: heart, liver, spleen
   Act: to open ostia, to repel con-
      tagion, to move Qi and blood
A&F: 0.3-0.5 gram as pill or
   powder; externally as burned
   scent
C&C: Yin deficiency with strong
   Fire
For: 101, 335

Sulfur

Liuhuang 硫磺

T&N: acid; warm; poisonous
   Act: to restore Fire and aid Yang,
      to heal ulcers
A&F: 1-5 grams as decoction;
   externally as ointment

Sus scrofus domesticus (pig)

Zhudanzhi 猪胆汁

P: bile
T&N: bitter; cold
   M: liver, gallbladder, lung, large
      intestine
   Act: to cool Heat, to moisten
      Dryness, to relieve poison
A&F: 3-6 grams as decoction or
   liquid mixture
For: 93b, 130

Syzygium aromaticum

Dingxiang 丁香

P: flower bud
T&N: acrid; warm

M: stomach, spleen, kidney
Act: central warming, kidney
warming and Yang aid, lowering of upstream Qi
A&F: 1–3 grams as decoction, pill,
powder
C&C: Heat diseases, Yin deficiency
with internal Heat
For: 3, 14, 75, 140, 261, 335

Tabanus bivittatus
Mengchong 虻虫
P: whole female insect
T&N: bitter; cool; poisonous
M: liver
Act: to release hematoma, effu-
sion, and accumulation, to
open meridians
A&F: 1–3 grams as decoction, 0.3–
0.6 gram as ground powder
C&C: pregnancy
For: 126

Talc
Huashi 滑石
T&N: sweet; cold
M: stomach, bladder
Act: to cool Heat, to excrete
Dampness, to facilitate open-
ings
A&F: 9–12 grams as decoction, pill,
powder
C&C: spleen deficiency, Qi weak-
ness, spontaneous emission,
Heat injuring fluids
For: 9, 15, 33, 43, 80, 86, 106,
110, 161, 218, 232, 261, 275,
296, 330

Taraxacum mongolicum (dandelion)
Pugongying 蒲公英
P: whole herb, including root

T&N: bitter and sweet; cold
M: liver, stomach
Act: to cool Heat and relieve poi-
son, to promote urine and
dissipate accumulation
A&F: 9–30 grams as decoction,
pressed juice, powder
For: 39, 145

Terminalia chebula
Hezi 诃子
P: fruit
T&N: bitter, acid, and astringent;
warm
M: lung, stomach, large intestine
Act: to pull in lung, to impede
intestinal flow, to lower Qi
A&F: 3–9 grams as decoction, pill,
powder
C&C: exterior not yet clear and
interior with Dampness and
Fire
For: 141, 193, 313

Tetrapanax papyriferus (rice-paper
tree)
Tongcao 通草
P: medullary covering of stalk
(pith)
T&N: sweet; cool
M: lung, stomach
Act: to purge lung, to induce
urine flow, to promote milk
flow
A&F: 2–5 grams as decoction, pill,
powder
C&C: Qi and Yin both deficient,
pregnancy
For: 15, 132, 264, 275, 296, 342

Toona sinensis
Chun(gen)baipi 椿 (根) 白皮
P: root skin

T&N: bitter and astringent; cool
M: hand and foot Bright Yang
Act: to eliminate fever, to dry
Dampness, to impede intestinal movement, to stop bleeding, to kill parasites
A&F: 6–12 grams as decoction, pill, powder
C&C: deficiency Cold of spleen and stomach
For: 281

Torreya grandis
Feizi 榧子

P: seed
T&N: sweet; neither warm nor cool
M: lung, stomach, large intestine
Act: to kill parasites, to dissipate accumulation, to moisten Dryness
A&F: 4–9 grams as decoction, pill, powder
C&C: not to be used with *Phaseolus*
For: 338

Trachelospermum jasminoides
(star jasmine)
Luoshiteng 络石藤

P: stalk, leaf
T&N: bitter; cool
M: liver, kidney
Act: to dispel Wind, to open meridians, to stop bleeding, to disperse effusion
A&F: 6–9 grams as decoction, elixir, powder
C&C: not to be used with ferrosic oxide, *Acorus*, *Fritillaria*
For: 121

Trachycarpus wagnerianus
(windmill palm)
Zongluhui 棕榈炭

P: (fired) ashes
T&N: bitter and astringent; neither warm nor cool
Act: to pull in and stop bleeding
A&F: 6–12 grams as decoction
C&C: bleeding with internal clots or hematoma
For: 13, 123

Tricosanthes kirilowii
Gualouzi 栝楼子

P: seed (kernel)
T&N: sweet; cold
M: lung, stomach, large intestine
Act: to lubricate lung, to dissolve sputum, to facilitate intestines
A&F: 9–12 grams as decoction, pill, powder
C&C: deficiency Cold in spleen and stomach; not to be used with *Zingiber*, *Achyranthes*, *Aconitum*
For: 34, 35, 81, 141, 148, 153, 186

Tricosanthes kirilowii
Gualoupi 栝楼皮

P: fruit peel
T&N: sweet; cold
M: lung, stomach
Act: to lubricate lung and dissolve sputum, to facilitate Qi and loosen chest
A&F: 9–12 grams as decoction or powder
C&C: spleen deficiency with Dampness and Phlegm; not to be used with *Zingiber*, *Achyranthes*, *Aconitum*
For: 81, 142, 148

Tricosanthes kirilowii
Tianhuafen 天花粉

P: root

T&N: sweet, bitter and acid; cool

M: lung, stomach

Act: to generate fluid and quench thirst, to lower Fire and moisten Dryness, to drain pus and suppress swelling

A&F: 9–12 grams as decoction, pill, powder; externally as ground powder or cream

C&C: deficiency Cold of spleen and stomach with diarrhea; not to be used with *Zingiber*, *Achyranthes*, *Aconitum*

For: 80, 81, 83, 113, 148, 155, 187, 188, 221, 251, 276

Triticum aestivum (wheat)

Fuxiaomai 浮小麦

P: dry grain that floats on water

T&N: sweet and salty; cool

Act: to treat Heat evil in the bones, to stop spontaneous perspiration and night sweats

A&F: 9–15 grams as decoction or ashes

Triticum aestivum (wheat)

Huaixiaomai 淮小麦

P: full grains

Act: to support heart, to sedate Otherwise as above.

For: 87, 114

Tussilago farfara (coltsfoot)

Kuandonghua 款冬花

P: flower bud

T&N: acrid; warm

M: lung

Act: to lubricate lung and lower Qi, to dissolve sputum and stop cough

A&F: 1–9 grams as decoction, gel, pill, powder

For: 5, 107, 156, 173, 336

Typha angustata, T. latifolia (cattail)

Puhuang 蒲黄

P: pollen

T&N: sweet and acrid; cool

M: liver, heart

Act: to cool blood, to stop bleeding, to mobilize blood, to disperse clot and hematoma

A&F: 4–9 grams as decoction, pill, powder

C&C: pregnancy

For: 14, 33, 54

Ulmus macrocarpa

Wuyi 芜荑

P: fruit kernel

T&N: bitter and acrid; warm

M: spleen, stomach

Act: to kill parasites, to dissolve accumulation

A&F: 4–9 grams as decoction, pill, powder

C&C: spleen and stomach deficiency

For: 48

Uncaria rhynchophylla, U. sinensis

Gouteng 钩藤

P: branch with thorn

T&N: sweet; cool

M: liver, heart

Act: to cool Heat and calm liver, to calm Wind and stop convulsion

A&F: 4–9 grams as decoction or powder

C&C: Qi deficiency

For: 53, 75, 121, 236

Urine

Renniao 人尿

P: midstream urine from a child under ten years of age

T&N: salty; cool

M: lung, liver, kidney

Act: to nourish Yin, to reduce Fire, to stop bleeding, to dissipate effusion

A&F: 1–2 cups fresh or mixed with other drug decoctions

C&C: deficiency Cold in spleen and stomach, diarrhea, Yang deficiency without Fire

For: 93b

Vaccaria segetalis (cowherd)

Wangbuliuxing 王不留行

P: seed

T&N: bitter; neither warm nor cool

M: liver, stomach

Act: to mobilize blood and improve circulation, to assist labor and milk flow

A&F: 4–9 grams as decoction, pill, powder

C&C: pregnancy, blood loss, uterine bleeding

For: 110

Venerupis philoppinarum

Geke 蛤壳

P: shell

T&N: salty; cold

Act: to cool lung and dissolve sputum

A&F: 9–15 grams as ground powder or decoction

For: 323

Veratrum nigrum (false hellebore)

Lilu 藜芦

P: root, root stalk

T&N: bitter and acrid; cold; poisonous

M: liver

Act: emesis of Wind and Phlegm, killing of parasites

A&F: 0.3–0.6 gram as ground powder or pill

C&C: weak constitution, Qi deficiency, pregnancy

Viola patrinii (violet)

Zihuadiding 紫花地丁

P: whole herb

T&N: bitter and acrid; cold

Act: to dispel Heat and relieve poison, to cool blood and reduce swelling

A&F: 9–15 grams (max. 60 grams) as decoction; externally as ground powder

For: 39

Zanthoxylum bungeanum (Japanese prickly ash)

Chuanjiao 川椒

Jiaomu 椒目

P: fruit (sometimes, seed)

T&N: acrid; warm; mildly poisonous

M: spleen, lung, kidney

Act: central warming, parasiticide, relief of fish poison

A&F: 1–5 grams as decoction, pill, powder; externally as cream or solution

C&C: Yin deficiency and strong Fire, pregnancy

For: 2, 22, 107, 191, 241, 253

Zingiber officinale (ginger)

Shengjiang 生姜

P: fresh root stalk

T&N: acrid; warm

M: lung, stomach, spleen

Act: to disperse the exterior, to expel Cold, to stop vomiting, to loosen sputum

A&F: 3–9 grams as decoction or pressed juice

C&C: Yin deficiency with internal Heat

For: 3, 23, 25, 30, 31, 32, 50, 54, 61, 68, 76, 88, 89, 105, 107, 108, 111, 117, 128, 149, 164, 175, 187, 190, 194, 205, 216, 238, 247, 256, 269, 270, 284, 290, 295, 297, 304, 317, 324, 334, 336, 339, 341

Zingiber officinale (ginger)

Ganjiang 干姜

P: dried root and stalk

T&N: acrid; hot

M: spleen, stomach, lung

Act: central warming, rescue of Yang, facilitation of circulation

A&F: 1–5 grams as decoction

C&C: Yin deficiency with internal Heat, Heat in blood with uncontrolled flow

For: 2, 22, 36, 55, 62, 70, 85, 93, 156, 162, 173, 178, 184, 191, 201, 206, 220, 233, 237, 253, 255, 271, 297

Zingiber officinale (ginger)

Shengjiangpi 生姜皮

P: skin of root stalk

T&N: acrid; neither warm nor cool

Act: to move water and reduce edema

A&F: 3–6 grams as decoction

For: 40, 96

Ziziphus jujuba (Chinese jujube)

Dazao 大枣

P: fruit

T&N: sweet; warm

M: spleen, stomach

Act: to restore spleen and mediate stomach, to nourish Qi and generate blood, to eliminate poison

A&F: 9–15 grams as decoction or pill

C&C: Dampness and Phlegm, accumulations, gingivitis, parasites

For: 12, 23, 25, 30, 31, 50, 51, 62, 65, 68, 76, 85, 87, 89, 108, 111, 128, 149, 160, 173, 175, 195, 208, 216, 220, 238, 244, 247, 267, 269, 270, 286, 290, 294, 295, 297, 317, 324, 336, 339, 341

Ziziphus jujuba (Chinese jujube)

(Suan)zaoren (酸) 枣仁

P: seed

T&N: sweet; neither warm nor cool

M: heart, spleen, liver, gallbladder

Act: to support liver, to calm heart, to sedate, to hold back perspiration

A&F: 6–15 grams as decoction, pill, powder

C&C: strength disease with blocked Fire, diarrhea

For: 198, 277, 283, 310, 311, 324

Ziziphus jujuba (Chinese jujube)

Zao(ren)he 枣 (仁) 核

P: seed kernel

T&N: bitter; neither warm nor cool

Act: to treat leg ulcers, to treat stomatitis

A&F: apply topically as ground powder

12

Formulas for Common Compound Drugs

All the basic prescriptions mentioned in the book are listed here by number. The numbering sequence is determined by the dictionary order of the Chinese names. Quantities and indications are omitted, but these can and should be derived by the principles described in the text and from the information given with each drug in chapter 11. New prescriptions not listed can be designed for specific purposes by the same principles. In general, the king is listed first. Where necessary, special instructions for preparation are given.

Ref: page (paragraph or case number) reference of application.

1. Yi guan jian 一贯煎
Yin-Generating Liver-Opening
  Prescription
Rehmannia glutinosa, fresh
Lycium chinense, ripe fruit
Adenophora vertillaria
Ophiopogon japonicus
Angelica sinensis
Melia toosendan
Ref: 157 (6), 164 (1), 295 (22),
  297 (24)

2. Yi hao qu chong tang 一号驱虫汤
First Decoction for Expelling
  Worms
Areca catechu, seed
Quisqualis indica
Melia azedarach
Prunus mume, unripe fruit
Saussurea lappa
Poncirus trifoliata
Zanthoxylum bungeanum, fruit
Asarum heterotropoides
Zingiber officinale, dry
Mirabilite
Ref: 157 (7)

3. Ding xiang shi di tang 丁香柿蒂汤
Clove and Persimmon Calyx
  Decoction

Syzygium aromaticum
Diospyros kaki
Codonopsis pilosula
Zingiber officinale, fresh
Ref: 157 (8), 167 (7)

4. Qi wei du qi wan 七味都气丸
Seven-Ingredient Qi-Restoring Pill

Rehmannia glutinosa, cooked
Cornus officinalis
Dioscorea opposita
Alisma plantago-aquatica
Poria cocos, body
Paeonia suffruticosa
Schisandra chinensis
Ref: 157 (6), 167 (5)

5. Jiu xian san 九仙散
Nine-Immortal Powder

Codonopsis pilosula
Equus asinus
Schisandra chinensis
Prunus mume, unripe fruit
Papaver somniferum, fried
Tussilago farfara, flower bud
Morus alba, fried root skin
Fritillaria
Platycodon grandiflorum
Ref: 158 (12)

6. Er xian tang 二仙汤
Two-Immortal Decoction

Curculigo orchioides
Epimedium grandiflorum
Morinda officinale
Angelica sinensis
Phellodendron amurense
Anemarrhena asphodeloides
Ref: 157 (6)

7. Er chen tang 二陈汤
Two-Cured Decoction

Citrus tangerina, fruit peel
Pinellia ternata, treated
Poria cocos, body
Glycyrrhiza uralensis, fried
Ref: 77, 157 (10), 164 (1),
    171 (9)

8. Ren shen xie fei tang 人参泻肺汤
Ginseng Lung-Clearing Decoction

Panax ginseng
Scutellaria baicalensis
Gardenia jasminoides
Poncirus trifoliata
Mentha haplocalyx
Glycyrrhiza uralensis
Forsythia suspensa, fruit
Prunus armeniaca, seed kernel
Morus alba, root skin
Rheum palmatum
Platycodon grandiflorum
Ref: 166 (4), 285 (1)

9. Ba zheng san 八正散
Eight-Right Powder for
    Rectification

Plantago asiatica, seed
Akebia quinata
Dianthus superbus
Polygonum aviculare
Talc
Glycyrrhiza uralensis
Gardenia jasminoides
Rheum palmatum
Juncus effusus
Ref: 157 (11), 168 (10), 169 (4), 304
    (39)

10. Ba zhen tang 八珍汤
Eight-Treasure Decoction
No. 66, plus No. 67
Ref: 157 (6)

11. Shi quan da bu tang 十全大补汤
Complete Restorative Decoction
No. 10, plus the following:
Astragalus, dried root
Cinnamomum, bark
Ref: 157 (6)

12. Shi zao tang 十枣汤
Ten-Jujube Decoction
Euphorbia pekinense
Daphne genkwa
Euphorbia kansui
Grind to powder. For each dose,
    use 1–3 grams and decoct with:
Ziziphus jujuba, fruit
Ref: 156 (3), 171 (11)

13. Shi hui san 十灰散
Ten-Ashes Powder
Cirsium japonicum, ash
Cephalanoplos segetum, ash
Trachycarpus wagnerianus, ash
Biota orientalis, leaf ash
Rheum palmatum, ash
Paeonia suffruticosa, ash
Gardenia jasminoides, ash
Rubia cordifolia, ash
Nelumbo nucifera, leaf ash
Imperata cylindrica, root ash
Equal amounts; grind and mix.
    Each dose 9 grams.
Ref: 157 (9)

14. Shi xiang zhi tong wan 十香止
痛丸
Ten-Fragrant Analgesic Pill
Cyperus rotundus
Corydalis yanhusuo
Lindera strychnifolia
Citrus medica
Magnolia officinalis, bark

Typha angustata, fresh pollen
Pleropus pselaphon
Boswellia carterii
Santalum album
Saussurea lappa
Dalbergia odorifera
Aquilaria agallocha
Lysimachia foenum-graceum
Eragrostis tenella
Amomum villosum
Syzygium aromaticum
Rheum palmatum, cooked
Alpinia officinarum
Ref: 167 (8), 294 (19)

15. San ren tang 三仁汤
Three-Nut Decoction
Prunus armeniaca
Coix lachryma-jobi
Amomum cardamomum
Magnolia officinalis, bark
Pinellia ternata
Phyllostachys nigra, leaf
Talc
Tetrapanax papyriferus
Ref: 156 (2), 159 (4), 170 (4), 291 (13)

16. San zi tang 三子汤
Three-Seed Decoction
Perilla frutescens, fruit
Brassica alba
Raphanus sativus
Ref: 157 (10)

17. San sheng yin 三生饮
Three-Fresh Drink
Arisaema consanguineum
Aconitum carmichaeli, root
Aconitum carmichaeli, secondary root
Saussurea lappa
Ref: 168 (1)

18. San jia fu mai tang 三甲复脉汤
Three-Skin Pulse-Restoring
　Decoction
Cannabis sativa
Glycyrrhiza urelensis
Rehmannia glutinosa fresh
Ophiopogon japonicus
Equus asinus
Paeonia lactiflora
Ostrea rivularis
Amyda sinensis
Chinemys reevesii
Ref: 169 (3)

19. Da cheng qi tang 大承气汤
Major Qi-Facilitating Decoction
Mirabilite
Magnolia officinalis, bark
Poncirus trifoliata, tiny fruit
Rheum palmatum
Ref: 156 (3), 159 (4), 161 (8), 163
　(11, 12), 170 (6), 289 (8)

20. Da an wan 大安丸
Major Settling Pill
Shenqu
Crataegus pinnatifida
Poria cocos, body
Citrus tangerina, fruit peel
Atractylodes macrocephala
Raphanus sativus
Forsythia suspensa, fruit
Ref: 165 (3), 171 (10)

21. Da ding feng zhu 大定风珠
Major Wind-Calming Pill
Paeonia lactiflora, white
Equus asinus
Chinemys reevesii
Rehmannia glutinosa
Cannabis sativa

Schisandra chinensis
Ostrea rivularis
Ophiopogon japonicus
Amyda sinensis
Artemisia argyi, fried
Gallus gallus, egg yolk
Ref: 164 (1), 168 (1), 296 (22)

22. Da jian zhong tang 大建中汤
Major Central-Supporting
　Decoction
Zanthoxylum bungeanum, fruit
Zingiber officinale, dry
Codonopsis pilosula
Make decoction, discard residue,
　then add
Grain syrup
Ref: 157 (5), 288 (5)

23. Da chai hu tang 大柴胡汤
Major Bupleurum Decoction
Bupleurum chinense
Scutellaria baicalensis
Pinellia ternata, treated
Zingiber officinale, fresh
Ziziphus jujuba, fruit
Rheum palmatum
Poncirus trifoliata, tiny fruit
Paeonia lactiflora, white
Ref: 157 (4), 162 (9)

24. Da xian xiong tang 大陷胸汤
Major Chest (Blockage)-Relieving
　Decoction
Rheum palmatum
Mirabilite
Euphorbia kansui
Ref: 161 (7)

25. Da qing long tang 大青龙汤
Major Green Dragon Decoction

Ephedra sinica
Cinnamomum cassia, branch
Prunus armeniaca
Glycyrrhiza uralensis
Zingiber officinale, fresh
Ziziphus jujuba, fruit
Gypsum
Ref: 160 (7), 171 (11)

26. Da huang mu dan pi tang 大黄牡丹皮汤

Rheum-Paeonia Decoction

Rheum palmatum
Paeonia suffruticosa
Prunus persica
Benincasa hispida, seed
Mirabilite
Ref: 157 (7), 168 (9)

27. Da huang huang lian xie xin tang 大黄黄连泻心汤

Rheum-Coptis Heart-Clearing Decoction

Rheum palmatum
Coptis chinensis
Ref: 161 (7)

28. Xiao er li pi tang 小儿理脾汤

(Infant) Spleen-Regulating Decoction

Alpinia katsumadai
Euryale ferox
Saussurea lappa
Poria cocos, body
Stove soil
Halloysite
Nelumbo nucifera, seed
Ref: 158 (12)

29. Xiao cheng qi tang 小承气汤

Minor Qi-Facilitating Decoction

Rheum palmatum
Magnolia officinale, bark
Poncirus trifoliata, tiny fruit
Ref: 156 (3), 161 (8), 163 (12)

30. Xiao jian zhong tang 小建中汤

Minor Central-Supporting Decoction

Paeonia lactiflora, white
Cinnamomum cassia, branch
Glycyrrhiza uralensis, fried
Zingiber officinale, fresh
Ziziphus jujuba, fruit
Grain syrup
Ref: 157 (5), 165 (3), 297 (25)

31. Xiao chai hu tang 小柴胡汤

Minor *Bupleurum* Decoction

Bupleurum chinense
Scutellaria baicalensis
Pinellia ternata, treated
Glycyrrhiza uralensis, fried
Zingiber officinale, fresh
Ziziphus jujuba, fruit
Codonopsis pilosula
Ref: 157 (4), 162 (9)

32. Xiao xu ming tang 小续命汤

Minor Life-Extending Decoction

Ephedra sinica
Stephania tetrandra
Panax ginseng
Astragalus, dried root
Cinnamomum cassia, branch heart
Glycyrrhiza uralensis
Paeonia lactiflora
Ligustinum wallichii
Prunus armeniaca
Aconitum carmichaeli
Saposhnikovia divaricata
Zingiber officinale, fresh
Ref: 168 (1)

33. Xiao ji yin zi 小蓟饮子
Cephalanoplos Drink

Rehmannia glutinosa, fresh
Cephalanoplos segetum
Talc
Akebia quinata
Typha angustata, fried pollen
Nelumbo nucifera, root node
Phyllostachys nigra, leaf
Angelica sinensis
Gardenia jasminoides
Glycyrrhiza uralensis
Ref: 157 (9), 158 (2)

34. Xiao luo zao wan 小萝皂丸
Minor *Gleditsia* Pill

Raphanus sativus
Gleditsia sinensis, thorn
Trichosanthes kirilowii, seed
Arisaema consanguineum
Mactra quandrangularis
Ref: 166 (4), 300 (31)

35. Xiao xian xiong tang 小陷胸汤
Minor Chest (Blockage)-Relieving
   Decoction

Coptis chinensis
Pinellia ternata
Trichosanthes kirilowii, seed
Ref: 161 (7)

36. Xiao qing long tang 小青龙汤
Minor Green Dragon Decoction

Ephedra sinica
Cinnamomum cassia, branch
Asarum heterotropoides
Zingiber officinale, dry
Pinellia ternata, treated
Schisandra chinensis
Paeonia lactiflora, white
Glycyrrhiza uralensis

Ref: 157 (10), 160 (7), 166 (4), 171
   (9, 11), 300 (31)

37. Dan zhi xiao yao san 丹栀逍遥散
Paeonia-Gardenia Care-free Powder

No. 190, plus:
Paeonia suffruticosa
Gardenia jasminoides
Ref: 157 (4)

38. Wu ren wan 五仁丸
Five-Seed Pill

Prunus persica, seed
Prunus armeniaca, seed
Biota orientalis, seed
Pinus koraiensis, seed
Prunus japonica, seed
Citrus tangerina, fruit peel
Ref: 168 (9)

39. Wu wei xiao du yin 五味消毒饮
Five-Ingredient Poison-Eliminating
   Drink

Lonicera japonica, flower
Taraxacum mongolicum
Viola patrinii
Chrysanthemum
Senecio nudicaulis
Ref: 157 (7)

40. Wu pi yin 五皮饮
Five-Skin Drink

Citrus tangerina, fruit peel
Poria cocos, fungal body skin
Zingiber officinale, fresh skin
Morus alba, root skin
Areca catechu, fruit peel
Ref: 157 (11)

41. Wu ji san 五积散
Five-Accumulation Powder

Nos. 7, 76, 175, and 249 combined
Ref: 77

42. Wu ling san 五苓散
Five-Ingredient Powder with Poria
Poria cocos, body
Polyporus umbellatus
Atractylodes macrocephala
Alisma plantago-aquatica
Cinnamomum cassia, branch
Ref: 157 (11), 160 (7), 165 (3), 169
  (4), 304 (38)

43. Liu yi san 六一散
Six-to-One Powder
Talc, 6 parts
Glycyrrhiza uralensis, 1 part
Ref: 157 (11), 165 (3)

44. Liu he ding zhong tang 六和定
中汤
Six Mediating-Settling Decoction
Agastache rugosa
Perilla frutescens, leaf
Elsholtzia splendens
Dolichos lablab
Saussurea lappa
Santalum album
Paeonia lactiflora, red
Poncirus trifoliata
Platycodon grandiflorum
Chaenomeles lagenaria
Citrus tangerina, fruit peel
Crataegus pinnatifida
Magnolia officinalis, bark
Glycyrrhiza uralensis
Hordeum vulgare
Oryza sativa, sprouting grain
Shenqu
Ref: 170 (4)

45. Liu jun zi tang 六君子汤
Six-Noble Decoction
No. 66, plus:
Citrus tangerina, fruit peel
Pinellia ternata
Ref: 157 (6), 165 (3), 297 (25)

45b. Jia wei liu jun zi tang 加味六君
子汤
Six-Noble Plus Decoction
No. 45, plus:
Acorus gramineus
Polygala tenuifolia
Ref: 165 (2)

46. Liu wei di huang wan 六味地黄丸
Six-Ingredient Pill with *Rehmannia*
Rehmannia glutinosa, cooked
Cornus officinalis
Dioscorea opposita
Alisma plantago-aquatica
Poria cocos, body
Paeonia suffruticosa
Ref: 157 (6), 165 (2), 166 (5)

47. Hua ban tang 化斑汤
Rash-Dissolving Decoction
Gypsum
Anemarrhena asphodeloides
Glycyrrhiza uralensis
Oryza sativa
Rhinoceros horn
Scrophularia ningpoensis
Ref: 160 (6)

48. Hua chong wan 化虫丸
Worm-Eliminating Pill
Carpesium abratanoides
Areca catechu, seed
Melia azedarach, root skin

Polyporus mylittae
Quisqualis indica
Ulmus macrocarpa
Pharbitis nil, black
Rheum palmatum
Use 120 grams each. Add
Mirabilite 240 grams
Make into pills. Take 3–6 grams at
bedtime.

Ref: 157 (7)

49. Sheng ya tang 升压汤

Pressure-Relieving Decoction

Panax ginseng, or
Codonopsis pilosula
Polygonatum spp.
Glycyrrhiza uralensis, fried

Ref: 157 (5)

50. Sheng yang yi wei tang 升阳益
胃汤

Yang-Raising Stomach-Benefiting
Decoction

Panax ginseng
Atractylodes macrocephala
Scutellaria baicalensis
Coptis chinensis
Pinellia ternata
Glycyrrhiza uralensis
Citrus tangerina, fruit peel
Poria cocos, body
Alisma plantago-aquatica
Saposhnikovia divaricata
Angelica sylvestris
Angelica pubescens
Bupleurum chinense
Paeonia lactiflora, white
Zingiber officinale, fresh
Ziziphus jujuba, fruit

Ref: 165 (3)

51. Tian wang bu xin dan 天王补
心丹

Divine Ruler Heart-Restoring Pill

Panax ginseng
Poria cocos, body
Scrophularia ningpoensis
Platycodon grandiflorum
Polygala tenuifolia
Angelica sinensis
Melaphis chinensis
Asparagus chochinchinensis
Ophiopogon japonicus
Salvia miltiorrhiza
Ziziphus jujuba, fruit
Rehmannia glutinosa, fresh
Biota orientalis, seed

Ref: 164 (2)

52. Tian tai wu yao san 天台乌药散

Lindera Hernia Powder

Lindera strychnifolia
Saussurea lappa
Foeniculum vulgare
Alpinia officinarum
Citrus tangerina, unripe peel
Areca catechu, seed
Melia toosendan
Croton tiglium

Ref: 157 (8)

53. Tian ma gou teng yin 天麻钩
藤饮

Gastrodia-Uncaria Drink

Gastrodia elata
Uncaria rhynchophylla
Haliotis diversicolor
Loranthus yadoriki
Eucommia ulmoides
Gardenia jasminoides
Scutellaria baicalensis
Cyathula officinalis, Szechuan

Leonurus heterophyllus
Poria cocos, grown on pine root
Polygonum multiflorum
Ref: 158 (14)

54. Shao fu zhu yu tang 少腹逐瘀汤

Lower Abdomen Blood-Mobilizing
  Decoction

Angelica sinensis
Ligustinum wallichii
Paeonia lactiflora, red
Typha angustata, pollen
Pleropus pselaphon, fried
Commiphora myrrha
Corydalis yanhusuo
Foeniculum vulgare
Zingiber officinale, toasted
Cinnamomum cassia
Ref: 157 (9)

55. Mu xiang shun qi tang 木香顺气汤

Saussurea Qi-Facilitating
  Decoction

Saussurea lappa
Alpinia katsumadai
Alpinia oxyphylla
Atractylodes, root stalk
Magnolia officinalis, bark
Citrus tangerina, unripe peel
Pinellia ternata
Evodia rutaecarpa
Zingiber officinale, dry
Poria cocos, body
Alisma plantago-aquatica
Cimicifuga foetida
Bupleurum chinense
Angelica sinensis
Ref: 163 (1b, 1d), 295 (21), 298 (26)

56. Mu tong san 木通散

Akebia Powder

Akebia quinata
Areca catechu, seed
Saiga tatarica
Paeonia lactiflora, red
Scutellaria baicalensis
Angelica sinensis
Plantago asiatica, seed
Glycyrrhiza uralensis
Ref: 167 (8)

57. Zhi sou san 止嗽散

Cough-Suppressing Powder

Schizonepeta tenuifolia
Aster tartaricus
Stemona japonica
Cynanchum stauntoni
Citrus tangerina, fruit peel
Platycodon grandiflorum
Glycyrrhiza uralensis
Ref: 157 (10)

58. Niu huang wan 牛黄丸

Bovine Gallstone Pill

Bos taurus, gallstone
Curcuma longa
Rhinoceros
Scutellaria baicalensis
Coptis chinensis
Gardenia jasminoides
Realgar
Cinnabar
Dryobalanops aromatica
Moschus moschiferus
Pteria margaritifera, pearl
Ref: 170 (6), 299 (29)

59. Jia wei wu wei yi gong san 加味五味异功散

Modified Five-Ingredient
  Unusually Effective Powder

Panax ginseng
Atractylodes macrocephala

Poria cocos, body
Glycyrrhiza uralensis
Citrus tangerina, fruit peel
Platycodon grandiflorum
Ref: 165 (3)

60. Jia jian fu mai tang 加减复脉汤
Modified Pulse-Restoring
  Decoction
Rehmannia glutinosa
Paeonia lactiflora, white
Ophiopogon japonicus
Cannabis sativa
Equus asinus
Glycyrrhiza uralensis, fried
Ref: 168 (1)

61. Ban xia hou po tang 半夏厚朴汤
Pinellia-Magnolia Decoction
Pinellia ternata
Magnolia officinalis, bark
Poria cocos, body
Perilla frutescens, leaf
Zingiber officinale, fresh
Ref: 157 (8)

62. Ban xia xie xin tang 半夏泻心汤
Pinellia Heart-Clearing Decoction
Pinellia ternata
Scutellaria baicalensis
Zingiber officinale, dry
Coptis chinensis
Codonopsis pilosula
Glycyrrhiza uralensis, fried
Ziziphus jujuba, fruit
Ref: 157 (4), 161 (7)

63. Ban xia bai zhu tian ma tang
  半夏白术天麻汤
Pinellia-Atractylodes-Gastrodia
  Decoction

No. 7, plus:
Atractylodes macrocephala
Gastrodia elata
Ref: 157 (10), 171 (9)

64. You gui yin 右归饮
Right Return Drink (Kidney Yang
  Deficiency)
Aconitum carmichaeli
Cinnamomum cassia
Rehmannia glutinosa, cooked
Dioscorea opposita
Cornus officinalis
Lycium chinense, ripe fruit
Eucommia ulmoides
Glycyrrhiza uralensis, fried
Ref: 157 (6), 169 (2)

65. Si qi tang 四七汤
Four-Seven Decoction
No. 61, plus:
Ziziphus jujuba, fruit
Ref: 157 (8), 171 (8)

66. Si jun zi tang 四君子汤
Four-Noble Decoction
Codonopsis pilosula, or
Panax ginseng
Poria cocos, body
Atractylodes macrocephala
Glycyrrhiza uralensis, fried
Ref: 157 (6), 158 (1), 164 (2), 166 (3)

67. Si wu tang 四物汤
Four-Ingredient Decoction
Rehmannia glutinosa, cooked
Paeonia lactiflora, white
Angelica sinensis
Ligustinum wallichii
Ref: 157 (6), 158 (2), 163 (1), 295
  (21), 298 (26, 27)

68. Si shen wan 四神丸

Four-Deity Pill

Psoralea corylifolia
Schisandra chinensis
Myristica fragrans, roasted
Evodia rutaecarpa
Zingiber officinale, fresh
Ziziphus jujuba, fruit
Ref: 158 (12), 166 (3), 167 (5), 303
   (36, 37)

69. Si ling san 四苓散

Four-Ingredient Powder with
   Poria

Poria cocos, body
Polyporus umbellatus
Atractylodes macrocephala
Alisma plantago-aquatica
Ref: 157 (11)

70. Si ni tang 四逆汤

Four-Contrary Decoction

Aconitum carmicheli, treated
Zingiber officinale, dry
Glycyrrhiza uralensis, fried
Ref: 157 (5), 162 (11), 163 (12), 164
   (2), 169 (2), 293 (16)

71. Si ni jia ren shen tang
   四逆加人参汤

Four-Contrary plus Ginseng
   Decoction

No. 70, plus:
Panax ginseng
Ref: 157 (5)

72. Si ni san 四逆散

Four-Contrary Powder

Bupleurum chinense
Paeonia lactiflora, white

Poncirus trifoliata, tiny fruit
Glycyrrhiza uralensis
Ref: 157 (8)

73. Zuo jin wan 左金丸

"Left Gold Pill" (Liver-Spleen
   Mediating Pill)

Coptis chinensis, 4 parts
Evodia rutaecarpa, 1 part
Make into pills. 1–3 grams two or
   three times daily.
Ref: 157 (4), 164 (1)

74. Ping ke he ji 平咳合剂

Cough-Suppressing
Soothing Preparation

Citrus tangerina, fruit peel
Pinellia ternata, treated
Atractylodes spp., root stalk
Magnolia officinalis, bark
Ref: 157 (10)

75. Ping gan shu luo wan 平肝舒
   络丸

Liver-Settling Circulation-
   Regulating Pill

This formula contains 43 ingredients:
Panax ginseng
Rehmannia glutinosa, cooked
Boswellia carterii
Commiphora myrrha
Citrus tangerina, fruit peel
Cyperus rotundus
Magnolia officinalis, bark
Corydalis yanhusuo
Poria cocos, body
Santalum album
Chinemys reevesii
Angelica sylvestris
Saposhnikovia divaricata
Alpinia katsumadai
Poncirus trifoliata

Amomum villosum
Agastache rugosa
Saussurea lappa
Lindera strychnifolia
Coptis chinensis
Atractylodes macrocephala
Polygonum multiflorum
Bletilla striata
Clematis chinensis
Citrus medica L. v. *sarcodactylis*
Chaenomeles lagenaria
Uncaria rhynchophylla
Bombyx mori, worm
Bupleurum chinense
Asarum heterotropoides
Angelica dahurica
Loranthus yadoriki
Achyranthes bidentata
Aquilaria agallocha
Citrus tangerina, unripe peel
Bambusa textilis
Cinnamomum cassia, bark
Ligustinum wallichii
Syzygium aromaticum
Arisaema consanguineum, treated
   with bovine bile
Dryobalanops aromatica
Cinnabar
Saiga tatarica
Ref: 164 (1)

76. Ping wei san 平胃散
Stomach-Settling Powder
Atractylodes, root stalk
Magnolia officinalis, bark
Citrus tangerina, fruit peel
Glycyrrhiza uralensis
Zingiber officinale, fresh
Ziziphus jujuba, fruit
Ref: 77, 157 (11), 165 (3), 169 (4)

77. Zhen qi san 正气散
Qi-Rectifying Powder

Agastache rugosa
Citrus tangerina, fruit peel
Poria cocos, body
Magnolia officinalis, bark
Areca catechu, fruit peel
Oryza sativa, sprouting grain
Atractylodes spp., root stalk
Ref: 169 (4)

78. Yu nu jian 玉女煎
Maiden's Fry
Gypsum
Rehmannia glutinosa, cooked
Ophiopogon japonicus
Anemarrhena asphodeloides
Achyranthes bidentata
Ref: 156 (2), 160 (6)

79. Yu ping feng san 玉屏风散
Jade Windscreen Powder
Astragalus spp., dried root
Atractylodes macrocephala
Saposhnikovia divaricata
Ref: 158 (12)

80. Yu lu san 玉露散
Jade Dew Powder
Gypsum
Talc
Mirabilite
Trichosanthes kirilowii, root
Glycyrrhiza uralensis
Ref: 169 (3)

81. Gua lou xie bai bai jiu tang 瓜楼
   薤白白酒汤
Tricosanthes-Allium Wine Decoction
Trichosanthes kirilowii, whole herb
Allium chinense
Decoct in white wine.
Ref: 157 (8), 165 (2)

82. Gua lou xie bai ban xia tang 瓜楼
薤白半夏汤

Tricosanthes-Allium-Pinellia
Decoction

No. 81, plus:
Pinellia ternata

Ref: 157 (8)

83. Gan han qing shang fa 甘寒清
上法

Sweet-Cold Upper Clearing
Prescription

Adenophoria tetraphylla
Ophiopogon japonicus
Polygonatum odoratum
Prunus armeniaca
Lilium brownii
Dendrobium nobile
Trichosanthes kirilowii, root
Gardenia jasminoides

Ref: 166 (4), 301 (32)

84. Gan cao tang 甘草汤

Glycyrrhiza Decoction

Glycyrrhiza uralensis, whole herb

Ref: 163 (11)

85. Gan cao xie xin tang 甘草泻心汤

Glycyrrhiza Heart-Clearing
Decoction

Pinellia ternata
Scutellaria baicalensis
Zingiber officinale, dry
Coptis chinensis
Glycyrrhiza uralensis, fried
Ziziphus jujuba, fruit

Ref: 157 (4), 161 (7)

86. Gan lu xiao du dan 甘露消毒丹

Sweet Dew Poison-Eliminating Pill

Agastache rugosa

Acorus gramineus
Myristica fragrans
Artemisia capillaris
Talc
Akebia quinata
Scutellaria baicalensis
Forsythia suspensa, fruit
Fritillaria spp.
Belamcanda chinensis
Mentha haplocalyx

Ref: 170 (4)

87. Gan mai da zao tang 甘麦大枣汤

Licorice, Wheat, and Jujube
Decoction

Glycyrrhiza uralensis, fried
Triticum aestivum
Ziziphus jujuba, fruit

Ref: 158 (13)

88. Sheng hua tang 生化汤

Generation and Transformation
Decoction

Angelica sinensis
Ligustinum wallichii
Prunus persica
Zingiber officinale, toasted
Glycyrrhiza uralensis, fried

Ref: 157 (9)

89. Sheng jiang xie xin tang 生姜泻
心汤

Fresh Ginger Heart-Clearing
Decoction

Pinellia ternata, treated
Scutellaria baicalensis
Zingiber officinale, fresh
Coptis chinensis
Codonopsis pilosula
Glycyrrhiza uralensis, fried
Ziziphus jujuba, fruit

Ref: 157 (3), 161 (7)

90. Sheng mai san 生脉散
Pulse-Generating Powder
Panax ginseng
Ophiopogon japonicus
Schisandra chinensis
Ref: 157 (6), 166 (4), 169 (3)

91. Bai hu tang 白虎汤
White Tiger Decoction
Gypsum, fresh
Anemarrhena asphodeloides
Glycyrrhiza uralensis
Oryza sativa
Ref: 156 (2), 159 (4), 160 (5), 161
   (8), 163 (12), 169 (3)

92. Bai hu jia ren shen tang 白虎加
   人参汤
White Tiger Plus Ginseng Decoction
No. 91, plus:
Panax ginseng
Ref: 156 (2), 289 (8)

93. Bai tong tang 白通汤
Allium Unblocking Decoction
Allium fistulosum
Zingiber officinale, dry
Aconitum carmichaeli
Ref: 169 (2)

93b. *Niao dan bai tong tang* 尿胆白
   通汤
Urine-Bile Unblocking Decoction
No. 93, plus:
Human urine
Sus scrofa (pig) bile
Ref: 169 (2)

94. Bai tou weng tang 白头翁汤
Pulsatilla Decoction

Pulsatilla chinensis
Fraxinus bungeana
Phellodendron amurense
Coptis chinensis
Ref: 156 (2), 163 (12), 168 (9), 171
   (7), 302 (34)

95. Jiao tai wan 交泰丸
Mutually Sedating Pill
Coptis chinensis
Cinnamomum cassia, bark
Ref: 165 (2)

96. Quan sheng bai zhu san 全生白
   朮散
All Fresh (Uncooked) *Atractylodes*
   Powder
Citrus tangerina, fruit peel
Poria cocos, skin
Zingiber officinale, fresh skin
Areca catechu, fruit peel
Atractylodes macrocephala

97. An gong niu huang wan 安宫牛
   黄丸
Gallstone Organ-Settling Pill
Bos taurus, gallstone
Rhinoceros horn
Pteria margaritiflora, pearl
Moschus moschiferus
Gardenia jasminoides
Coptis chinensis
Curcuma longa, root
Realgar
Dryobalanops aromatica, camphor
Make into pills. Take 0.6–1.2 grams
   as needed.
Ref: 159 (5), 169 (3)

98. Zhu sha an shen wan 朱砂安神丸
Cinnabar Sedating Pill
Cinnabar

Coptis chinensis
Rehmannia glutinosa, fresh
Angelica sinensis
Glycyrrhiza uralensis, fried
Grind and make into pills. Take 3–9
  grams at bedtime.
Ref: 158 (13), 164 (2), 294 (18)

99. Bai he gu jin tang 百合固金汤

Lilium Lung-Preserving Decoction

Rehmannia glutinosa, fresh
Rehmannia glutinosa, cooked
Ophiopogon japonicus
Fritillaria spp.
Lilium brownii
Angelica sinensis
Paeonia lactiflora, white
Scrophularia ningpoensis
Platycodon grandiflorum
Glycyrrhiza uralensis

Ref: 166 (4)

100. Zhu ye dou gao tang 竹叶豆
  膏汤

Phyllostachys-Gypsum Decoction

Phyllostachys nigra, leaf
Gypsum
Ophiopogon japonicus
Pinellia ternata
Panax ginseng, or
  Codonopsis pilosula
Oryza sativa
Glycyrrhiza uralensis

Ref: 156 (2)

101. Zhi bao dan 至宝丹

Greatest Treasure Special Precious
  Pill

Rhinoceros horn
Eretmochelys imbricata
Amber
Cinnabar

Realgar
Dryobalanops aromatica, treated
  parts
Moschus moschiferus
Bos taurus, gallstone
Styrax benzoin
Native gold
Native silver

Ref: 159 (5), 168 (9), 170 (6),
  171 (7)

102. Zhou che wan 舟车丸

Vessel and Vehicle (Diuretic) Pill

Pharbitis nil, black
Euphorbia kansui, roasted
Daphne genkwa, vinegar treated
Euphorbia pekinensis, vinegar
  treated
Rheum palmatum
Citrus tangerina, unripe peel
Citrus tangerina, ripe peel
Saussurea lappa
Areca catechu, seed
6 grams on arising in the morning
  before food.

Ref: 156 (3)

103. Xue fu zhu yu tang 血府逐
  瘀汤

Contusion-Clearing Decoction

Angelica sinensis
Paeonia lactiflora, red
Rehmannia glutinosa, fresh
Ligustinum wallichii
Prunus persica
Carthamus tinctorius
Bupleurum chinense
Poncirus trifoliata, fruit
Platycodon grandiflorum
Glycyrrhiza uralensis
Achyranthes bidentata

Ref: 157 (9), 158 (2)

104. Xing jun san 行军散

March Powder

Bos taurus, gallstone
Moschus moschiferus
Pteria margaritifera, pearl
Dryobalanops aromatica, camphor
Borax
Realgar
Niter

Ref: 169 (3)

105. Fang feng tang 防风汤

Saposhnikovia Decoction

Saposhnikiovia divaricata
Gentiana macrophylla
Angelica sylvestris
Cinnamomum cassia, branch
Pueraria lobata
Angelica sinensis
Poria cocos, pink part near outer
  skin
Prunus armeniaca
Scutellaria baicalensis
Glycyrrhiza uralensis
Zingiber officinale, fresh

106. Fang feng tong shen san 防风
  通圣散

Saposhnikovia High-Efficacy
  Powder

Saposhnikovia divaricata
Schizonepeta tenuifolia
Forsythia suspensa, fruit
Ephedra sinica
Mentha haplocalyx
Ligustinum wallichii
Angelica sinensis
Paeonia lactiflora, white
Atractylodes macrocephala
Gardenia jasminoides
Rheum palmatum
Mirabilite

Gypsum
Scutellaria baicalensis
Platycodon grandiflorum
Glycyrrhiza uralensis
Talc

Ref: 168 (1)

107. Leng xiao wan 冷哮丸

Cold Wheeze Pill

Ephedra sinica
Aconitum carmichaeli, root
Asarum heterotropoides
Zanthoxylum bungeanum, fruit
Alunite
Gleditsia sinensis
Pinellia ternata
Arisaema consanguineum, bile
  treated
Prunus armeniaca
Glycyrrhiza uralensis
Aster tartaricus
Tussilago farfara
Zingiber officinale, juice
Shenqu

Ref: 165 (4), 300 (31)

108. Wu zhu yu tang 吴茱萸汤

Evodia Decoction

Evodia rutaecarpa
Codonopsis pilosula
Zingiber officinale, fresh
Ziziphus jujuba, fruit

Ref: 157 (5), 162 (11), 163 (12), 167
  (7, 8), 294 (19)

109. Ren shen lan wei yan tang 妊娠
  阑尾炎汤

Pregnancy Appendicitis Decoction

Poria cocos, body
Spatholobus suberectus
Salvia miltiorrhiza
Angelica sinensis

Lonicera japonica, flower
Forsythia suspensa, fruit
Scutellaria baicalensis, alcohol
treated
Paeonia lactiflora, red
Paeonia lactiflora, white
Benincasa hispida, seed
Citrus tangerina, fruit peel
Glycyrrhiza uralensis

Ref: 157 (7)

110. Niao dao pai shi tang 尿道排
石汤

Urinary Stone-Expelling Decoction

Glechoma longituba
Lygodium japonicum
Pyrrosia lingua
Sparganium stoloniferum
Pseudosciaena crocea
Prunus persica
Talc
Cyathula officinalis
Vaccaria segetalis

Ref: 157 (7)

111. Xing su san 杏苏散

Prunus-Perilla Powder

No. 7, plus:
Perilla frutescens
Prunus armeniaca
Peucedanum praeruptorum
Platycodon grandiflorum
Poncirus trifoliata, tiny fruit
Zingiber officinale, fresh
Ziziphus jujuba, fruit

Ref: 157 (10), 159 (3), 168 (1),
171 (9)

112. Qi ju di huang wan 杞菊地黄丸

*Lycium-Chrysanthemum-
Rehmannia* Pill

No. 46, plus:

Lycium chinense, ripe fruit
Chrysanthemum

Ref: 157 (6), 163, 164 (1)

113. Sha shen mai dong tang 沙参麦
冬汤

Glehnia-Ophiopogon Decoction

Glehnia littoralis
Polygonatum odoratum
Ophiopogon japonicus
Trichosanthes kirilowii, root
Dolichos lablab, seed
Morus alba, leaf
Glycyrrhiza uralensis

Ref: 156 (2), 166 (4), 170 (5)

114. Mu li san 牡蛎散

Oyster Shell Powder

Ostrea rivularis, raw
Ephedra sinica
Triticum aestivum
Astragalus spp., root stalk

Ref: 158 (12)

115. Shao yao tang 芍药汤

Peony Decoction

Paeonia lactiflora, white
Coptis chinensis
Scutellaria baicalensis
Rheum palmatum
Areca catechu, seed
Angelica sinensis
Glycyrrhiza uralensis
Saussurea lappa
Cinnamomum cassia, bark

Ref: 156 (2)

116. Shao yao gan cao fu zi tang
芍药甘草附子汤

Paeonia-Glycyrrhiza-Aconitum
Decoction

Paeonia lactiflora, white
Glycyrrhiza uralensis
Aconitum carmichaeli
Ref: 161 (7)

117. Chen sha miao xiang san 辰砂妙香散

Cinnabar Wonder Powder

Cinnabar
Astragalus spp., dried root
Panax ginseng
Glycyrrhiza uralensis
Platycodon grandiflorum
Dioscorea opposita
Polygala tenuifolia
Zingiber officinale, fresh
Poria cocos, grown on pine root
Poria cocos, body
Saussurea lappa
Moschus moschiferus
Ref: 164 (2)

118. Fu zi tang 附子汤

Aconitum Decoction

Aconitum carmichaeli
Poria cocos, body
Panax ginseng
Atractylodes macrocephala
Paeonia lactiflora
Ref: 169 (2)

119. Fu zi xie xin tang 附子泻心汤

Aconitum Heart-Clearing Decoction

Rheum palmatum
Coptis chinensis
Scutellaria baicalensis
Aconitum carmichaeli
Ref: 161 (7)

120. Fu zi li zhong tang 附子理中汤

Aconitum Central-Regulating Decoction

No. 233, plus:
Aconitum carmichaeli
Ref: 157 (5), 165 (3), 166 (7), 171 (7), 303 (36, 37)

121. E jiao ji zi huang tang 阿胶鸡子黄汤

Gelatin-Egg Yolk Decoction

Equus asinus
Paeonia lactiflora, white
Haliotis diversicolor
Uncaria rhynchophylla
Rehmannia glutinosa, fresh
Poria cocos, grown on pine root
Gallus gallus, egg yolk
Ostrea rivularis
Trachelospermum jasminoides
Glycyrrhiza uralensis
Ref: 164 (1), 168 (1)

122. E jiao huang qin tang 阿胶黄芩汤

Gelatin-*Scutellaria* Decoction

Equus asinus
Paeonia lactiflora, white, fresh
Coptis chinensis
Rehmannia glutinosa, fresh
Scutellaria baicalensis
Ref: 170 (5)

123. Gu chong tang 固冲汤

Vaginal Bleeding Decoction

Atractylodes macrocephala
Astragalus spp., fresh dried root
Fossil bones, fired
Ostrea rivularis
Cornus officinalis
Paeonia lactiflora, white
Sepiella maindroni
Rubia cordifolia
Trachycarpus wagnerianus
Melaphis chinensis
Ref: 158 (12)

124. Gu jing wan 固精丸

Semen-Conserving Pill

Astragalus complanatus
Euryale ferox
Nelumbo nucifera, stamen and
    pistils
Fossil bones, fired
Ostrea rivularis, fired

Ref: 158 (12)

125. Yi gan xie fei fang 抑肝泄肺方

Liver-Supporting Lung-Clearing
    Prescription

Citrus tangerina, unripe peel
Prunus armeniaca
Eriobotrya japonica
Bupleurum chinense
Scutellaria baicalensis
Pinellia ternata
Glycyrrhiza uralensis
Morus alba, root skin

Ref: 164 (1)

126. Di dang tang 抵当汤

Resistance Decoction

Hirudo nipponica
Tabanus bivittatus
Prunus persica
Rheum palmatum

Ref: 160 (7), 168 (10)

127. Mi niao xi gan ran he ji 泌尿系
    感染合剂

Diuretic Prescription

Bupleurum chinense
Scutellaria baicalensis
Phellodendron amurense
Plantago asiaticus, seed
Schisandra chinensis

Ref: 157 (11)

128. Zhi gan cao tang 炙甘草汤

Roast *Glycyrrhiza* Decoction

Glycyrrhiza uralensis
Codonopsis pilosula
Ziziphus jujuba, fruit
Zingiber officinale, fresh
Cinnamomum cassia, branch
Rehmannia glutinosa, fresh
Equus asinus
Ophiopogon japonicus
Cannabis sativa

Ref: 157 (6), 164 (1, 2), 291 (12)

129. Zhi bai di huang wan 知柏地
    黄丸

*Anemarrhena-Phellodendron-
    Rehmannia* Pill

No. 46, plus:
Anemarrhena asphodeloides
Phellodendron amurense

Ref: 157 (6), 170 (6)

130. Fei er wan 肥儿丸

Infant-Fattening Pill

Shenqu
Coptis chinensis
Myristica fragrans
Quisqualis indica
Hordeum vulgare
Areca catechu, seed
Saussurea lappa
Sus scrofa domestica, bile

Ref: 171 (12)

131. Wo long dan 卧龙丹

Sleeping Dragon Pill

Bos taurus, gallstone
Native gold
Dryobalanops aromatica
Schizonepeta tenuifolia, whole herb

Rhododendron sinense
Moschus moschiferus
Cinnabar
Gleditsia sinensis
Juncus effusus
Ref: 171 (7)

132. Fang siang dan shen fa fang 芳香淡渗法方

Agastache Dampness-Eliminating
   Prescription

Amomum cardamomum
Agastache rugosa
Eupatorium fortunei
Glycine max, sprouting seed
Coix lachryma-jobi
Tetrapanax papyriferus
Stachys baicalensis
Eriobotrya japonica
Ref: 170 (4)

133. Jin gui shen qi wan 金匮肾气丸

Kidney Qi Pill from the *Golden Cabinet*

Aconitum carmichaeli
Cinnamomum cassia, cooked
Dioscorea opposita
Cornus officinalis
Alisma plantago-aquatica
Poria cocos, body
Paeonia suffruticosa
Ref: 157 (6), 166 (5)

134. Jin ling zi san 金铃子散

Melia Powder

Melia toosendan
Corydalis yanhusuo
Ref: 157 (8), 164 (1)

135. Jin suo gu jing wan 金销固精丸

Gold Lock Semen-Conserving Pill

Astragalus complanatus
Euryale ferox
Fossil bones
Ostrea rivularis
Nelumbo nucifera, stamen and pistils
Nelumbo nucifera, seed
Ref: 167 (5), 302 (35)

136. Qing zhou bai wan zi 青州白丸子

Shandong White Pill

Arisaema consanguineum
Aconitum carmichaeli, secondary roots
Pinellia ternata
Aconitum carmichaeli, tuberous root
Ref: 171 (9)

137. Qing hao bie jia tang 青蒿鳖甲汤

Artemisia-Amyda Decoction

Artemisia apiacea, whole herb
Amyda sinensis
Rehmannia glutinosa, fresh
Anemarrhena asphodeloides
Paeonia suffruticosa
Ref: 156 (2), 170 (6)

138. Bao he wan 保和丸

Stomach-Regulating Pill

Crataegus pinnatifida
Shenqu
Raphanus sativus
Poria cocos, body
Citrus tangerina, fruit peel
Pinellia ternata
Forsythia suspensa, fruit
Grind and make into pills. 6–9
   grams twice daily.
Ref: 157 (7), 167 (7), 171 (10),
   286 (2)

139. Guan xin pian 冠心片

(Blood-Mobilizing Contusion-Dissolving) Heart-Crown Flake

Paeonia lactiflora, red
Carthamus tinctorius
Salvia miltiorrhiza
Ligustinum wallichii
Dalbergia odorifera
Ref: 157 (9), 165 (2)

140. Hou po san 厚朴散

Magnolia Powder

Magnolia officinalis, bark
Fossil bones
Coptis chinensis
Syzygium aromaticum
Angelica sinensis
Saussurea lappa
Atractylodes macrocephala
Myristica fragrans
Ref: 167 (8)

141. Ke xue fang 咳血方

Coughing of Blood Formula

Isatis indigotica
Trichosanthes kirilowii, kernel
Pumice
Gardenia jasminoides
Terminalia chebula
Ref: 157 (9), 166 (4)

142. Xuan bai cheng qi tang 宣白承气汤

Qi-Facilitating Decoction

Gypsum
Rheum palmatum
Trichosanthes kirilowii, fruit peel
Prunus armeniaca
Ref: 167 (4)

143. Xuan fei shu feng fa fang 宣肺疏风法方

Lung-Facilitating Wind-Dissipating Prescription

Mentha haplocalyx
Arctium lappa
Platycodon grandiflorum
Fritillaria spp.
Peucedanum praeruptorum
Citrus tangerina, red scraping from peel
Morus alba, leaf
Ref: 168 (1)

144. Gong wai yun tang 宫外孕汤

Ectopic Pregnancy Decoction

Scutellaria baicalensis
Boswellia carterii, fresh
Commiphora myrrha, fresh
Paeonia lactiflora, red
Prunus persica
Ref: 157 (9)

145. Ji xing lan wei yan tang 急性阑尾炎汤

Acute Appendicitis Decoction

Rheum palmatum
Paeonia lactiflora, red
Taraxacum mongolicum
Lonicera japonica, flower
Forsythia suspensa, fruit
Coix lachryma-jobi
Benincasa hispida, seed
Patrinii villosa
Glycyrrhiza uralensis, fresh
Ref: 157 (7)

146. Zhi shi dao zhi wan 枳实导滞丸

Poncirus Obstruction-Removing Pill

Rheum palmatum
Poncirus trifoliata, fried fruit

Shenqu
Poria cocos, body
Scutellaria baicalensis
Coptis chinensis
Atractylodes macrocephala
Alisma plantago-aquatica
Pill or decoction, 6 grams twice
  daily.
Ref: 157 (7), 171 (10)

147. Zhi zhu wan 枳术丸
Poncirus-Atractylodes Pill
Atractylodes macrocephala
Poncirus trifoliata, fruit
Pill, 6–9 grams twice daily.
Ref: 157 (7)

148. Zhi shi xie bai gui zhi tang 枳实
  薤白桂枝汤
Poncirus-Allium-Cinnamomum
  Decoction
Trichosanthes kirilowii, whole herb
Allium chinense
Poncirus trifoliata
Magnolia officinalis, bark
Cinnamomum cassia, branch
Ref: 157 (8)

149. Chai hu gui zhi tang 柴胡桂
  枝汤
Bupleurum-Cinnamomum Decoc-
  tion
Bupleurum chinense
Scutellaria baicalensis
Pinellia ternata
Cinnamomum cassia, branch
Paeonia lactiflora, white
Zingiber officinale, fresh
Glycyrrhiza uralensis
Ziziphus jujuba, fruit
Ref: 162 (9), 289 (7)

150. Chai hu shu gan san
  柴胡疏肝散
Bupleurum Liver-Clearing Powder
Bupleurum chinense
Paeonia lactiflora, white
Glycyrrhiza uralensis
Poncirus trifoliata, almost ripe fruit
Ligustinum wallichii
Cyperus rotundus
Ref: 157 (8), 158 (1), 164 (1)

151. Zhi zi bai pi tang 栀子柏皮汤
Gardenia-Phellodendron Decoction
Gardenia jasminoides
Phellodendron amurense
Glycyrrhiza uralensis
Ref: 162 (8)

152. Zhi zi chi tang 栀子豉汤
Gardenia-Glycine Decoction
Gardenia jasminoides
Glycine max, seed
Ref: 161 (7)

153. Huo xue san yu tang 活血散
  瘀汤
Blood-Mobilizing Decoction
Ligustinum wallichii
Angelica sinensis
Paeonia lactiflora, red
Caesalpinia sappan
Paeonia suffruticosa
Poncirus trifoliata, fruit
Trichosanthes kirilowii, kernel
Prunus persica
Areca catechu, seed
Rheum palmatum
Ref: 168 (9)

154. Huo luo xiao zhi dan 活络效
  灵丹
Circulation-Enhancing Pill

Salvia miltiorrhiza
Angelica sinensis
Boswellia carterii, fresh
Commiphora myrrha, fresh
Ref: 157 (9)

155. Shen xi dan 神犀丹
Magical Rhinoceros Special Pill
Rhinoceros horn
Acorus gramineus
Rehmannia glutinosa, fresh
Scutellaria baicalensis
Lonicera japonica, flower
Fecal filtrate
Forsythia suspensa, fruit
Clerodendron cyrtophyllum,
  root
Glycine max
Scrophularia ningpoensis
Trichosanthes kirilowii, root
Lithospermum erythrorhizon
Ref: 171 (7)

156. Hu jiao li zhong wan 胡椒理
  中丸
Piper-Centrally Regulating Pill
Piper nigrum
Tussilaga farfara
Artemisia argyi, fried
Piper longum
Alpinia officinarum
Asarum heterotropoides
Citrus tangerina, fruit peel
Zingiber officinale, dry
Atractylodes macrocephala
Ref: 171 (9)

157. Wei ling tang 胃苓汤
Fungi Stomach Decoction
Nos. 42 and 76 combined
Ref: 157 (11)

158. Dan dao pai shi tang 胆道排
  石汤
Gallstone-Expelling Decoction
Glechoma longituba
Artemisia capillaris
Curcuma longa, root
Poncirus trifoliata, fruit
Saussurea lappa
Rehmannia glutinosa, fresh
Ref: 157 (7)

159. Ling gui zhu gan tang 苓桂朮
  甘汤
*Poria-Cinnamomum-Atractylodes-
  Glycyrrhiza* Decoction
Poria cocos, body
Cinnamomum cassia, branch
Atractylodes macrocephala
Glycyrrhiza uralensis, fried
Ref: 157 (10), 171 (9)

160. Ling gui gan zao tang 苓桂甘
  枣汤
*Poria-Cinnamomum-Glycyrrhiza-
  Zizyphus* Decoction
Poria cocos, body
Cinnamomum cassia, branch
Glycyrrhiza uralensis
Ziziphus jujuba, fruit
Ref: 161 (7)

161. Ku xin tong xiang fa fang 苦辛
  通降法方
Acrid-Bitter Reduction Prescription
Agastache rugosa, stalk
Gardenia jasminoides
Scutellaria baicalensis
Coptis chinensis
Phragmites communis, fresh
Citrus tangerina, red scraping from
  peel

Poncirus trifoliata, tiny fruit
Talc
Ref: 170 (4)

162. Chu han qu shi fa fang 除寒祛
湿法方
Cold-Dampness-Eliminating Pre-
scription
Artemisia capillaris
Poria cocos, body
Atractylodes macrocephala
Atractylodes spp., root stalk
Glycyrrhiza uralensis
Zingiber officinale, dry
Aconitum carmichaeli
Ref: 169 (4)

163. Chu shi qiang huo tang 除湿羌
活汤
Angelica Dampness-Eliminating
Decoction
Angelica sylvestris
Ligusticum sinense
Cimicifuga foetida
Bupleurum chinense
Saposhnikovia divaricata
Atractylodes spp., root stalk
Ref: 169 (4)

164. Chu shi juan wei tang 除湿蠲
痹汤
Dampness-Eliminating Stomach-
Healing Decoction
Atractylodes spp., root stalk
Atractylodes macrocephala
Poria cocos, body
Angelica sylvestris
Alisma plantago-aquatica
Citrus tangerina, fruit peel
Glycyrrhiza uralensis
Zingiber officinale, juice

Phyllostachys nigra, liquid from
roasting stalk

165. Xiang sha liu wei tang 香砂六
味汤
Six Plus *Saussurea-Amomum*
Decoction
No. 45, plus:
Saussurea lappa
Amomum villosum
Ref: 157 (6)

166. Xiang sha ping wei wan 香砂平
胃丸
Saussurea-Amomum Stomach-
Settling Pill
No. 76, plus:
Saussurea lappa
Amomum villosum
Ref: 157 (11)

167. Xiang sha zhi zhu wan 香砂枳
术丸
*Saussurea-Amomum-Poncirus-
Atractylodes* Pill
No. 147, plus:
Saussurea lappa
Amomum villosum
Ref: 157 (7)

168. Xiang ru yin 香薷饮
Elsholtzia Drink
Elsholtzia splendens
Magnolia officinalis, bark
Dolichos lablab, seed
Coptis chinensis
Ref: 164 (1), 169 (3)

169. Xiang su cong chi tang 香苏葱
豉汤

Cyperus-Perilla-Allium-Glycine
Decoction

Cyperus rotundus
Citrus tangerina, fruit peel
Allium fistulosum
Perilla frutescens
Glycine max, seed
Artemisia argyi, fried
Ref: 170 (5)

170. Xiang su yin 香苏饮
Cyperus-Perilla Drink

Cyperus rotundus
Perilla frutescens, leaf
Citrus tangerina, fruit peel
Glycyrrhiza uralensis
Ref: 168 (1)

171. Xiang lian wan 香连丸
Saussurea-Coptis Pill

Coptis chinensis
Evodia rutaecarpa
Saussurea lappa
Ref: 170 (4)

172. Lian ge san 凉膈散
Diaphragm-Cooling Powder

Rheum palmatum
Mirabilite
Glycyrrhiza uralensis
Gardenia jasminoides
Scutellaria baicalensis
Mentha haplocalyx
Forsythia suspensa, fruit
Make into powder. 9–18 grams
  each dose. Wrap and decoct.
Ref: 156 (3), 170 (4)

173. She gan ma huang tang 射干麻
黄汤
Belamcanda-Ephedra Decoction

Ephedra sinica
Asarum heterotropoides
Pinellia ternata
Schisandra chinensis
Belamcanda chinensis
Aster tartaricus
Tussilago farfara
Zingiber officinale
Ziziphus jujuba, fruit
Ref: 157 (10)

174. Jie geng tang 桔梗汤
Platycodon Decoction

Glyccyrrhiza uralensis, fresh
Platycodon grandiflorum
Ref: 163 (11)

175. Gui zhi tang 桂枝汤
Cinnamomum Decoction

Cinnamomum cassia, branch
Paeonia lactiflora, white
Zingiber officinale, fresh
Glycyrrhiza uralensis, fried
Ziziphus jujuba, fruit
Ref: 77, 156 (1), 160 (7), 168 (1)

176. Gui zhih jia ge gen tang 桂枝加
葛根汤
Cinnamomum-Pueraria Decoction

No. 175, plus:
Pueraria lobata
Ref: 156 (1), 286 (3)

177. Gui zhi gan cao tang 桂枝甘
草汤
Cinnamomum-Glycyrrhiza Decoction

Cinnamomum cassia, branch
Glycyrrhiza uralensis
Ref: 161 (7)

178. Gui zhi jiang fu tang 桂枝姜附汤

Cinnamomum-Zingiber-Aconitum Decoction

Cinnamomum cassia, branch
Zingiber officinale, dry
Aconitum carmichaeli
Atractylodes macrocephala
Ref: 169 (4)

179. Gui gan long mu tang 桂甘龙牡汤

Cinnamomum-Glycyrrhiza-Fossil Bone-*Ostrea* Decoction

Cinnamomum cassia, branch
Glycyrrhiza uralensis
Fossil bones
Ostrea rivularis
Ref: 158 (13)

180. Sang xing tang 桑杏汤
Mulberry and Apricot Decoction

Morus alba, leaf
Prunus armeniaca
Adenophora tetraphylla
Fritillaria spp.
Glycine max, seed
Gardenia jasminoides
Pear peel
Ref: 159 (3), 170 (5)

181. Sang ju yin 桑菊饮
Mulberry and Chrysanthemum Drink

Morus alba, leaf
Chrysanthemum
Mentha haplocalyx
Prunus armeniaca
Platycodon grandiflorum
Glycyrrhiza uralensis, fresh
Forsythia suspensa, fruit

Phragmites communis
Ref: 156 (1), 159 (3), 168 (1), 290 (10)

182. Sang piao xiao san 桑螵蛸散
Paratenodera Powder

Paratenodera sinensis
Polygala tenuifolia
Acorus gramineus
Fossil bones
Codonopsis pilosula
Poria cocos, grown on pine root
Angelica sinensis
Chinemys reevesii
Ref: 158 (12)

183. Tao ren cheng qi tang 桃仁承气汤
Prunus Qi-Regulating Decoction

Prunus persica
Cinnamomum cassia, branch
Rheum palmatum
Mirabilite
Glycyrrhiza uralensis
Ref: 160 (7), 168 (10)

184. Tao hua tang 桃花汤
Peach Blossom (Dysentery) Decoction

Halloysite
Zingiber offficinale, dry
Oryza sativa
Ref: 162 (11)

185. Tao hong si wu tang 桃红四物汤
Four-Substance Decoction with Safflower and Peach Pit

No. 67, plus:
Prunus persica
Carthamus tinctorius
Ref: 157 (6), 158 (2)

186. Xiao he wan 消核丸
Tubercle-Dissolving Pill

Citrus tangerina, orange scraping
Paeonia lactiflora, red
Forsythia suspensa, fruit
Scutellaria baicalensis
Gardenia jasminoides
Scrophularia ningpoensis
Ostrea rivularis
Glycyrrhiza uralensis
Trichosanthes kirilowii, seed
Pinellia ternata
Bombyx mori
Rheum palmatum, roasted
Ref: 171 (8)

187. Xiao ke fang 消渴方
Dryness-Eliminating Prescription

Coptis chinensis
Trichosanthes kirilowii, root
Rehmannia glutinosa, fresh
Nelumbo nucifera, juice
Bos taurus, milk
Zingiber officinale, juice
Ref: 167 (7)

188. Xiao chuang yin 消疮饮
Furuncle(Boil)-Dissolving Drink

Lonicera japonica, flower
Manis pentadactyla, fried scales
Trichosanthes kirilowii, root
Angelica dahurica
Angelica sinensis
Paeonia lactiflora, red
Fritillaria verticillata
Saposhnikovia divaricata
Boswellia carterii
Commiphora myrrha
Gleditsia sinensis, thorn
Citrus tangerina, fruit peel
Glycyrrhiza uralensis
Ref: 157 (7)

189. Xiao luo wan 梢瘰丸
Scrofula-Dissolving Pill

Scrophularia ningpoensis
Ostrea rivularis
Fritillaria verticillata
Grind together, form pill with
    honey. 9 grams twice daily.
Ref: 157 (10)

190. Xiao yao san 消遥散
Carefree (Liver-Unblocking
    Spleen-Restoring) Powder

Bupleurum chinense
Angelica sinensis
Paeonia lactiflora, white
Atractylodes macrocephala
Poria cocos, body
Glycyrrhiza uralensis, fried
Zingiber officinale, fresh, roasted
Mentha haplocalyx
Ref: 157 (4), 164 (1)

191. Wu mei wan 乌梅丸
Mume Pill

Prunus mume, unripe fruit
Coptis chinensis
Phellodendron amurense
Codonopsis pilosula
Angelica sinensis
Aconitum carmichaeli
Cinnamomum cassia, branch
Zanthoxylum bungeanum, fruit
Zingiber officinale, dry
Asarum heterotropoides
Ref: 157 (7), 163 (12), 171 (12)

192. Wu tou tang 乌头汤
Aconitum-Ephedra Decoction

Aconitum carmichaeli
Ephedra sinica
Paeonia lactiflora

Astragalus spp., dried root
Glycyrrhiza uralensis
Ref: 169 (2)

193. Zhen ren yang zang tang 真人养脏汤

Genuine Zang-Nourishing
Decoction

Papaver somniferum
Terminalia chebula
Myristica fragrans
Saussurea lappa
Cinnamomum cassia, bark
Panax ginseng
Atractylodes macrocephala
Angelica sinensis
Paeonia lactiflora, white
Glycyrrhiza uralensis
Ref: 168 (9)

194. Zhen wu tang 真武汤

Kidney-Warming Spleen-
Strenghtening Decoction

Poria cocos, body
Atractylodes macrocephala
Paeonia lactiflora, white
Zingiber officinale, fresh
Aconitum carmichaeli
Ref: 157 (11), 162 (11), 166 (3),
304 (38)

195. Zhen zhu mu wan 真珠母丸

Mother-of-Pearl Pill

Pteria magaritifera, shell
Angelica sinensis
Panax ginseng
Rehmannia glutinosa, cooked
Ziziphus jujuba
Biota orientalis, kernel
Rhinoceros horn
Poria cocos, grown on pine root

Aquilaria agallocha
Fossil teeth
Ref: 164 (1)

196. Qin jiao bie jia san 秦艽鳖甲散

Gentiana-Amyda Powder

Gentiana macrophylla
Amyda sinensis
Lycium chinense, root skin
Anemarrhena asphodeloides
Bupleurum chinense
Angelica sinensis
Prunus mume, unripe fruit
Ref: 156 (2), 170 (6)

197. Fu tu wan 茯菟丸

Poria-Cuscuta Pill

Cuscuta chinensis
Schisandra chinensis
Nelumbo nucifera, seed
Poria cocos, body
Dioscorea opposita
Ref: 167 (5)

198. Fu shen san 茯神散

Poria Powder

Poria cocos, grown on pine root
Ophiopogon japonicus
Dictamnos dasycarpus
Lycium chinense, root skin
Ziziphus jujuba, seed
Adenophora tetraphylla
Saiga tatarica
Glycyrrhiza uralensis
Ref: 167 (6)

199. Yin chen wu ling san 茵阵五苓散

Artemisia and Five-Ingredient
Powder with Poria

No. 42, plus:
Artemisia capillaris
Ref: 156 (2), 165 (3)

200. Yin chen hao tang 茵陈蒿汤
Artemisia Decoction
Artemisia capillaris
Gardenia jasminoides
Rheum palmatum
Ref: 156 (2), 162 (8), 164 (1), 165 (3)

201. Yin chen fu zi gan jiang tang 茵陈附子干姜汤
Artemisia-Aconitum-Zingiber Decoction
Artemisia capillaris
Atractylodes macrocephala
Aconitum carmichaeli
Zingiber officinale, dry
Ref: 156 (1)

202. Hui xiang ju he wan 茴香橘核丸
Foeniculum-Citrus Pill
Foeniculum vulgare
Citrus tangerina, seed
Cyperus rotundus
Manis pentadactyla
Citrus tangerina, unripe peel
Psoralea corylifolia
Litchi chinensis
Laminaria japonica
Melia toosendan
Saussurea lappa
Prunus persica
Areca catechu, seed
Curcuma zeodaria
Corydalis yanhusuo
Cinnamomum cassia
Ref: 167 (8)

203. Jing fang bai du san 荆防败毒散
Schizonepeta-Saposhnikovia Poison-Eliminating Powder
Schizonepeta tenuifolia
Saposhnikovia divaricata
Angelica sylvestris
Angelica pubescens
Ligustinum wallichii
Bupleurum chinense
Peucedanum praeruptorum
Platycodon grandiflorum
Poncirus trifoliata, tiny fruit
Poria cocos, body
Glycyrrhiza uralensis
Mentha halpcalyx
Ref: 156 (1)

204. Zhui chong wan 追虫丸
Worm-Expelling Pill
Pharbitis nil, black
Areca catechu, seed
Polyporus mylittae
Saussurea lappa
Artemisia capillaris
Gleditsia sinensis, thorn
Melia toosendan, root skin
Ref: 171 (12)

205. Gao liang jiang tang 高良姜汤
Alpinia Decoction
Alpinia officinarum
Magnolia officinalis, bark
Angelica sinensis
Cinnamomum cassia, center of branch
Zingiber officinale, fresh
Ref: 167 (7)

206. Gan jiang huang qin huang lian ren shen tang 干姜黄芩黄连人参汤

Zingiber-Scutellaria-Coptis-
  Ginseng Decoction

Zingiber officinale, dry
Scutellaria baicalensis
Coptis chinensis
Panax ginseng
Ref: 163 (12)

207. Shen zhu jian pi tang 参术健
  脾汤

Ginseng-*Atractylodes* Spleen-
  Strengthening Decoction
Panax ginseng
Atractylodes macrocephala
Citrus tangerina, fruit peel
Poncirus trifoliata, tiny fruit
Crataegus pinnatifida
Shenqu
Hordeum vulgare
Ref: 165 (3)

208. Shen ling bai zhu san 参苓白
  术散

Codonopsis-Poria-Atractylodes
  Powder
Codonopsis pilosula
Poria cocos, body
Atractylodes macrocephala
Glycyrrhiza uralensis, fried
Dolichos lablab, seed
Dioscorea opposita
Coix lachryma-jobi
Nelumbo nucifera, seed
Citrus tangerina, fruit peel
Amomum villosum
Platycodon grandiflorum
Ziziphus jujuba, fruit
Ref: 157 (6), 165 (3), 298 (27)

209. Shen ge san 参蛤散
Ginseng-Gecko Powder
Gekko gecko, one pair

Panax ginseng, 9 grams
Grind into powder. Use 1 gram two
  or three times daily.
Ref: 158 (12)

210. Shen fu tang 参附汤
Ginseng-*Aconitum* Decoction
Panax ginseng
Aconitum carmichaeli, treated
Ref: 157 (5), 164 (2)

211. Shen fu long mu jiu ni tang
  参附龙牡救逆汤

Ginseng-*Aconitum*-Fossil Bone-
  Ostrea Rescue Decoction
Panax ginseng
Aconitum carmichaeli, treated
Fossil bones
Ostrea rivularis
Ref: 157 (5)

212. Kong ye dan 控涎丹
Fluid-Control Pill
Euphorbia pekinensis
Euphorbia kansui
Brassica alba
Take at bedtime with bland ginger
  decoction.
Ref: 156 (3), 171 (9)

213. Pai nong san 排脓散
Pus-Dissolving Powder
Poncirus trifoliata, tiny fruit
Paeonia lactiflora
Platycodon grandiflorum
Ref: 168 (9)

214. Bai du san 败毒散
Poison-Eliminating Powder
Schizonepeta tenuifolia, whole herb

Saposhnikovia divaricata
Panax ginseng
Glycyrrhiza uralensis
Poria cocos, body
Bupleurum chinense
Peucedanum praeruptorum
Ligustinum wallichii
Poncirus trifoliata, fruit
Platycodon grandiflorum
Ref: 171 (7)

215. Xuan fu hua tang 旋复花汤
Inula Decoction
Inula brittanica
Ref: 164 (1)

216. Xuan fu dai zhe tang 旋复代
赭汤
Inula-Hematite Decoction
Inula brittanica
Hematite
Zingiber officinale, fresh
Pinellia ternata
Glycyrrhiza uralensis, fried
Ziziphus jujuba, fruit
Codonopsis pilosula
Ref: 157 (8), 161 (7)

217. Qing yan ning fei tang 清咽
宁肺汤
Throat-Clearing Lung-Calming
Decoction
Platycodon grandiflorum
Gardenia jasminoides
Scutellaria baicalensis
Morus alba, root skin
Glycyrrhiza uralensis
Peucedanum praeruptorum
Fritillaria
Anemarrhena asphodeloides
Ref: 166 (4), 170 (6)

218. Qing yi shi re fa fang 清宣湿热
法方
Dampness-Heat-Cooling
Prescription
Artemisia apiacea, fruit
Amomum cardamomum
Prunus armeniaca
Coix lachryma-jobi
Atractylodes spp., root stalk
Magnolia officinalis, bark
Eriobotrya japonica
Talc
Ref: 170 (4)

219. Qing ying tang 清营汤
Encampment-Clearing Decoction
Rhinoceros horn
Rehmannia glutinosa, fresh
Scrophularia ningpoensis
Ophiopogon japonicus
Lonicera japonica, flower
Forsythia suspensa, fruit
Salvia miltiorrhiza
Phyllostachys nigra, leaf
Coptis chinensis
Ref: 156 (2), 158 (2), 159 (5), 291
(11)

220. Qing shu yi qi tang 清暑益气汤
Heat-Cooling Qi-Enhancing
Decoction
Astragalus spp., dried root
Panax ginseng
Atractylodes macrocephala
Atractylodes spp., root stalk
Shenqu
Citrus tangerina, unripe peel
Citrus tangerina, ripe peel
Glycyrrhiza uralensis
Ophiopogon japonicus
Schisandra chinensis
Angelica sinensis

Phellodendron amurense
Alisma plantago-aquatica
Cimicifuga foetida
Pueraria lobata
Zingiber officinale
Ziziphus jujuba, fruit
Ref: 169 (3)

221. Qing qi hua tan wan 清气化痰丸

Qi-Clearing Phlegm-Dissolving Pill
Citrus tangerina, fruit peel
Pinellia ternata, treated
Poria cocos, body
Scutellaria baicalensis
Trichosanthes kirilowii
Arisaema consanguineum, bile treated
Poncirus trifoliata, tiny fruit
Prunus armeniaca
Ref: 157 (10), 166 (4), 171 (9), 285 (1), 300 (30)

222. Qing zao jiu fei tang 清燥救肺汤

Dryness-Cooling Lung-Saving Decoction
Morus alba, leaf
Gypsum
Adenophora tetraphylla
Glycyrrhiza uralensis
Cannabis sativa
Equus asinus
Ophiopogon japonicus
Prunus armeniaca
Eriobotrya imbricata
Ref: 157 (10), 166 (4), 170 (5)

223. Qing re shen shi tang 清热渗湿汤

Heat-Cooling Dampness-Mobilizing Decoction

Phellodendron amurense
Coptis chinensis
Poria cocos, body
Alisma plantago-aquatica
Atractylodes spp., root stalk
Atractylodes macrocephala
Glycyrrhiza uralensis
Ref: 170 (4)

224. Qing re jie du san 清热解毒散

Heat-Cooling Poison-Eliminating Powder
Angelica sylvestris
Paeonia lactiflora, white
Gypsum
Panax ginseng
Astragalus spp., dried root
Anemarrhena asphodeloides
Cimicifuga foetida
Pueraria lobata
Glycyrrhiza uralensis
Coptis chinensis
Rehmannia glutinosa, fresh
Ref: 170 (7)

225. Qing gong tang 清宫汤

Pericardium-Heat-Dissipating Decoction
Scrophularia ningpoensis, heart of root
Nelumbo nucifera, sprout
Phyllostachys nigra
Forsythia suspensa, seed
Rhinoceros horn
Ophiopogon japonicus
Ref: 159 (5)

226. Qing wei san 清胃散

Stomach-Cooling Powder
Coptis chinensis
Rehmannia glutinosa, fresh
Paeonia suffruticosa

Cimicifuga foetida
Angelica sinensis
Ref: 167 (7), 170 (6), 299 (29)

227. Qing wen bai du yin 清瘟败
    毒饮
Poison-Eliminating Cooling Drink
Gypsum
Rehmannia glutinosa, fresh
Rhinoceros horn
Coptis chinensis
Gardenia jasminoides
Scutellaria baicalensis
Anemarrhena asphodeloides
Forsythia suspensa, fruit
Paeonia suffruticosa
Paeonia lactiflora, red
Scrophularia ningpoensis
Platycodon grandiflorum
Glycyrrhiza uralensis
Phyllostachys nigra, fresh leaf
Ref: 156 (2), 160 (6), 164 (1), 170
    (7)

228. Qing gu san 清骨散
Hyperthermia-Cooling Powder
Stellaria dichotoma
Picrorrhiza kurrooa
Gentiana macrophylla
Amyda sinensis
Lycium chinense, root skin
Artemisia apiacea, whole herb
Anemarrhena asphodeloides
Glycyrrhiza uralensis
Ref: 156 (2)

229. Xi jiao di huang tang 犀角地
    黄汤
Rhinoceros Horn and *Rehmannia*
    Decoction
Rhinoceros horn

Rehmannia glutinosa, fresh
Paeonia lactiflora, red
Paeonia suffruticosa
Ref: 156 (2), 160 (6)

230. Qian niu wan 牵牛丸
Pharbitis Pill
Pharbitis nil
Rheum palmatum
Areca catechu, seed
Realgar
Ref: 171 (12)

231. Qian zhen san 牵正散
Hemiplegia-Reversing (Wind-
    Eliminating) Powder
Aconitum carmichaeli
Bombyx mori, larva
Buthus martensi
Grind equal amounts into powder.
    Use 3 grams as needed.
Ref: 158 (14)

232. Zhu ling tang 猪苓汤
Poria-Polyporus Decoction
Poria cocos, body
Polyporus umbellatus
Alisma plantago-aquatica
Equus asinus
Talc
Ref: 157 (11), 163 (11)

233. Li zhong tang 理中汤
Central-Regulating Decoction
Codonopsis pilosula
Zingiber officinale, dry
Atractylodes macrocephala
Glycyrrhiza uralensis
Ref: 157 (5), 162 (10), 169 (2), 293
    (16)

234. Yi gong san 异功散
Spleen-Qi-Strengthening and
  Regulating Powder
No. 66, plus:
Citrus tangerina, fruit peel
Ref: 157 (6)

235. Ling qiao jie du wan 羚翘解
毒丸
Saiga Horn-*Lonicera* Poison-
  Relieving Pill
No. 305, plus:
Saiga tatarica, horn powder
Ref: 249 (1)

236. Ling yang gou teng tang 羚羊
钩藤汤
Saiga-Uncaria Decoction
Saiga tatarica
Uncaria rhynchophylla
Morus alba, leaf
Fritillaria cirrhosa
Rehmannia glutinosa, fresh
Chrysanthemum
Paeonia lactiflora, white, fresh
Glycyrrhiza uralensis
Phyllostachys nigra, fresh inner
  stalk lining
Poria cocos, grown on pine root
Ref: 158 (14), 164 (1), 168 (1)

237. Tong mai si ni tang 通脉四逆汤
Circulation-Facilitating Decoction
Zingiber officinale, dry
Aconitum carmichaeli
Glycyrrhiza uralensis
Ref: 162 (11), 169 (2), 290 (9)

238. Tong qiao huo xue tang 通窍活
血汤

Conduit-Opening Circulation-
  Enhancing Decoction
Paeonia lactiflora, red
Ligustinum wallichii
Prunus persica
Carthamus tinctorius
Agastache rugosa
Zingiber officinale, fresh
Ziziphus jujuba, fruit
Allium fistulosum
Ref: 157 (9)

239. Zhu han san 逐寒散
Cold-Repelling Powder
Cnidium monnieri
Ligusticum sinense
Cornus officinalis
Saposhnikovia divaricata
Ref: 168 (10)

240. Lian po yin 连朴饮
Coptis-Magnolia Drink
Coptis chinensis
Magnolia officinalis, bark
Acorus gramineus
Pinellia ternata
Glycine max, seed
Gardenia jasminoides
Phragmites communis
Ref: 159 (4), 170 (4)

241. Lian mei an hui tang 连梅安
蛔汤
Roundworm Decoction
Picrorhiza kurrooa
Zanthoxylum bungeanum, fruit
Polyporus mylittae
Prunus mume, unripe fruit
Phellodendron amurense, Szechuan
Areca catechu, seed
Ref: 171 (12)

242. Lian li tang 连理汤

Coptis Central-Regulating
Decoction

No. 233, plus:
Coptis chinensis
Ref: 157 (5)

243. Mai wei di huang wan 麦味地黄丸

Lung-Kidney Deficiency Cough
Pill

No. 46, plus:
Ophiopogon japonicus
Schisandra chinensis
Ref: 157 (6), 166 (4)

244. Mai men dong tang 麦门冬汤

Ophiopogon Decoction

Ophiopogon japonicus
Pinellia ternata
Codonopsis pilosula
Oryza sativa, grain
Glycyrrhiza uralensis
Ziziphus jujuba, fruit
Ref: 157 (10), 166 (4), 167 (7), 285
(1), 299 (29)

245. Ma zi ren wan 麻子仁丸

Cannabis pill

Cannabis sativa, seed
Prunus armeniaca
Rheum palmatum
Poncirus trifoliata, tiny fruit
Magnolia officinalis, bark
Paeonia lactiflora, white
Make into pills with honey. Take 6–
12 grams twice daily.
Ref: 156 (3)

246. Ma xing shi gan tang 麻杏石甘汤

Ephedra-Prunus-Gypsum-
Glycyrrhiza Decoction

Ephedra sinica
Prunus armeniaca
Gypsum
Glycyrrhiza uralensis
Ref: 156 (1), 159 (4), 166 (4), 292
(14)

247. Ma huang lian qiao chi xiao
dou tang 麻黄连翘赤小豆汤

Ephedra-Forsythia-Phaseolus
Decoction

Ephedra sinica
Prunus armeniaca
Glycyrrhiza uralensis
Forsythia suspensa, root
Morus alba, root skin
Phaseolus calcaratus
Zingiber officinale, fresh
Ziziphus jujuba, fruit
Ref: 195 (4), 162 (8)

248. Ma huang fu zi xi xin tang 麻黄
附子细辛汤

Ephedra-Aconitum-Asarum
Decoction

Ephedra sinica
Aconitum carmichaeli
Asarum heterotropoides
Ref: 163 (11)

249. Ma huang tang 麻黄汤

Ephedra Decoction

Ephedra sinica
Cinnamomum cassia, branch
Prunus armeniaca
Glycyrrhiza uralensis
Ref: 76, 77, 156 (1), 160 (7), 169
(2), 286 (3)

250. Fu fang da cheng qi tang 复方
大承气汤
Double Action Qi-Facilitating
  Decoction
Mirabilite
Magnolia officinalis, bark
Poncirus trifoliata, fruit
Prunus persica
Paeonia lactiflora, red
Raphanus sativus
Rheum palmatum
Ref: 156 (3)

251. Fu yuan huo xue tang 复元活
血汤
Circulation-Enhancing Decoction
Bupleurum chinense
Trichosanthes kirilowii, root
Angelica sinensis
Carthamus tinctorius
Glycyrrhiza uralensis
Manis pentadactyla, toasted scales
Rheum palmatum
Prunus persica
Ref: 157 (9)

252. Pu ji qing du yin 普济清毒饮
General Poison-Eliminating Drink
Scutellaria baicalensis
Coptis chinensis
Clerodendron cyrtophyllum, leaf
Forsythia suspensa, fruit
Lasiophaera fenzlii
Arctium lappa
Mentha haplocalyx
Bombyx mori, larva
Scrophularia ningpoensis
Glycyrrhiza uralensis
Citrus tangerina, fruit peel
Cimicifuga foetida
Bupleurum chinense
Platycodon grandiflorum
Ref: 156 (2), 170 (7)

253. Jiao mei wan 椒梅丸
Zanthoxylum-Mume Pill
Zanthoxylum bungeanum
Prunus mume, unripe fruit
Poncirus trifoliata, tiny fruit
Saussurea lappa
Cinnamomum cassia, bark
Magnolia officinalis Szechuan, bark
Zingiber officinale, dry
Coptis chinensis
Areca catechu, seed
Amomum villosum
Ref: 171 (12)

254. Wen dan tang 温胆汤
Gallbladder-Warming Decoction
No. 7, plus:
Poncirus trifoliata, tiny fruit
Phyllostachys nigra, inner stalk
  lining
Ref: 157 (10), 165 (2)

255. Wen pi tang 温脾汤
Spleen-Warming Decoction
Rheum palmatum
Aconitum carmichaeli
Zingiber officinale, dry
Codonopsis pilosula
Glycyrrhiza uralensis, fried
Ref: 156 (3)

256. Wen jing tang 温经汤
Meridian-Warming Decoction
Evodia rutaecarpa
Cinnamomum cassia, branch
Angelica sinensis
Ligustinum wallichii
Paeonia lactiflora, white
Paeonia suffruticosa
Equus asinus
Ophiopogon japonicus

Codonopsis pilosula
Glycyrrhiza uralensis
Pinellia ternata
Zingiber officinale
Ref: 157 (9)

257. Tong feng wan 痛风丸
Pain and Wind Pill

Angelica sylvestris
Atractylodes spp.
Cinnamomum cassia, branch
Carthamus tinctorius
Ligustinum wallichii
Prunus persica
Phellodendron amurense
Arisaema consanguineum
Shenqu
Gentiana scabra
Angelica dahurica
Clematis chinensis
Stephania tetrandra
Ref: 169 (1)

258. Tong xie yao fang 痛泻要方
Dysentery Prescription

Atractylodes macrocephala
Paeonia lactiflora, white
Citrus tangerina, fruit peel
Saposhnikovia divaricata
Ref: 157 (4), 164 (1), 295 (21)

259. Xi ye san 稀涎散
Saliva-Reducing Powder

Gleditsia sinensis, thorn
Alunite
Ref: 168 (1)

260. Cheng shi juan bi tang 程氏蠲
痹汤
Master Cheng's Wind-Dampness
(Rheumatism) Decoction

Angelica sylvestris
Angelica pubescens
Cinnamomum cassia, branch
Gentiana macrophylla
Angelica sinensis
Ligustinum wallichii
Glycyrrhiza uralensis, fried
Piper kadsura
Morus alba, branch
Boswellia carterii
Saussurea lappa
Ref: 157 (5)

261. Zi xue dan 紫雪丹
Purple Snow Special (Epidemic-
   Preventing) Pill

Talc
Gypsum
Mirabilite
Saiga tartarica
Saussurea lappa
Rhinoceros horn
Aquilaria agallocha
Syzygium aromaticum
Cimicifuga foetida
Scrophularia ningpoensis
Moschus moschiferus
Cinnabar
Gold (native)
Ref: 168 (9), 169 (3), 171 (7)

262. Zi wan tang 紫菀汤
Aster Decoction

Aster tartaricus
Anemarrhena asphodeloides
Fritillaria
Panax ginseng
Poria cocos, body
Schisandra chinensis
Equus asinus
Platycodon grandiflorum
Glycyrrhiza uralensis
Ref: 166 (4)

263. Shen qi wan 肾气丸
Kidney Qi Pill

Aconitum carmichaeli
Cinnamomum cassia, bark
Rehmannia glutinosa, cooked
Dioscorea opposita
Cornus officinalis
Alisma plantago-aquatica
Poria cocos, body
Paeonia suffruticosa

264. Bei xie shen shi tang 草薢渗
湿汤

Dioscorea Dampness-Dissolving
Decoction

Dioscorea hypoglauca
Coix lachryma-jobi
Phellodendron amurense
Paeonia lactiflora, red
Paeonia suffruticosa
Alisma plantago-aquatica
Gypsum
Tetrapanax papyriferus

265. Bu zhong yi qi tang 补中益气汤
Central Restoration and Qi-
Enhancing Decoction

Astragalus spp., dried root
Codonopsis pilosula
Atractylodes macrocephala
Glycyrrhiza uralensis, fried
Angelica sinensis
Citrus tangerina, fruit skin
Cimicifuga foetida
Bupleurum chinense
Ref: 157 (6), 165 (2, 3), 170 (6)

266. Bu yang huan wu tang 补阳还
五汤

Yang-Restoring Decoction

Astragalus spp., fresh roots
Angelica sinensis

Paeonia lactiflora, red
Ligustinum wallichii
Prunus persica
Carthamus tinctorius
Pheretima aspergillum
Ref: 157 (9)

267. Bu xin dan 补心丹
Heart (Yin)-Restoring Pill

Panax ginseng, or
    Codonopsis pilosula
Scrophularia ningpoensis
Salvia miltiorrhiza
Poria cocos, body
Polygala tenuifolia
Platycodon grandiflorum
Angelica sinensis
Asparagus chochinchinensis
Ophiopogon japonicus
Biota orientalis, kernel
Ziziphus jujuba, red
Schisandra chinensis
Rehmannia glutinosa, fresh
Make into pills with honey; coat
    with cinnabar; 9 grams each.
    Take one twice daily.
Ref: 158 (13), 164 (2), 299 (28)

268. Bu fei tang 补肺汤
Lung (Qi)-Restoring Decoction

Panax ginseng
Morus alba, root skin
Astragalus spp., dried root
Rehmannia glutinosa, cooked
Schisandra chinensis
Aster tartaricus
Ref: 166 (4), 301 (33)

269. Yue bi jia zhu tang 越婢加朮汤
Atractylodes Wind-Dissipating
    Decoction

Ephedra sinica
Gypsum
Zingiber officinale, fresh
Glycyrrhiza uralensis
Ziziphus jujuba, fruit
Atractylodes macrocephala

270. Yue bi tang 越婢汤

Wind-Dissipating Decoction

Ephedra sinica, stalk
Gypsum
Glycyrrhiza uralensis
Zingiber officinale, fresh
Ziziphus jujuba, fruit
Ref: 169 (1)

271. Yang he tang 阳和汤

Yang-Warming Decoction

Rehmannia glutinosa, cooked
Brassica alba
Cervus nippon, antler gelatin
Cinnamomum cassia, bark
Ephedra sinica, stalk
Zingiber officinale, toasted ash
Glycyrrhiza uralensis
Ref: 157 (7)

272. Lu rong da bu tang 鹿茸大补汤

Cervus Velvet Major Restorative

Cervus nippon, antler velvet
Cistanche salsa
Eucommia ulmoides
Paeonia lactiflora, white
Atractylodes macrocephala
Aconitum carmichaeli
Cinnamomum cassia, bark
Panax ginseng
Schisandra chinensis
Dendrobium nobile
Pinellia ternata
Astragalus spp., dried root
Poria cocos, body

Angelica sinensis
Rehmannia glutinosa, cooked
Glycyrrhiza uralensis
Ref: 166 (5)

273. Huang tu tang 黄土汤

Yellow Earth Decoction

Stove soil
Glycyrrhiza uralensis
Atractylodes macrocephala, fried
Aconitum carmichaeli
Rehmannia glutinosa, cooked
Equus asinus
Scutellaria baicalensis
Ref: 157 (9)

274. Huang qi jian zhong tang 黄芪建中汤

Astragalus Central-Strengthening Decoction

No. 30, plus:
Astragalus spp., dried root
Ref: 157 (5)

275. Huang qin hua shi tang 黄芩滑石汤

Scutellaria-Talc Decoction

Scutellaria baicalensis
Talc
Poria cocos, body
Areca catechu, fruit peel
Amomum cardamomum
Tetrapanax papyriferus
Polyporus umbellatus
Ref: 170 (4)

276. Huang lian shang qing wan 黄连上清丸

Coptis Upper Cooling Pill

Coptis chinensis
Scutellaria baicalensis

Phellodendron amurense
Gardenia jasminoides
Chrysanthemum, white
Angelica sinensis
Platycodon grandiflorum
Pueraria lobata
Mentha haplocalyx
Scrophularia ningpoensis
Trichosanthes kirilowii
Ligustinum wallichii
Curcuma longa, root stalk
Forsythia suspensa, fruit
Rheum palmatum
Ref: 168 (1)

277. Huang lian qing xin yin 黄连清
    心饮
Coptis Heart-Clearing Drink
Coptis chinensis
Rehmannia glutinosa, fresh
Angelica sinensis
Glycyrrhiza uralensis
Ziziphus jujuba, seed
Poria cocos, grown on pine root
Polygala tenuifolia
Panax ginseng
Nelumbo nucifera, seed
Ref: 166 (5), 302 (35)

278. Huang lian jie du tang 黄连解
    毒汤
Coptis Poison-Eliminating
    Decoction
Coptis chinensis
Scutellaria baicalensis
Phellodendron amurense
Gardenia jasminoides
Ref: 156 (2), 170 (6)

279. Huang lian e jiao tang 黄连阿
    胶汤
Coptis-Gelatin Decoction

Coptis chinensis
Equus asinus
Scutellaria baicalensis
Paeonia lactiflora, white
Ref: 158 (13), 162 (11)

280. Huang lian e jiao ji zi huang
    tang 黄连阿胶鸡子黄汤
Coptis-Gelatin-Egg Yolk Decoction
Coptis chinensis
Scutellaria baicalensis
Paeonia lactiflora
Equus asinus
Gallus gallus, egg yolk
Ref: 165 (2)

281. Yu dai wan 愈带丸
Vaginitis Pill
Toona sinensis
Paeonia lactiflora, white
Alpinia officinarum, ash
Phellodendron amurense, ash
Ref: 158 (12)

282. Xin jia xiang ru yin 新加香薷饮
Newly Augmented Elsholtzia Drink
Elsholtzia splendens
Lonicera japonica, flower
Dolichos lablab, fresh flower
Magnolia officinalis, bark
Forsythia suspensa, fruit
Ref: 159 (3)

283. Hua shi bu gan san 滑氏补肝散
Liver-Restoring Powder
Ziziphus jujuba, seed
Rehmannia glutinosa, cooked
Atractylodes macrocephala
Angelica sinensis
Cornus officinalis
Dioscorea opposita

Ligustinum wallichii
Chaenomeles lagenaria
Angelica pubescens
Schisandra chinensis

Ref: 163 (1)

284. Nuan gan jian 暖肝煎
Liver-Warming Fry

Angelica sinensis
Lycium chinense, ripe fruit
Foeniculum vulgare
Cinnamomum cassia, bark
Lindera strychnifolia
Aquilaria agallocha
Poria cocos, body
Zingiber officinale, fresh

Ref: 157 (8), 163 (1)

285. Zi zao yang ying tang 滋燥养营汤
Moistening Encampment-Restoring Decoction

Angelica sinensis
Rehmannia glutinosa, fresh
Paeonia lactiflora
Scutellaria baicalensis
Gentiana macrophylla
Saposhnikovia divaricata
Glycyrrhiza uralensis

Ref: 170 (5)

286. Dang gui si ni tang 当归四逆汤
Angelica Four Contrary Decoction

Angelica sinensis
Cinnamomum cassia, branch
Paeonia lactiflora, white
Asarum heterotropoides
Glycyrrhiza uralensis, fried
Akebia quinata, or
    Spatholobus suberectus
Ziziphus jujuba, fruit

Ref: 157 (5), 163 (12)

287. Dang gui jian zhong tang 当归建中汤
Angelica Central Strengthening Decoction

No. 30, plus:
Angelica sinensis

Ref: 157 (5)

288. Dang gui bu xue tang 当归补血汤
Angelica Blood-Restoring Decoction

Astragalus spp., dried root
Angelica sinensis

Ref: 157 (6), 158 (2)

289. Dang gui long hui wan 当归龙荟丸
Angelica-Gentiana-Aloe Pill

Gentiana scabra
Scutellaria baicalensis
Gardenia jasminoides
Angelica sinensis
Coptis chinensis
Phellodendron amurense
Rheum palmatum
Aloe vera
Isatis indigotica
Saussurea lappa
Moschus moschiferus

Ref: 156 (2), 164 (1), 295 (20)

290. Ge gen tang 葛根汤
Pueraria Decoction

Ephedra sinica, stalk
Cinnamomum cassia, branch
Glycyrrhiza uralensis
Pueraria lobata
Paeonia lactiflora, white
Zingiber officinale, fresh
Ziziphus jujuba, fruit

Ref: 160 (7)

291. Ge gen huang qin huang lian tang 葛根黄芩黄连汤

Kudzu, *Coptis*, and *Scutellaria* Decoction

Pueraria lobata
Scutellaria baicalensis
Coptis chinensis
Glycyrrhiza uralensis
Ref: 156 (2)

292. Wan ying wan 万应丸

All-Purpose Worm-Eliminating Pill

Pharbitis nil, black
Areca catechu, seed
Sparganium stoloniferum
Curcuma zeodaria
Saussurea lappa
Polyporus mylittae
Ref: 171 (12)

293. Cong chi tang 葱豉汤
Allium-Glycine Decoction

Allium fistulosum, or *Nelumbo nucifera*, pistils or stamen
Glycine max, seed
Ref: 156 (1), 168 (1)

294. Ting li da zao xie fei tang 葶苈大枣泻肺汤

Lepidium-Ziziphus Lung-Clearing Decoction

Lepidium apetalum
Ziziphus jujuba, fruit
Ref: 157 (10), 171 (11)

295. Da yuan yin 达原饮
Purifying Drink

Scutellaria baicalensis
Paeonia lactiflora, white
Magnolia officinalis, bark

Amomum tsao-ko
Anemarrhena asphodeloides
Glycyrrhiza uralensis
Areca catechu, seed
Zingiber officinale, fresh
Ziziphus jujuba, fruit
Ref: 170 (7)

296. Lei shi qing lian di shu fa fang 雷氏清凉涤暑法方

Master Lei's Cooling Heat-Cleansing Prescription

Talc
Glycyrrhiza uralensis, powder
Artemisia apiacea, fruit
Forsythia suspensa, fruit
Poria cocos Yunnan
Tetrapanax papyriferus, Szechuan
Dolichos lablab, seed
Ref: 169 (3)

297. Shi pi yin 实脾饮
Spleen-Strengthening Decoction

Atractylodes macrocephala
Magnolia officinalis, bark
Chaenomeles lagenaria
Saussurea lappa
Amomum tsao-ko
Areca catechu, fruit peel or seed
Poria cocos, body
Zingiber officinale, dry
Aconitum carmichaeli
Glycyrrhiza uralensis, stir-fried
Zingiber officinale, fresh
Ziziphus jujuba, fruit
Ref: 157 (11)

298. Man xing lan wei yan tang 慢性阑尾炎汤

Chronic Appendicitis Decoction
Paeonia lactiflora, red
Spatholobus suberectus

Angelica sinensis
Paeonia suffruticosa
Lindera strychnifolia
Citrus tangerina, fruit peel
Melia toosendan
Ref: 157 (7)

299. Huai hua san 槐花散
Sophora Powder

Sophora japonica, fried flower
Biota orientalis, fried leaf
Schizonepeta tenuifolia, fried
Poncirus trifoliata, fried fruit
Ref: 157 (9)

300. Huai jiao wan 槐角丸
Sophora Pill

Sophora japonica, fruit
Saposhnikovia divaricata
Sanguisorba officinalis
Angelica sinensis
Poncirus trifoliata, almost ripe fruit
Scutellaria baicalensis
Ref: 157 (9)

301. Ge xia zhu yu tang 隔下遂瘀汤
Subdiaphragmatic Blood-
    Mobilizing Decoction
Angelica sinensis
Ligustinum wallichii
Paeonia lactiflora, red
Prunus persica
Carthamus tinctorius
Pleropus pselaphon, fried
Paeonia suffruticosa
Lindera strychnifolia
Corydalis yanhusuo
Cyperus rotundus
Poncirus trifoliata, almost ripe fruit
Glycyrrhiza uralensis
Ref: 157 (9)

302. Wei jing tang 苇茎汤
Phragmites Decoction

Phragmites communis
Coix lachryma-jobi
Prunus persica
Benincasa hispida, seed
Ref: 157 (7), 166 (4)

303. Cang zhu bai hu tang 苍朮白
    虎汤
Atractylodes White Tiger
    Decoction

No. 91, plus:
Atractylodes macrocephala
Ref: 156 (2), 170 (4)

304. Yuan zhi tang 远志汤
Polygala Decoction

Polygala tenuifolia
Rehmannia glutinosa, cooked
Saposhnikovia divaricata
Panax ginseng
Chrysanthemum morifolium
Atractylodes macrocephala
Poria cocos, grown on pine root
Peucedanum praeruptorum
Poncirus trifoliata, almost ripe
    fruit
Zingiber officinale, fresh
Cinnamomum cassia
Ref: 167 (6)

305. Yin qiao jie du wan 银翘解
    毒丸
Lonicera Poison-Relieving Pill

Lonicera japonica, bud
Forsythia suspensa, fruit
Arctium lappa
Mentha haplocalyx
Schizonepeta tenuifolia, ear
Glycine max, seed

Platycodon grandiflorum
Glycyrrhiza uralensis
Phyllostachys nigra, leaf
Ref: 156 (1)

306. Yin qiao san 银翘散
Lonicera Powder
No. 305, plus:
Phragmites communis
Ref: 156 (1), 159 (3), 168 (1), 290 (10)

307. Zeng ye cheng qi tang 增液承气汤
Moistening Qi-Regulating Decoction
Rheum palmatum
Mirabilite
Scrophularia ningpoensis
Ophiopogon japonicus
Rehmannia glutinosa, fresh
Ref: 156 (3), 170 (5)

308. Run chang wan 润肠丸
Intestine-Lubricating Pill
Rheum palmatum
Angelica sinensis
Angelica sylvestris
Prunus persica
Cannabis sativa
Ref: 156 (3)

309. Tiao wei cheng qi tang 调胃承气汤
Stomach- and Qi-Regulating Decoction
Rheum palmatum
Mirabilite
Glycyrrhiza uralensis
Ref: 156 (3), 161 (8)

310. Suan zao ren tang 酸枣仁汤
Ziziphus Decoction
Ziziphus jujuba, seed
Anemarrhena asphodeloides
Poria cocos, body
Ligustinum wallichii
Glycyrrhiza uralensis, fried
Ref: 158 (13), 164 (1)

311. Yang xin tang 养心汤
Heart-Strengthening Decoction
Astragalus, dried root
Poria cocos, body
Angelica sinensis
Ligustinum wallichii
Pinellia ternata, treated
Glycyrrhiza uralensis
Biota orientalis, seed
Ziziphus jujuba, seed
Polygala tenuifolia
Schisandra chinensis
Panax ginseng
Cinnamomum cassia, bark
Ref: 164 (2), 293 (16)

312. Yang yin qing fei tan 养阴清肺汤
Yin-Generating Lung-Clearing Decoction
Rehmannia glutinosa, fresh
Ophiopogon japonicus
Scrophularia ningpoensis
Paeonia suffruticosa
Fritillaria cirrhosa
Glycyrrhiza uralensis, fresh
Mentha haplocalyx
Paeonia lactiflora, white
Ref: 156 (2), 166 (4)

313. Yang zang tang 养脏汤
Zang-Strengthening Decoction
Terminalia chebula

Myristica fragrans
Papaver somniferum
Codonopsis pilosula
Atractylodes macrocephala
Glycyrrhiza uralensis, fried
Cinnamomum cassia, bark
Angelica sinensis
Paeonia lactiflora, white
Saussurea lappa
Ref: 158 (12)

314. Dao chi san 导赤散

Heat-Reducing Diuretic

Rehmannia glutinosa, fresh
Akebia quinata
Glycyrrhiza uralensis, terminal root
Phyllostachys nigra, leaf

Ref: 156 (2), 164 (2), 167 (8), 170
  (6), 293 (17), 294 (18)

315. Dao tan ding zhi fa fang 导痰定
  志法方

Phlegm-Wind-Reducing Sedating
  Prescription

Gastrodia elata
Buthus martensi
Pinellia ternata
Arisaema consanguineum, treated
  with bile
Citrus tangerina, red scraping from
  fruit peel
Acorus gramineus
Poncirus trifoliata, tiny fruit
Poria cocos, body
Phyllostachys nigra, inner stalk
  lining

Ref: 165 (2), 169 (1), 171 (9)

316. Dao tan tang 导痰汤

Phlegm-Reducing Decoction
  No. 7, plus:

Atractylodes macrocephala
Gastrodia elata
Ref: 157 (10)

317. Ju pi zhu ru tang 橘皮竹茹汤

Citrus-Phyllostachys Decoction

Citrus tangerina, fruit peel
Phyllostachys nigra, inner stalk
  lining
Zingiber officinale, fresh
Ziziphus jujuba, fruit
Glycyrrhiza uralensis
Codonopsis pilosula

Ref: 157 (8)

318. Du shen tang 独参汤

Ginseng Decoction

Panax ginseng
Ref: 157 (5)

319. Du huo ji sheng tang 独活寄
  生汤

Angelica Liver-Kidney-
  Strengthening and Evil-
  Dissipating Decoction

Angelica pubescens
Gentiana macrocephala
Saposhnikovia divaricata
Ligustinum wallichii
Asarum heterotropoides
Loranthus yadoriki
Achyranthes bidentata
Eucommia ulmoides
Angelica sinensis
Paeonia lactiflora, white
Rehmannia glutinosa, cooked
Poria cocos, body
Codonopsis pilosula
Cinnamomum cassia, branch
Glycyrrhiza uralensis

Ref: 157 (5)

320. Long dan xie gan tang 龙胆泻肝汤

Gentiana Liver-Clearing Decoction

Gentiana scabra
Scutellaria baicalensis
Gardenia jasminoides
Alisma plantago-aquatica
Akebia quinata
Plantago asiatica, seed
Angelica sinensis
Rehmannia glutinosa, fresh
Bupleurum chinense
Glycyrrhiza uralensis

Ref: 156 (2), 164 (1), 167 (6), 170 (6)

321. Ji sheng shen qi wan 济生肾气丸

Kidney-Yang-Restoring Edema-
Reducing Pill

No. 263, plus:
Achyranthes bidentata
Plantago asiatica, seed

Ref: 157 (6), 167 (5)

322. Suo quan wan 缩泉丸

Urine-Reducing Pill

Alpinia oxyphylla
Lindera strychnifolia
Dioscorea opposita

Ref: 167 (5)

323. Dai ge san 黛蛤散

Isatis-Venerupis Powder

Isatis indigotica, 1 part
Venerupis phillipinarum, 10 parts
Each dose 9 grams.

Ref: 157 (10)

324. Gui pi tang 归脾汤

Codonopsis Spleen-Restoring
Decoction

Codonopsis pilosula
Atractylodes macrocephala
Poria cocos, grown on pine root
Astragalus, dried root
Glycyrrhiza uralensis
Angelica sinensis
Ziziphus jujuba, seed
Euphoria longan
Polygala tenuifolia
Saussurea lappa
Zingiber officinale, fresh
Ziziphus jujuba, fruit

Ref: 157 (6), 165 (2)

325. Xie xin tang 泻心汤

Strength Heat-Eliminating
Decoction

Rheum palmatum
Coptis chinensis
Scutellaria baicalensis

Ref: 156 (3)

326. Xie fei san 泻肺散

Lung Heat-Eliminating Powder

Morus alba, root skin
Lycium chinense, root skin
Glycyrrhiza uralensis, fresh
Oryza sativa, grain

Ref: 156 (2), 166 (4), 170 (6), 285
(1), 300 (30)

327. Xie qing wan 泻青丸

(Liver) Fire Cathartic Pill

Gentiana scabra
Gardenia jasminoides
Rheum palmatum
Ligustinum wallichii
Angelica sinensis
Angelica sylvestris
Saposhnikovia divaricata
Phyllostachys nigra, leaf

Ref: 170 (6)

328. Xie huang san 泻黄散

(Spleen) Fire Cathartic Powder

Saposhnikovia divaricata
Agastache rugosa
Gardenia jasminoides
Gypsum
Glycyrrhiza uralensis
Ref: 170 (6)

329. Zhen gan xi feng tang 镇肝熄
风汤

Liver-Controlling Wind-
Extinguishing Decoction

Hematite
Achyranthes bidentata
Fossil bones
Ostrea rivularis
Chinemys reevesii
Paeonia lactiflora, white, fresh
Scrophularia ningpoensis
Asparagus chochinchinensis
Melia toosendan
Hordeum vulgare
Artemisia apiacea, whole herb
Glycyrrhiza uralensis

Ref: 158 (14), 164 (1), 296 (23)

330. Shuan jie san 双解散

Double (Interior and Exterior)
Dissipation Powder

Schizonepeta tenuifolia, whole herb
Saposhnikovia divaricata
Gardenia jasminoides
Scutellaria baicalensis
Angelica sinensis
Paeonia lactiflora, white
Platycodon grandiflorum
Glycyrrhiza uralensis
Ephedra sinica, stalk
Mentha haplocalyx
Ligustinum wallichii
Forsythia suspensa, fruit

Gypsum
Talc
Atractylodes macrocephala
Ref: 170 (7)

331. Meng shi gun tan wan 礞石滚
痰丸

Chlorite Phlegm-Eliminating Pill
Chlorite
Aquilaria agallocha
Rheum palmatum
Scutellaria baicalensis
Ref: 171 (9)

332. Huo po xia ling tang 藿香夏
苓汤

Agastache-Magnolia-Pinellia-Poria
Decoction

Agastache rugosa
Magnolia officinalis, bark
Pinellia ternata
Poria cocos, body
Prunus armeniaca
Coix lachryma-jobi
Amomum cardamomum
Polyporus embellatus
Alisma plantago-aquatica
Glycine max, seed
Ref: 169 (4)

333. Huo xiang zhen qi san 藿香正
气散

Agastache Qi-Restoring Powder

Agastache rugosa
Perilla frutescens, leaf
Angelica dahurica
Areca catechu, fruit peel
Poria cocos, body
Atractylodes macrocephala, or
other species
Citrus tangerina, fruit skin
Pinellia ternata, treated

Magnolia officinalis, bark
Platycodon grandiflorum
Glycyrrhiza uralensis
Ref: 157 (11), 159 (3), 169 (1, 2, 3), 170 (7)

334. Su zi jiang qi tang 苏子降气汤
Perilla Qi-Lowering Decoction

Perilla frutescens, fruit
Pinellia ternata, treated
Glycyrrhiza uralensis, fried
Peucedanum praeruptorum
Magnolia officinalis, bark
Citrus tangerina, peel scraping
Angelica sinensis
Cinnamomum cassia, bark
Zingiber officinale, fresh
Ref: 157 (8), 166 (4)

335. Su he xiang wan 苏合香丸
Liquidambar Pill

Liquidambar orientalis
Styrax benzoin
Rhinoceros horn
Dryobalanops aromatica, resin
Cyperus rotundus
Saussurea lappa
Atractylodes macrocephala
Aquilaria aggallocha
Syzygium aromaticum
Moschus moschiferus
Cinnabar
Ref: 164 (1)

336. Zhong ru bu fei tang 钟乳补肺汤
Stalactite Lung-Strengthening Decoction

Panax ginseng
Ophiopogon japonicus
Schisandra chinensis
Tussilago farfara

Aster tartaricus
Morus alba, root skin
Stalactite
Quartz
Oryza sativa var. *glutinosa*
Zingiber officinale, fresh
Ziziphus jujuba, fruit
Cinnamomum cassia, tender branch
Ref: 166 (4)

337. Qu tao tang 驱绦汤
Tapeworm Decoction

Cucurbita moschata
Areca catechu, seed
Do not use in pregnancy.
Ref: 157 (7)

338. Qu gou tang 驱钩汤
Hookworm Decoction

Torreya grandis
Areca catechu, seed
Sargentodoxa cureata
Dryopteris crassirhizoma
Take twice daily for 3 days; each time follow with 3 petals of fresh *Allium sativum*.
Ref: 157 (7)

339. Bie jia yin zi 鳖甲饮子
Purifying and (Spleen) Swelling-Reducing Drink

Amyda sinensis, fried in vinegar
Atractylodes macrocephala, root stalk
Astragalus, dried root
Ligustinum wallichii
Paeonia lactiflora, white
Areca catechu, seed
Amomum tsao-ko
Magnolia officinalis, bark
Citrus tangerina, ripe peel

Glycyrrhiza uralensis
Zingiber officinale, fresh
Ziziphus jujuba, fruit
Prunus mume, unripe fruit, slight amount
Ref: 157 (7)

340. Juan bi tong luo fa fang 蠲痹通络法方

Dampness-Dissolving Circulation-Enhancing Prescription

Angelica pubescens
Clematis chinensis
Cinnamomum cassia, tender branch
Angelica sinensis
Loranthus yadoriki
Piper kadsura
Homalomena occulta
Saposhnikovia divaricata
Commiphora myrrha
Asarum heterotropoides
Aconitum carmichaeli, root
Astragalus, raw root
Piper wallichii
Angelica sylvestris
Boswellia carterii
Atractylodes, root stalk

Ref: 169 (4)

341. Juan bi tang 蠲痹汤

Dampness-Dissolving (Qi-Enhancing) Decoction

Angelica sylvestris
Saposhnikovia divaricata
Curcuma longa, stalk
Angelica sinensis
Paeonia lactiflora, red
Astragalus, dried root
Glycyrrhiza uralensis, fried
Zingiber officinale, fresh
Ziziphus jujuba, fruit

Ref: 157 (5)

342. Can shi tang 蚕矢汤

Bombyx Droppings Decoction

Coptis chinensis
Scutellaria baicalensis
Gardenia jasminoides
Evodia rutaecarpa
Pinellia ternata
Glycine max, sprouting seed
Coix lachryma-jobi
Tetrapanax papyriferus
Chaenomeles lagenaria
Bombyx mori, larval droppings

Ref: 171 (7)

Appendix: Illustrative Cases

Case 1: LB, 22-year-old male

LB was chilled on arising, with heaviness in the body, headache, generalized body aching, nasal congestion, and fever. He continued to work. The following day he developed a cough, productive of yellow sputum. He no longer felt cold, but high fever persisted, with thirst and desire for cold drinks, dry constipation, and scanty and dark yellow urine. When examined, he was febrile, had a red complexion, a red tongue with a dry yellow coating, and a smooth and rapid pulse.

Analysis. The presence of both chills and fever indicated that the illness was in the exterior. The heaviness of the body could be due to Cold in the exterior. However, the loss of chills but rise in fever the next day indicated that the disease was leaving the exterior and interiorizing. The thirst with desire for cold drink, dry constipation, scanty and dark yellow urine, red complexion, red tongue with dry yellow coating, and smooth and rapid pulse were all symptoms of interior Heat. In combination with a cough that was productive of yellow sputum, these clearly indicated that the illness was caused by Heat strength in the lung.

Diagnosis. Heat strength in the lung.

Treatment. Use formulas 221 and 326 for the Heat in the lung. As the Heat becomes dissipated from the lung, if there is any further symptom of Cold, then follow with formulas 8 and 244.

Case 2: LC, 43-year-old male

For years, LC had had repeated epigastric pain, generally after eating foods of a cold nature or when the weather was changing. The pain was lessened either by pressure or by applying heat over the area of pain. His appetite was chronically poor, and there was gradual but steady weight loss, with generalized weakness and fatigue. Urination and defecation were both normal. When examined, the pulse was deep, small, but stringy; the tongue was pale and its coating thin and white.

Analysis. Because the epigastric pain had lasted for years, the illness was in the interior and was of deficiency. The precipitation by foods of a cold nature and the preference for epigastric pressure or heat indicated Cold and deficiency. A weak stomach did not accept food well, hence the poor appetite, consequent weight loss, and weakness. The deep pulse also reflected an interior illness, the smallness reflecting deficiency, and the stringiness pain. The pallor of the tongue and the thin whiteness of the coating both suggested Cold in deficiency.

Diagnosis. Interior Cold and deficiency with stomach pain.

Treatment. Use formula 138, without *Forsythia*, but with added *Aconitum carmichaeli* and *Zingiber officinale*.

Case 3: CA, 65-year-old male

CA had a chronically weak constitution, marked cold intolerance, and chronically cold hands and feet. Even slight activity produced perspiration and shortness of breath. One night he stayed out until very late. The next morning he had headache, nasal congestion, increased cold intolerance, and fever. When examined, his pulse was faint and small and his tongue pale with a thin white coating.

Analysis. The chronically weak constitution, cold intolerance, cold hands and feet, and lack of exercise tolerance all pointed to deficiency of Yang Qi. The fever, increase in cold intolerance, headache, and nasal congestion were all due to Cold in the exterior. Nevertheless, because of the chronic Yang deficiency, the pulse was faint and small rather than superficial and tight, as might be expected for an exterior illness, and similarly the tongue was pale.

Diagnosis. Exterior strength in Yang deficiency.

Treatment. Start with formula 176, and follow with formula 249.

Case 4: WB, 25-year-old male

WB overindulged one day and subsequently had abdominal bloating and diarrhea. He consulted a physician, who thought he had diarrhea from interior deficiency and prescribed formula 233 with added halloysite and limonite to warm internally and to stop diarrhea. The diarrhea did stop, but the distention worsened. The patient became drowsy and dull, with periodic agitation, cold hands and feet, dry and red lips, and scanty yellow urine. When examined, the pulse was elusive at moderate depth, but forceful when palpated deeply. The tongue was red, with a dry and black coating.

Analysis. The patient was young and strong. His illness began with excessive eating, with subsequent distention and diarrhea; such symptoms usually result from Heat strength. The other physician mistakenly treated him with a formula designed to warm and restore, thus aggravating the illness. Although the diarrhea did stop, the Heat strength became trapped internally, so that the patient's hands and feet became cold and his sensorium became clouded. The elusive pulse suggested a Cold disease, but the lips were red and dry, the urine scanty and yellow, the pulse forceful on deep palpation, and the tongue coating black and dry. These all indicated internal Heat strength. The erroneous use of a warming and restorative drug caused further increase in the internal Heat with blockage of Yang Qi.

Diagnosis. Genuine Heat internally with false Cold externally.

Treatment. Formula: cooked *Rehmannia glutinosa, Anemarrhena asphodeloides, Phellodendron amurense, Alisma plantago-aquatica, Mentha haplocalyx, Phragmites communis,* and *Chrysanthemum indicum.*

Case 5: TK, 45-year-old male

TK had chronic diarrhea, which gradually responded to warming and restorative drugs. Recently, he repeatedly felt hot but without thirst, preferred to sleep with blankets, and had fatigue with no desire to move around. He self-diagnosed Cold injury and self-administered drugs for acrid-warming diaphoresis. Following that, he developed persistent heavy sweating, high fever yet no thirst, the desire to wrap himself completely in a blanket, a weak voice, shallow respirations, and scanty pale urine. When examined, his pulse was rapid, large, but weak, and his tongue pale, moist, and without coating.

Analysis. Chronic diarrhea responding to warming restoratives was due to deficiency Cold. As the diarrhea resolved the Yang Qi recovered, hence the hot feeling. The absence of thirst indicated that the hot feeling was not due to interior Heat. The preference for blankets and the fatigue with no desire to move about were because the patient had not completely recovered from the deficiency Cold. The patient mistook his condition (improving, but incomplete recovery from deficiency Cold) to be due to Cold injury in the exterior and thus took acrid-warming diaphoretic drugs. In a body that still had Yang deficiency, this method of treatment resulted in persistent heavy perspiration and further weakening of Yang Qi, hence the weak voice, shallow respirations, rapid, large, but weak pulse, and the symptoms of impending collapse. Yang deficiency led to interior Cold, hence his desire to wrap himself in blankets. The pale and moist tongue without coating also indicated deficiency Cold. The rise in fever following diaphoresis was due to trapping of Yin Cold internally and externalization of Yang Qi.

Diagnosis. Genuine Cold internally with false Heat externally.

Treatment. Use formula 22, with added *Pueraria lobata*, *Bupleurum chinense*, and *Cimicifuga foetida.* Add *Phragmites communis* and *Lonicera japonica*, bud, for fever.

Case 6: WD, 21-year-old male

WD took a cold-water bath. That night he developed cold intolerance and fever. He took one pill of formula 305. The fever persisted and the cold intolerance worsened. He had no perspiration but developed generalized body aching, headache with nasal congestion, a pale tongue with thin white coating, and a tight and superficial pulse.

Analysis. This case demonstrated very typical features. The illness resulted from external Cold, being localized in the exterior of Greater Yang; it was thus a case of exterior Cold. Cold in the exterior caused the cold intolerance and absence of perspiration. The nature of Cold is to congeal, and impedance in the function of the sinews and muscles caused the body aching. The nose is the exterior opening of the lung, so that impedance of the lung Qi produced nasal congestion. The tongue and pulse findings also indicated exterior strength disease caused by Wind and Cold. Formula 305 was acrid-cooling and was therefore inappropriate. The proper treatment was dispersion of the exterior by diaphoresis, using an acrid-warming diaphoretic.

Diagnosis. Cold strength in the exterior.

Treatment. Formula: *Ephedra sinica*, *Perilla frutescens*, *Angelica sylvestris*, *Taraxacum mongolicum*, and fresh root stalk of *Zingiber officinale*. Following a dose, instruct the patient to stay under a blanket.

Case 7: LD, 57-year-old male

LD was exposed to cold and developed cold intolerance and fever. Two days later, he developed alternating chills and fever, with bitter taste, chest tightness and discomfort, and loss of appetite. His tongue coating was slightly yellow and dry, and his pulse stringy and moderately rapid.

Analysis. At the outset the illness was due to exterior damage by Wind and Cold. The development of recurrent chills and fever, chest tightness, and so on indicated that the disease evil was progressing internally. The absence of such interior symptoms as diaphoresis, thirst, or large pulses indicated that the illness had not reached the interior. Thus, the disease evil was in the Lesser Yang region, with symptoms that were half exterior and half interior.

Diagnosis. Cold strength in Lesser Yang.

Treatment. Use forumula 149.

Case 8: CC, 27-year-old male

CC had a strong constitution and was well developed. Four days previously he had been exposed to the Heat evil and had developed high fever, worsening dizziness, and loss of consciousness. He had been given formula 101 and formula 91, to no avail. When examined, he was still feverish, with deep red flushing of the face and dryness of the lips. He was alternately unconscious and delirious. His abdomen was distended, and he had been constipated for days. His pulse was deep and strong.

Analysis. This illness resulted from Heat strength in the Bright Yang Fu organs. The Heat evil was strong, hence the fever and facial flushing. The abdominal distention, constipation, and deep and strong pulse indicated that the disease was in the Bright Yang Fu organs. The Heat damaged the body fluids, causing dryness of the lips. The Heat evil invading the heart caused delirium and intermittent coma. Because the illness arose from the internal transmission of the Heat evil rather than internal accumulation of poison blocking the openings, such drugs as formula 101, which unblock conduits, would be ineffective. In the absence of severe thirst, parching, or profuse perspiration, formula 91 would be inappropriate. The proper treatment consisted of eliminating the internal Heat evil by catharsis, using, for example, formula 19. Following elimination of the Heat evil, the body fluids could recover and the symptoms resolve. Following a good response, one should generally continue with cooling drinks and fluid-producing foods.

Diagnosis. Heat in Bright Yang, with damage to body fluids.

Treatment. Use formula 92.

Case 9: CJ, 36-year-old male

CJ was chronically weak. Because of dietary indiscretion, he developed sudden abdominal pain, vomiting, and diarrhea. He took an unidentified drug, and the vomiting stopped. The abdominal pain and diarrhea persisted, however, and over the following week he further developed abdominal distention and loss of taste and the desire for drink. Just before his arrival, his condition deteriorated, with cold intolerance, generalized aching with body heaviness, and cold hands and feet. His tongue coating was white and greasy and his pulse deep and faint.

Analysis. Vomiting and diarrhea due to dietary indiscretion in a chronically weak patient should belong in the Greater Yin region, with chronic deficiency of the spleen. Inadequate treatment permitted progression of the illness (into Lesser Yin) to produce symptoms of generalized deficiency Cold. Weakness of the kidney Yang in the Lesser Yin did not allow warming of the spleen, so that the Yang Qi deteriorated, allowing the symptoms of cold intolerance, cold extremities, deep and faint pulse, and so forth. The pale and greasy tongue coating indicated spleen deficiency. If not treated promptly and adequately, the Yang Qi in the Lesser Yin region would deteriorate further, with the risk of collapse due to Yang destruction.

Diagnosis. Deficiency of Yang Qi in Lesser Yin, resulting from chronic spleen deficiency.

Treatment. Use formula 237, with added *Panax ginseng* and *Astragalus* spp. (moist-stir-fried).

Case 10: SF, 30-year-old male

SF had fever and headache for two days, with mild aversion to wind and cold, nasal congestion, and mild cough. His tongue coating was thin and white, the tongue red along the sides and at the tip, and his pulse was superficial and rapid.

Analysis. The fever and cold aversion are symptoms of the guard level. The mild aversion to wind and cold, the thin and white tongue coating, and the superficial and rapid pulse indicate the illness was due to Wind and Heat.

Diagnosis. Wind and Heat at the guard level.

Treatment. Use formula 181. (For more severe cases, formula 306 may be more potent.)

Case 11: LK, 5-year-old female

LK developed acute high fever in midsummer, with headache, thirst with desire for cold drinks, restlessness, and diaphoresis. Two days later, the sensorium became clouded and she showed somnolence, with persistent high fever. The tongue was deep red and the coating yellow. The pulse was tidal and rapid.

Analysis. At midsummer, the Heat evil tends to invade and progress rapidly. The precipitous development of high fever, headache, thirst, and diaphoresis were all symptoms of marked Heat. The disturbed sensorium, somnolence, and dark red tongue all pointed to disease at the encampment level in the middle position. The yellow tongue coating and the tidal and rapid pulse indicated that Heat was still strong at the pneuma level.

Diagnosis. Heat at both pneuma and encampment levels.

Treatment. Use formula 219.

Case 12: YA, 28-year-old female

YA had high fever and disturbed sensorium that improved with cooling drugs. A week later, she developed trembling of her extremities, fatigue, and weight loss. The tongue was dark red and without coating, and the pulse small and rapid.

Analysis. Although the early symptoms of fever and disturbed sensorium seemed to respond to treatment, the fatigue, weight loss, dark red and coatless tongue, and small, rapid pulse all indicated that the liver and kidney Yin was damaged by the Heat evil. Because the liver and kidney Yin was deficient, the sinews were not adequately nourished, leading to the trembling of the extremities, which was a symptom of internal movement of deficiency Wind.

Diagnosis. Damage of liver and kidney Yin, with internal movement of deficiency Wind.

Treatment. Use formula 128.

Case 13: WK, 35-year-old male

WK had prolonged fever for about two weeks, especially in the afternoon. In addition, his limbs were weak, and he had generalized fatigue. There was tightness in the chest with impeded inspiration. There was no thirst, but stools were watery and urine was scanty and dark yellow. The complexion was pale yellow, the tongue coating greasy and slightly yellow, and the pulse limp and mildly rapid.

Analysis. The fever, weak limbs, fatigue, chest tightness, and watery diarrhea without thirst were symptoms of Dampness immobilized in the interior. The illness was thus one of Dampness and Heat tarrying at the pneuma level. The greasy and slightly yellow tongue coating and the limp and mildly rapid pulse indicated that there was more Dampness than Heat.

Diagnosis. Dampness and Heat at the pneuma level, more Dampness than Heat.

Treatment. Dissolving Dampness and cooling Heat. Use Formula 15 with added raw *Glycyrrhiza uralensis*.

Case 14: LL, 36-year-old female

Three days before, LL developed a sudden chill followed by fever and headache. The next day, the chill gradually cleared but high fever persisted. She started coughing, producing mucous and yellow sputum. There was also left chest pain that was aggravated by coughing, restlessness, and thirst. She was constipated and had scanty and dark urine for the three days. The tongue coating was yellow and greasy, and the pulse smooth and rapid.

Analysis. The sudden onset, chills, fever, and headache all indicated that the disease was at the guard level. The subsequent loss of chills and rise in fever, thirst, and restlessness indicated progression into the pneuma level. The cough and yellow mucous sputum indicated localization in the lung. The chest pain, aggravated by coughing, was due to Phlegm and Heat obstructing the meridians and disharmony of the lung Qi. The constipation and scanty and dark urine indicated interior Heat. The yellow greasy tongue coating and the smooth and rapid pulse were symptoms of Phlegm and Heat trapped internally.

Diagnosis. Heat evil trapped in the lung.

Treatment. Cooling the lung and dissolving Phlegm. Use formula 246 with *Trichosanthes kirilowii*, *Arctium lappa*, and the orange scraping from the peel of *Citrus tangerina*.

Case 15: CK, 35-year-old female

CK had had a miscarriage some six weeks previously, at which time she had lost considerable amounts of blood. Subsequently, she had frequent palpitations, irritability, and insomnia with increased dreaming, and she was easily startled. During the past week, she had overworked herself to the extent that all these symptoms worsened and she became restless, nervous, and unable to sleep at all. Her mouth became dry, her palms and soles hot, her stools dry, her urine yellow, her cheeks flushed red, her tongue tip red with scant coating, and her pulse small and rapid.

Analysis. The blood loss associated with the miscarriage and the subsequent symptoms were clearly due to heart blood insufficiency. During the previous week, excessive activity caused further damage of heart blood, progressing to deficiency of heart Yin, with consequent restless anxiety and other symptoms of burning Fire due to Yin deficiency.

Diagnosis. Heart blood insufficiency; strong Fire due to Yin deficiency.

Treatment. Nourishing Yin to reduce Fire; generating blood to calm Shen. Formula: raw and cooked *Rehmannia glutinosa*, white *Paeonia lactiflora*, *Paeonia suffruticosa*, *Ophiopogon japonicus*, *Angelica sinensis*,

Scutellaria baicalensis, Polygonum multiflorum stalk, fried *Ziziphus jujuba* seed, and fresh *Ostrea rivularis*.

Case 16: ZY, 54-year-old male

For about a year, ZY had periodic tightness in the chest and obstructed respiration. This was aggravated by exertion and alleviated by resting. He often had shortness of breath and palpitations of the heart. In the last three months, the chest congestion and respiratory obstruction worsened to the point of precordial pain on any exertion. This pain lasted three to five minutes each time and occurred three or four times daily. The previous day, the weather had suddenly turned cold, and his chest pain worsened precipitously and came repeatedly. The patient was obese, with pale complexion, fat tongue with milky coating, and a small and stringy pulse.

Analysis. Deficiency of heart Qi caused palpitation of the heart and shortness of breath. Impedance of Qi caused chest tightness and obstructed respiration. Upon exertion, the heart Qi became more deficient, so that it was less able to move. The Qi and blood then became stagnant, causing blockage of the heart meridian and therefore precordial pain. On cold exposure, Qi became congealed, worsening the precordial pain. The fat tongue with creamy coating indicated Dampness and Phlegm.

Diagnosis. Insufficiency of heart Qi, with Cold invasion of the interior and obstruction of the heart meridian.

Treatment. To restore Qi and liven blood, to disperse Cold and release obstruction. Use formula 311, supplemented with formula 233. If interior Cold symptoms persist, may need to use formula 70 in place of formula 233.

Case 17: SG, 30-year-old male

For three days, SG had sores in his mouth and tongue, as well as restlessness, thirst, dark urine with burning sensation during urination, red tongue with a thin yellow coating, and rapid pulse.

Analysis. Mouth sores, restlessness, thirst, red tongue with thin yellow coating, and rapid pulse were all symptoms of Fire. The heart opens to the exterior through the tongue, hence when heart Fire rose to the upper position, the tongue turned red and sores developed. The Fire damaged the body fluids, hence thirst. The Fire heated the heart, hence restlessness. The heart Fire transferred to the small intestine, hence dark urine with burning sensation on urination.

Diagnosis. Heart Fire rising.

Treatment. To cool heart and reduce Fire. Use formula 314.

Case 18: TZ, 29-year-old female

About a week previously, TZ abruptly became hyperactive and excessively talkative, not stopping all day, and developed marked insomnia. She frequently wandered about aimlessly. Her salivation increased dramatically, but her stools became very dry and constipated. The tongue was red with yellow greasy coating, and the pulse was smooth and rapid.

Analysis. The patient showed abnormal activity of Shen. Since the heart houses Shen, the disease was located in the heart. The increased salivation, greasiness of the tongue coating, and smooth pulse reflected Dampness and Phlegm in the interior. The dry stools, yellowness of the tongue coating and redness of the tongue, and rapidity of the pulse reflected Heat strength. This illness thus resulted from the interaction of Phlegm and Heat, both disturbing the heart.

Diagnosis. Disturbance of the heart by Phlegm and Fire.

Treatment. Use formulas 98 and 314 together, with added *Agastache rugosa* and *Eupatorium fortunei.*

Case 19: LM, 18-year-old male

The day before, LM ate cold and raw food. Soon after, he developed abdominal cramps, which improved with application of a hot-water bottle to the abdomen. Appetite and both excretory functions were normal. The tongue coating was thin and the pulse stringy and tight.

Analysis. Cold and raw diet brought on congealment by Cold and impedance of Qi, so that the functions of the small intestine became disturbed. This led to cramping. Warmth improved the circulation of Qi and blood and hence relieved the symptoms. The stringy and tight configuration of the pulse was due to the pain.

Diagnosis. Cold-induced congelation and Qi impedance in the small intestine.

Treatment. Use formula 108. Add formula 14 if pain is not relieved.

Case 20: CN, 35-year-old male

CN was well developed and in good health, but of an impatient and quick-tempered disposition. Four days previously, he was emotionally upset and suddenly developed fluctuating headaches and dizziness, which persisted. When the headaches worsened, his face and head were red and hot, with bloodshot eyes and occasional twitching of the face. He also had ringing in the ears, restlessness, a bitter taste, thirst with desire for cold drinks, dark urine, and dry stools; and he was irascible. His tongue coating was yellow, and his pulse stringy, rapid, and forceful.

Analysis. The patient's impatient and quick-tempered disposition indicated a generally strong liver. The emotional upset caused liver damage by the pent-up anger, which transformed into Fire. Rise of the liver Fire into the head caused the headaches, dizziness, and red and hot face and head. The liver Fire further followed the gallbladder (Lesser Yang) meridian to the ears, causing ringing there. The liver governs anger, thus when liver Fire became strong internally, the patient became irascible and had a bitter taste, dark urine, dry stools, thirst, and a desire for cold drinks. The occasional facial twitching indicated that the liver Fire was already transforming into Wind and moving internally. The yellow tongue coating and the stringy and rapid pulse were also manifestations of liver Fire.

Diagnosis. Fire strength in the liver meridian; internal movement of liver Wind.

Treatment. Use formula 289.

Case 21: LN, 25-year-old female

LN was of quiet and reserved disposition, tending to keep frustrations inside. For some six months, she had frequently felt fluctuating pain in her ribs and chest tightness. She sighed often and was emotionally depressed; she had loss of appetite and gastric fullness, and her menses became scanty. Her tongue coating was thin and her pulse stringy but small.

Analysis. The chronic penting-up of frustrations caused liver damage from congelation of liver Qi, producing rib pains, chest tightness, and frequent sighing. Because liver by its nature tends to move and disperse, liver obstruction influenced the ability of the spleen and stomach to accept and digest, hence her gastric fullness and loss of appetite. Also, blood became deficient, leading to decrease in menses. The thin tongue coating and the small, stringy pulse also reflected liver obstruction and blood insufficiency.

Diagnosis. Liver obstruction with blood deficiency; disharmony of liver and spleen.

Treatment. Use formulas 67 and 258. Formula 55 is also effective but contains *Pinellia ternata* and *Zingiber officinale*, which are contraindicated in pregnancy.

Case 22: HH, 60-year-old male

HH was of a weak constitution and impatient disposition, with frequent dizziness, headache, ringing in the ears, and high blood pressure. The previous day, he had suddenly lost consciousness. He regained consciousness quickly, but the left half of the body felt numb and heavy, with difficulty moving. The tongue was red and the coating white. The pulse was small, stringy, and rapid, and had no force at the "foot" position.

Analysis. The chronically weak constitution reflected Yin deficiency and liver overactivity. The exacerbation caused further Yin deficiency and rise of liver Yang, allowing internal movement of liver Wind, rushing up of Qi and blood, and blocking of conduits, hence the sudden loss of consciousness. To bypass the block, the Yang Wind entered the meridians, thus causing the hemiparesis. The red tongue with white coating and the stringy, small, and rapid pulse, especially with no force at the "foot" position, were all symptoms of Yin deficiency in the liver and kidney.

Diagnosis. Yin deficiency in the liver and kidney; upward movement of liver Wind.

Treatment. Use formula 1 to increase Yin and formula 21 for the Wind.

Case 23: RT, 20-year-old female

RT had developed high fever acutely three days previously, with nausea and vomiting, right flank pain, a bitter taste, and dry mouth but no thirst. Her stools became dry, her urine scanty and dark, and her sclerae jaundiced; the tongue was red with a yellow and greasy coating, and the pulse was stringy and rapid.

Analysis. When liver and gallbladder were damaged by Dampness and Heat, bile dispersed and caused scleral jaundice. As Dampness and Heat invaded the stomach, nausea and vomiting resulted. Because of the strong Heat in liver and gallbladder, fever, bitter taste, dry mouth, constipation, dark urine, flank pain, and stringy and rapid pulse developed. There was Dampness in the Heat, hence no thirst despite a dry mouth. The yellow and greasy tongue coating also reflected accumulation of Dampness and Heat.

Diagnosis. Dampness and Heat in the liver and gallbladder; jaundice due to excess liver Yang.

Treatment. Use formula 329. This formula contains *Achyrantes* and *Hordeum*, both of which are contraindicated in pregnancy.

Case 24: LP, 50-year-old male

LP had been ill for over a year, with frequent elusive pain in the ribs on both sides associated with dizziness and blurring of vision. There was aching and weakness in his waist and legs. He was impatient and restless. Stools were dry and urine dark. The tongue was red with scanty coating, and the pulse stringy, small, and rapid.

Analysis. This illness had become chronic, implying that there was some deficiency. Aching and weakness of the flanks and legs, dizziness with blurring of vision, restlessness, and impatience all reflected insufficiency of liver and kidney, with Yin deficiency and thus rise in liver Yang. Yin deficiency produced internal Heat, hence the restlessness, constipation, dark urine, red tongue with scanty coating, and small and rapid pulse. Because the liver meridian traverses the side ribs, deficiency of liver Yin caused pain in those areas.

Diagnosis. Deficiency of liver and kidney Yin.

Treatment. Use formula 1.

Case 25: YC, 48-year-old female

YC had chronic deficiency Cold in the spleen and stomach. For several days she overindulged, with consequent epigastric pain (which was somewhat relieved by pressure and local heat application), nausea and vomiting of some fluids, bubbly sounds in the abdomen, abdominal distention and watery diarrhea, and coldness in all four extremities. Her tongue was pale with a creamy coating, and her pulse deep and small.

Analysis. The dietary indiscretion caused a relapse of this patient's chronic deficiency Cold in the spleen and stomach. Epigastric pain, nausea and vomiting, abdominal distention, and watery diarrhea all indicated that the disease was in the spleen and stomach. Epigastric pain, alleviated by local heat and pressure, and cold limbs were symptoms of deficiency Cold. As the spleen Yang weakened, fluids could not mobilize, and water and Dampness accumulated in the stomach. Dampness then blocked the middle sphincter, leading to abnormal movement of spleen and stomach Qi, hence nausea and vomiting. The pale tongue and deep and small pulse both indicated deficiency, while the creamy tongue coating indicated congelation of water and Dampness.

Diagnosis. Deficiency Cold in spleen and stomach; internal stagnation of water and Dampness.

Treatment. Use either formula 45 or formula 30 with added *Aconitum carmichaeli.* (Formula 45 contains *Pinellia*, whereas formula 30 contains *Cinnamomum* and *Zingiber.*) Add *Myristica fragrans* and halloysite for chronic diarrhea.

Case 26: WL, 30-year-old male

WL had frequent right flank pain for over a year, accompanied by abdominal distention and watery diarrhea. He gradually developed generalized tiredness and weakness with sallow complexion and emaciated body. The tongue was pale, and the pulse stringy and small.

Analysis. This patient showed flank pain, stringy pulse, and other symptoms of liver meridian disease, as well as abdominal distention, watery diarrhea, and other symptoms of spleen deficiency. His liver and spleen were thus in disharmony. The chronicity of the illness, deficiency of the spleen, and weakness of the stomach led to inadequate digestion and absorption of food and water. The source for generating Qi and blood was thus inadequate, causing weakness and tiredness, sallow complexion, and bodily emaciation. The pallor of the tongue and smallness and stringiness of the pulse were symptoms of deficiency.

Diagnosis. Blood deficiency and liver blockage; disharmony of liver and spleen.

Treatment. Use formulas 55 and 67, with added *Astragalus* spp.

Case 27: LR, 20-year-old female

For over three years, LR frequently had early menses that flowed for over ten days, producing large quantities of light-colored blood. She also often had purpuric spots on her skin, dizziness, blurring of vision, insomnia with excessive dreaming, loss of appetite, abdominal distention following eating, watery diarrhea upon eating any greasy foods, frequent numbness of the limbs and body, dry, scaly skin, sallow and dry complexion, lethargy, and emaciation. Her tongue was pale with a thin coating, and her pulse was small.

Analysis. This patient's numerous and complicated symptoms could be grouped according to three causes: spleen deficiency, blood loss, and blood deficiency. Excessive menses and skin purpura were probably related to the inability of the weakened spleen to command blood. Repeated blood loss led to blood deficiency, which in turn caused malnourishment of the heart and liver. With deficiency of blood, the sinews and skin could not flourish, hence numbness of the limbs and body and the drying and scaling of the skin. The tongue and pulse also reflected insufficiency of Qi and blood.

Diagnosis. Spleen unable to command blood; malnourishment of heart and liver.

Treatment. Use formulas 67 and 208, but note that the latter contains *Pinellia* and *Zingiber*.

Case 28: SH, 37-year-old female

For about a year, SH had been anxious and restless, with frequent insomnia and excessive dreaming, shortness of breath, and weakness. She was able to eat, but the foods were tasteless, and her abdomen often bloated. She also had night sweats. Menses were normal, but she had profuse vaginal discharge. The tongue was swollen and had indentation marks from the teeth. It was red with a thin white coating. The pulse was small and rapid.

Analysis. When heart Yin was insufficient, heart Yang increased, and there were anxiety and restlessness. With deficiency of heart Yin, Shen could not remain secure, hence the insomnia and excessive dreaming. Night perspiration, red tongue, and small and rapid pulse were symptoms of interior Heat due to Yin deficiency. Spleen deficiency disturbed digestion, so that food became tasteless and the abdomen distended. Sinking of water and Dampness then caused increased vaginal discharge. Spleen deficiency also disturbed metabolism, causing shortness of breath and weakness, symptoms of Qi deficiency.

Diagnosis. Heart and spleen both deficient.

Treatment. Use formula 267 with added Euphorbia longan.

Case 29: LS, 32-year-old male

LS had a hankering for acrid and hot spicy foods, so that he generally had foul mouth odor and gum swelling and was constipated. He self-administered formula 58 often, with improvement, but did not persist in the treatment. Over the previous two weeks, he had developed burning epigastric pain, loss of appetite, bloating following eating, dry mouth and lips, and constipation. The tongue was red with scant coating, and the pulse was small and rapid.

Analysis. The excessive hot and spicy foods transformed into Heat and generated Fire. Fire damage to the stomach caused halitosis, gingivitis, and constipation. Formula 58 was appropriate but was not used extensively enough. The chronicity of Heat in the stomach eventually led to damage of stomach Yin, hence the burning epigastric pain, dryness of lips and mouth, constipation, red tongue with scant coating, and small and rapid pulse. Insufficiency of stomach Yin allowed deterioration of stomach function, hence the loss of appetite and distention following eating.

Diagnosis. Chronic stomach Heat, with insidious exhaustion of stomach Yin.

Treatment. For Heat in the stomach, use formula 226. For the Yin deficiency, use formula 244, with added Phragmites communis, Dendrobium nobile, Tricosanthes kirilowii, root, Polygonatum odoratum, Adenophora verticillata, and Gallus gallus domesticus.

Case 30: CP, 10-year-old male

CP had fever, coughing, and shortness of breath with rapid breathing for two days. The fever reached 40 degrees Centigrade. He had no chills, but did sweat. The coughing produced yellow sputum. He had thirst, dark urine, and dry stools. The tongue was red, the coating yellow and dry, and the pulse tidal and rapid.

Analysis. The symptoms of fever, cough, shortness of breath, and rapid respiration indicated the lung as the site of disease. Because the patient did not have cold aversion but had fever, cough productive of yellow sputum, thirst, dark urine, dry stools, and other symptoms of interior Heat, the illness was thus one of Heat invasion of the lung.

Diagnosis. Lung Heat with cough.

Treatment. Use either formula 221 or 326; 221 is somewhat better at reducing sputum.

Case 31: SJ, 45-year-old female

SJ was of weak constitution and was sickly. Some ten years previously, she had developed a persistent cough following exposure to the weather. During the past two years, the cough had flared up frequently, producing a thin and clear sputum with foaming. Three days previously, she was chilled. The cough recurred, with copious clear sputum, shortness of breath, headache, and fever without sweating. The tongue coating was white and smooth and the pulse superficial and tight.

Analysis. In this patient with weak constitution, the Qi of the guard level was not secure, hence the sickliness. Because the lung and the skin are related as an interior-exterior dyad, the lung Qi also became insufficient. The ten years of coughing and the thin foamy sputum indicated the presence of Phlegm and Dampness in the lung with water accumulation. Three days previously, the patient was injured by Wind and Cold, hence the fever without perspiration, headache, and superficial and tight pulse. As the Wind and Cold extended to the lung, the lung Qi failed; the cough worsened, and chest tightness developed. The Cold evil activated the Phlegm and water in the lung, hence the thin sputum and white, smooth tongue coating.

Diagnosis. Lung Cold with cough; persistent evil in the exterior.

Treatment. Start with formula 36, with added *Aster tartaricus* and *Stemona japonica*, together with formula 34. For longer-term treatment, use formula 107 with 34. Note that all three formulas contain ingredients that are contraindicated in pregnancy. Fortunately, pregnancy is unlikely in a 45-year-old.

Case 32: LT, 10-year-old female

LT had developed high fever and cough two weeks previously. Following treatment, the fever broke, but the coughing persisted and became very frequent. There was scanty sputum, and the throat was dry. The tongue was red and the coating clean. The pulse was small and rapid.

Analysis. Although the fever broke with treatment, the lung Yin had already been damaged, hence the persistent symptoms.

Diagnosis. Lung Yin deficiency, with cough.

Treatment. Use formula 83, with added *Stemona japonica* and *Uncaria rhynchophylla*.

Case 33: CR, 58-year-old male

CR had had coughing and shortness of breath for over ten years. Two days previously, he was caught in the rain and overexerted himself rushing home. The coughing and shortness of breath worsened, so that his cough became weak, his respirations short and rapid, and his sputum thin and clear but difficult to cough out. Whenever he coughed he sweated, with fatigue and weakness. The complexion was pallid, the tongue pale with white coating, the pulse deficient and elusive.

Analysis. The patient had been coughing for over ten years. Because chronic cough can damage Qi, it was clear that he had chronic Qi deficiency. The deterioration started after his hurrying in the rain. He did not show any chills or fever or other exterior symptoms, so the deterioration was not due to Cold injury but instead to exhaustion, which further damaged lung Qi. The subsequent symptoms were all manifestations of Qi deficiency.

Diagnosis. Lung Qi deficiency, with shortness of breath.

Treatment. Use formula 268.

Case 34: YH, 40-year-old male

YH had developed chills and fever three days previously. When examined, the patient had a temperature of 40 degrees Centigrade. He had bloody and purulent diarrhea over ten times daily associated with severe cramping and pain, scanty and dark urine, and marked thirst with desire for cold drinks. All four limbs were cold and clammy. The tongue coating was yellow and the pulse rapid.

Analysis. This is an example of Dampness and Heat in the large intestine. Dampness and Heat accumulating in the large intestine caused blood and Qi to become obstructed, so that the Qi of the visceral organs also became impeded, hence the abdominal cramping and pain and the bloody and purulent diarrhea. The fever, thirst with desire for cold drinks, and scanty and dark urine were symptoms of interior Heat. The cold and clammy limbs were symptoms of false Cold in the interior.

Diagnosis. Dampness and Heat with dysentery; genuine Heat, false Cold.

Treatment. Use formula 94, with added *Lonicera japonica, Forsythia suspensa, Saussurea lappa,* and *Paeonia lactiflora.*

Case 35: WY, 25-year-old male

WY had had flank aches, limb weakness, frequent spontaneous semen emission, and nervousness. These symptoms had been getting worse over the past year or so. Recently, he also developed forgetfulness, dizziness, blurred vision, insomnia with excessive dreaming, dry mouth, and restlessness. His urine became dark; his tongue coating sloughed, leaving a red denuded tongue; and his pulse was small, rapid, and somewhat stringy.

Analysis. The flank is the residence of the kidney, and the kidney stores Jing. When kidney Yin was deficient, Jing storage became inadequate, and the patient developed flank aches and limb weakness. Yin deficiency with subsequent rise in Yang activated Fire, and that led to spontaneous semen emission. The emotional burden and anxiety caused further deficiency of kidney Yin. The deficiency of kidney water caused heart Fire to rise and the liver to lose its nourishment, resulting in the symptoms of these two organs, such as insomnia, forgetfulness, increased dreaming, dizziness, blurring of vision, stringy pulse, and so forth.

Diagnosis. Kidney Yin deficiency with abnormal movement of kidney Fire and spontaneous emission.

Treatment. Use formula 277, with added *Lycium chinense* and *Chrysanthemum.* If necessary, add formula 135 for semen emission.

Case 36: CY, 25-year-old male

CY had decreased urine and ankle swelling starting two years previously. He improved with treatment, but the treatment was stopped too soon, so he continued to have these symptoms. During the past week his condition had worsened, with scant urine, frank swelling, abdominal distention, watery diarrhea, cold intolerance and cold limbs, pain with cold feeling in the back and waist, fatigue, and weakness. His face was pallid, his tongue pale and fat with teeth marks, his tongue coating white and greasy, and his pulse deep and small—especially weak in the "foot" position.

Analysis. This patient's disease had started two years ago but at that time was not treated adequately. The mobilization and excretion of water principally depends on the spleen and kidney. In this case, the long duration of water accumulation and Dampness and the daily worsening of swelling and decrease in urine clearly indicated severe decline in the Yang Qi of the spleen and kidney. Kidney Yang deficiency produced Cold, hence cold intolerance and cold limbs, cold feeling, and pain in the back and waist. Spleen Yang deficiency led to abdominal distention and watery diarrhea as well as cold limbs. The pallid face, fatigue and weakness, pale, fat tongue with teeth marks, and deep and small pulse especially weak in the "foot" position all reflected Yang deficiency in the spleen and kidney. The white and greasy tongue coating reflected Dampness and water accumulation in the interior.

Diagnosis. Yang deficiency in spleen and kidney; water accumulation in kidney deficiency.

Treatment. Use formulas 68 and 120.

Case 37: TM, 26-year-old female

For three years, TM had abdominal bloating and watery stools more frequently than usual. Recently, she further developed diarrhea at predawn, flank pain, cold intolerance, abdominal distention with loss of appetite, pale tongue with white coating, and deep and small pulse.

Analysis. The bloating and watery stools for three years indicated the spleen as the site of this illness. Watery diarrhea indicated spleen deficiency. As spleen deficiency persisted, the kidney became damaged, injuring kidney Yang. This in turn caused kidney Fire to decrease, hence the flank pain and cold intolerance. The weakened kidney Fire was unable to warm the spleen to aid digestion and fluid movement, so the patient developed diarrhea at predawn when Yang was normally weak and Yin strong. Insufficiency of spleen Yang led to abdominal distention and loss of appetite. The tongue and pulse findings were symptoms of deficiency Cold in the interior.

Diagnosis. Yang deficiency in the spleen and kidney; deficiency Cold with diarrhea.

Treatment. Use formulas 68 and 120. Both contain *Zingiber*, and formula 120 also contains *Aconitum*, which are contraindicated in pregnancy.

Case 38: SM, 50-year-old male

SM had chronic cough with sputum; the cough flared up whenever he was exposed to cold. Winter was especially difficult. The previous winter he had had many episodes, with cough and sputum and shortness of breath. Each time he was treated with formula 36; each time he improved, but relapsed again on discontinuing the medication. He developed swelling of the lower limbs that gradually extended to the entire body, loss of appetite, scanty urine, watery stools, fatigue and weakness, cold body and limbs, pallid complexion, white and smooth tongue, and deep, slow, and weak pulse.

Analysis. Formula 36 is intended for dispersion of Cold and dissolution of Phlegm. The patient had chronic cough with sputum not cleared by formula 36; thus, he had more than Cold injury. Deficiency of either spleen or kidney could generate sputum, and could further cause accumulation of water and Dampness with overflow into the somatic body in the form of swelling. The cold body and limbs, fatigue and weakness, pallid complexion, white and smooth tongue, and deep, slow, and weak pulse were all symptoms of deficiency Cold.

Diagnosis. Yang deficiency of the spleen and kidney; immobilization of water and Dampness, with overflow as swelling.

Treatment. Use formulas 42 and 194.

Case 39: YK, 24-year-old female

YK acutely developed frequency of urination, having to urinate more than ten times daily. Furthermore, she had urgency, hesitancy, and burning pain on urination, and the urine was red. She had a dry mouth but no thirst. The lower abdomen was distended and painful with cramps. She felt warm, but her temperature was 37 degrees Centigrade. The tongue was normal, the tongue coating mildly yellow and greasy, and the pulse stringy, rapid, and somewhat smooth.

Analysis. The acuteness of the symptoms indicated that this was a new illness. The symptoms were mainly those of Heat. The urinary frequency, burning pain, and red urine all pointed to the bladder as the site. The tongue coating and pulse indicated the presence of Dampness as well.

Diagnosis. Dampness and Heat trapped in the bladder.

Treatment. Use formula 9, with added *Rehmannia glutinosa, Cirsium japonicum, Melia toosendan,* and *Lindera strychnifolia.* Formula 9 contains *Dianthus,* contraindicated in pregnancy.

Select Bibliography

Beijing Medical School, Committee on the Foundations of Clinical Chinese Medicine 北京医学院《中医临证基础》编写组. *Zhongyi Linzheng Jichu* 中医临证基础 (Foundations of Clinical Chinese Medicine). Beijing: People's Educational Publishing Company 人民教育出版社, 1975.

Bensky, Dan, and Randall Barolet, comp. and trans. *Chinese Herbal Medicine: Formulas and Strategies*. Seattle: Eastland Press, 1990.

Commercial Press 商務印書館. *Changyong Zhongcaoyao Shouce* 常用中草药手册 (Handbook of Commonly Used Chinese Herbs). Hong Kong: Commercial Press, 1970; reissued 1972.

Hopei New School of Medicine 河北新医大学编. *Zhongyi Yi-an Bashili* 中医医案八十例 (Eighty Case Records in Chinese Medicine). Beijing: People's Educational Publishing Company 人民教育出版社, 1976.

Hunan School of Chinese Medicine 湖南中医学院编. *Linchuang Changyong Zhongyao Shouce* 临床常用中药手册 (Handbook of Common Bedside Herbs). Beijing: People's Health Publishing Company 人民卫生出版社, 1972.

Jianwen Book Company 建文書局. *Zhongguo Yiyao Dacidian* 中國醫藥大辭典 (Encyclopedic Dictionary of Chinese Medicines). Jianwen Book Company, 1977.

Jiangsu New School of Medicine 江苏新医学院编. *Zhongyao Dacidian* 中药大辞典 (Encyclopedic Dictionary of Chinese Medicines). Hong Kong: Commercial Press, 1978.

Qian, Letian 錢樂天, Zhongyuan Guo 郭中元, and Tongxuan Sun 孫桐軒. *Zhongyi Jiejing* 中醫捷徑 (Shortcuts in Chinese Medicine). Hong Kong: Taiping Book Company 太平書局, 1962.

Qin, Baiwei 秦伯未. *Zhongyi Rumen* 中醫入門 (Introduction to Chinese Medicine). Hong Kong: Taiping Book Company, 1963.

Ren, Yingqiu 任應秋. *Zhongyi Maixue Shijian* 中醫脈學十講 (Ten Lectures on the Pulse in Chinese Medicine). Hong Kong: Taiping Book Company, 1963.

Shanghai School of Chinese Medicine 上海中医学院编. *Zhen jiuxue* 针灸学 (Acupuncture and Moxibustion). Shanghai: People's Publishing Company 人民出版社, 1974.

—————. *Neikexue* 内科学 (Internal Medicine). Shanghai: People's Publishing Company, 1975.

Taiping Book Company 太平書局. *Zhongyi Zhenduan Zhiliao Yaozhi* 中醫診斷治療要旨 (Essentials of Diagnosis and Treatment in Chinese Medicine). Hong Kong: Taiping Book Company, 1962.

—————. *Zhongyi Changyong Xiaofang Shouce* 中醫常用效方手冊 (Handbook of Frequently Used Formulas of Chinese Herbs). Hong Kong: Taiping Book Company, 1963.

—————. *Zhongyi Mingci Cidian* 中醫名詞辭典 (Dictionary of Chinese Medical Terms). Hong Kong: Taiping Book Company, 1964.

Tienjin School of Chinese Medicine, Department of Internal Medicine 天津市中医医院内科编著]. *Zhongyi Neike* 中医内科 (Chinese Internal Medicine). Tienjin: People's Press 天津人民出版社, 1974.

Index

Numbers preceded by the letter f refer to formula numbers in chapter 12.

Nanguazi. *See* Cucurbita
nature of drugs 72
Nelumbo 152, 153, 210, 211
Newly-Augmented Elsholtzia Decoction. *See* f282
Niao dan bai tong tang. *See* f93b
Niao dao pai shi tang. *See* f110
Nine-Immortal Decoction. *See* f5
Niter 211
Niubangzi. *See* Arctium
Niuhuang. *See* Bos
Niu huang wan. *See* f58
Niuqi. *See* Achyranthes
Niuru. *See* Bos
nose diseases 129
Nourish the Heart Decoction. *See* Heart-Strengthening Decoction
Nourish the Yin and Clear the Lungs Decoction. *See* Yin-Generating Lung-Clearing Decoction
Nuan gan jian. *See* f284
nutmeg. *See* Myristica
Nuzhenzi. *See* Ligustrum

obesity 121
odor 42, 124
olfaction 42
Ophicalcite 166, 211
Ophiopogon 153, 154, 163, 211, 292
Ophiopogon Decoction. *See* f244
opisthotonus 121
opium poppy. *See* Papaver
orange, trifoliate. *See* Poncirus
Oryza 165, 212
Ostrea 67, 153, 154, 162, 166, 212, 293
Ou(zhi). *See* Nelumbo
oyster. *See* Ostrea
oyster, pearl. *See* Pteria
Oyster Shell Powder. *See* f114

Paeonia 75, 148, 150, 152, 155, 156, 168, 212, 292, 302
Paeonia-Gardenia Care-free Powder. *See* f37
Paeonia-Glycyrrhiza-Aconitum Decoction. *See* f116
pagoda tree. *See* Sophora
pain, body and limb 141
Pain and Wind Pill. *See* f257

Pai nong san. *See* f213
palpation 44–47
Panax 75, 152, 155, 159, 161, 162, 213, 290
Pangdahai. *See* Sterculia
Papaver 213
paralysis 121
parasites 39; diseases of 107; treatment of diseases of 171
Paratenodera 213
Paratenodera Powder. *See* f182
passions 38; diseases of 104; treatment of diseases of 171
Patrinii 152, 213
peach. *See* Prunus
Peach Blossom (Dysentery) Decoction. *See* f184
Peach-Pit Decoction to Order the Qi. *See* Prunus Qi-Regulating Decoction
Peilan. *See* Eupatorium
Pengsha. *See* Borax
peony. *See* Paeonia
Peony Decoction. *See* f115
pepper. *See* Piper
Pericardium-Heat-Dissipating Decoction. *See* f225
Perilla 149, 151, 166, 214, 288
Perilla Fruit Decoction for Directing Qi Downward. *See* Perilla Qi-Lowering Decoction
Perilla Qi-Lowering Decoction. *See* f334
persimmon. *See* Diospyros
perspiration 43, 125. *See also* diaphoresis
Peucedanum 151, 214
Pharbitis 75, 148, 150, 214
Pharbitis Pill. *See* f230
Phaseolus 75, 214, 215
Phellodendron 74, 150, 154, 155, 166, 215, 287
Pheretima 160, 215
Phlegm 38; diseases of 105; treatment of diseases of 171
Phlegm-Reducing Decoction. *See* f316
Phlegm-Wind-Reducing and Sedating Prescription. *See* f315

Phragmites 150, 155, 167, 215, 287, 288, 299
Phragmites Decoction. See f302
Phyllostachys 150, 151, 155, 165, 167, 215, 216
Phyllostachys-Gypsum Decoction. See f100
Phytolacca 150, 216
Picrorhiza 216
Picrorhiza and Mume Decoction to Calm Roundworm. See Roundworm Decoction
pig. See Sus
Pinellia 67, 72, 74, 75, 148, 151, 155, 165, 166, 216, 295, 297, 298
Pinellia, Atractylodes Macrocephala and Gastrodia Decoction. See Pinellia-Atractylodes-Gastrodia Decoction
Pinellia-Atractylodes-Gastrodia Decoction. See f63
Pinellia and Magnolia Bark Decoction. See Pinellia-Magnolia Decoction
Pinellia-Magnolia Decoction. See f61
Pinellia Decoction to Drain the Epigastrium. See Pinellia Heart-Clearing Decoction
Pinellia Heart-Clearing Decoction. See f62
Ping gan shu luo wan. See f75
Ping ke he ji. See f74
Ping wei san. See f76
Pinus 217
Pipaye. See Eriobotrya
Piper 149, 169, 217
Piper-Centrally Regulating Pill. See f156
Pishi. See Arsenolite
Plantago 150, 217
Platycodon 151, 218
Platycodon Decoction. See f174
Pleropus 75, 152, 155, 218
pneuma 62
Poison-Eliminating Cooling Drink. See f227
Poison-Eliminating Powder. See f214
poisoning 39
pokeweed. See Phytolacca
Polygala 153, 167, 218
Polygala Decoction. See f304

Polygonatum 167, 169, 218, 299
Polygonum 68, 150, 152, 218, 219, 293
Polyporus 150, 153, 219
Polyporus Decoction from the Comprehensive Recording. See Poria-Polyporus Decoction
pomegranate. See Punica
Poncirus 152, 155, 156, 164, 219
Poncirus-Allium-Cinnamomum Decoction. See f148
Poncirus-Atractylodes Pill. See f147
Poncirus Obstruction-Removing Pill. See f146
Poria 74, 150, 153, 220
Poria, Cinnamon Twig, Atractylodes Macrocephala, and Licorice Decoction. See Poria-Cinnamomum-Atractylodes-Glycyrrhiza Decoction
Poria-Cinnamomum-Atractylodes-Glycyrrhiza Decoction. See f159
Poria-Cinnamomum-Glycyrrhiza-Zizyphus Decoction. See f160
Poria-Cuscuta Pill. See f197
Poria-Polyporus Decoction. See f232
Poria Powder. See f198
positions, three 60–64
praying mantis. See Paratenodera
pregnancy, drugs contraindicated in 148
Pregnancy Appendicitis Decoction. See f109
premature ejaculation 167
Prepared Aconite Decoction. See Aconitum Decoction
Prepared Aconite Decoction to Drain the Epigastrium. See Aconitum Heart-Clearing Decoction
Prepared Aconite Pill to Regulate the Middle. See Aconitum Central-Regulating Decoction
prescriptions: catharsis 156; cooling 156; dispersion of exterior 156; dissipation 157; elimination of Dampness 157; elimination of Phlegm 157; mediation 157; regulation of blood 157; regulation of Qi 157; restoration 157; sedation 158; solidification 158; warming 157; Wind extinction 158